PET in the Evaluation of Alzheimer's Disease and Related Disorders

Daniel H.S. Silverman
Editor

PET in the Evaluation of Alzheimer's Disease and Related Disorders

Springer

Editor
Daniel H.S. Silverman, M.D., Ph.D.
Head, Neuronuclear Imaging Section
Associate Chief, Division of Biological Imaging
Associate Professor, Department of Molecular and Medical Pharmacology
Associate Director, UCLA Alzheimer's Disease Center Imaging Core
David Geffen School of Medicine
University of California
Los Angeles, CA
USA

ISBN 978-0-387-76419-1 e-ISBN 978-0-387-76420-7
DOI 10.1007/978-0-387-76420-7

Library of Congress Control Number: 2008940848

Printed on acid-free paper

springer.com

Preface

Among all the clinical indications for which radiologists, nuclear medicine physicians, neurologists, neurosurgeons, psychiatrists (and others examining disorders of the brain) order and read brain PET scans, demand is greatest for those pertaining to dementia and related disorders. This demand is driven by the sheer prevalence of those conditions, coupled with the fact that the differential diagnosis for causes of cognitive impairment is wide and often difficult to distinguish clinically.

The conceptual framework by which evaluation and management of dementia is guided has evolved considerably during the last decade. Although we still are far from having ideal tests or dramatic cures for any of the established causes of dementia, our options have expanded with respect to both the diagnostic and therapeutic tools now available. In the first chapter of this book, the contribution and limitations of different elements of the clinical examination for diagnosis of cognitive symptoms are described, and the roles of structural and functional neuroimaging in the clinical workup are given context.

The clinical utility of brain positron emission tomography (PET), as with other imaging modalities, depends in part on how accurately and fully the information inherently represented in the scans is appreciated and relayed in the interpretation of the images. Even highly trained imaging specialists are challenged by this since, for example, neuroradiologists are generally far more familiar with computed tomography (CT) and magnetic resonance (MR) studies of the brain than with PET studies, and specialists in PET and PET/CT facilities tend to be much more experienced with oncology studies than with dedicated brain studies performed for the evaluation of neurologic disorders. To help meet this challenge, the second chapter offers practical instruction on adopting a systematic method for visual analysis of scans, describes how quantification with clinically available and friendly software tools can be employed to assist with analysis, and then illustrates a straightforward approach for integrating the qualitative and quantitative findings in meaningful interpretations. An Atlas in the final section of this book complements Chapter 2 by providing interpretive practice for many real (and clinically realistic) cases, to which the tools outlined in the second chapter can be directly applied.

The most frequent causes of dementia are neurodegenerative disorders, with Alzheimer's disease being the most common. By the time patients are symptomatic with these disorders, they have undergone significant distinct alterations in brain metabolism. The increasing use of brain PET stems from the high sensitivity of this imaging tool in identifying those alterations. The third chapter looks at the full spectrum of changes in glucose metabolism detectable with PET in monitoring the course of cognitive decline, beginning before the emergence of the first neurologic symptoms, in people who are predisposed to developing problems, in some cases many years into the future. Progressive changes observed with PET in the brains of patients who experience very mild symptoms, to those who meet criteria for having mild cognitive impairment, to those suffering from full-blown dementia, are described, as is the role of PET in the differential diagnosis of the underlying cause for the dysfunction.

Neurodegenerative diseases often impact not only on cognitive function, but also on motor function. The two neurologic domains can be affected in isolation, but frequently a mixed presentation of symptoms occurs. For example, approximately one third of Alzheimer's patients eventually experience parkinsonian symptoms and, conversely, a similar proportion of patients with Parkinson's disease develop significant cognitive impairment. Other conditions, such as dementia with Lewy bodies, may be characterized at an early stage by both motor and cognitive problems. Chapter 4 examines neuronuclear imaging studies explicitly aimed at illuminating changes in the brain associated with movement disorders. Their potential utility with respect to drug development, as well as in direct clinical application, is explained.

Although the most commonly performed clinical PET studies by far are carried out with [^{18}F]fluorodeoxyglucose (FDG) as the imaged radiotracer, substantial advances have occurred in the development of other radiotracers with which to probe brain processes associated with neurodegenerative disease. Chapter 5 describes work that is making it possible to observe and measure the molecular participants of such processes as they accumulate, or are lost from, living brain tissue. In the setting of Alzheimer-related changes, one molecular participant in particular, the β-amyloid of extracellular plaques constituting one of the histopathologic hallmarks of Alzheimer's disease, has attracted substantial attention in both industry and academic scientific settings. Following the introduction of this area of investigation in the fifth chapter, Chapter 6 is devoted to expanding on the scientific implications and clinical potential of radiotracers being developed to localize and measure β-amyloid deposits occurring in the brain. In the latter chapter, particular attention is given to characterizing β-amyloid deposition in older people who would not be considered cognitively impaired by standard clinical criteria.

PET scans, particularly with FDG, have demonstrated diagnostic and prognostic utility in evaluating patients with cognitive impairment and in distinguishing among primary neurodegenerative disorders and other etiologies for cognitive decline. Since the diagnostic capabilities of this medical technology have outpaced therapeutic advances, a look into the future of PET requires concomitant consideration of the future of therapeutic strategies for addressing the underlying conditions. As preventive and specific disease-modifying treatments are developed, early detection of accurately diagnosed neuropathologic processes, facilitated by appropriate use of PET and other neuroimaging technologies, can be expected to increasingly impact on the enormous human toll currently exacted by these disorders.

Daniel H.S. Silverman, M.D., Ph.D.

Acknowledgments

There are many to whom much is owed for their roles in the creation of the present work, moving it from the realm of abstract ideas into its present reality. I would like to thank Rob Albano who, representing the publisher (at a time when Springer was still Springer-Verlag), was present from its inception and first invited me to consider a project along these lines. I felt fairly sure at the time that taking on this project was a bad move, but he managed not to let me talk him (or myself) out of it prematurely. I also wish to thank developmental editor Margaret Burns who, working with me from almost the earliest days of the project, managed to stay perfectly poised on the fine line between helpful prodding to keep the project moving forward and patient understanding when that forward motion may have seemed imperceptible to an external observer (particularly as obstacles to our originally anticipated timeline arose and had to be creatively overcome). Thanks are also due to Springer's book production manager Frank Ganz, and associate editor Katherine Cacace, for ably guiding this project through the final stretch and across the finish line. I am indebted to all of my colleagues who contributed as authors and co-authors to the final work: my friends and colleagues at UCLA, Linda Ercoli, Gary Small, Vladimir Kepe, Henry Huang, Saty Satyamurthy, and Jorge Barrio, with whom I have been fortunate to collaborate over the past decade on a wide range of imaging-related projects; Lisa Mosconi, who has shared her considerable experience on changes in brain metabolism associated with the earliest stages of Alzheimer's disease; John Seibyl, a friend of many years who has always sportingly accepted my invitations to participate in any number of forums of symposia and writing projects and has once again offered his insights into the movement side of the neurodegenerative coin, much to the benefit of this text; Bill Klunk, for readily agreeing at the outset to take responsibility, along with Chet Mathis and colleagues Julie Price, Steve DeKosky, Brian Lopresti, Nicholas Tsopelas, Judith Saxton, and Robert Nebes, for their excellent contribution on amyloid imaging; my colleague Karl Herholz, for his insights in attempting the impossible task of forecasting the future; and Vicky Lau, Cheri Geist, and Erin Siu, who applied their trained eyes, creative talents, and organizational skills to successfully bringing to life reams of clinical data and images into cogent clinical cases. Finally, I wish to express my appreciation to those who have played roles less directly related to this actual text, but no less important to its realization: Johannes Czernin, with whom I literally worked alongside since my first day on the Nuclear Medicine Service at UCLA, and Mike Phelps, whose pioneering work with PET served as a major source of my inspiration to enter the nuclear medicine field to begin with, for the nearly one and a half decades of friendship and support they have offered personally and, in addition, professionally in their roles heading the Ahmanson Biological Imaging Division, and Department of Molecular and Medical Pharmacology, respectively; and my family—my wife Wei, our kids, our parents Donna and Robert and Pei and Robert, and my sibs Anne, Beth, and Mikhael, whose contributions of friendship, love, understanding of my professional commitments (and over-commitment), as well as the many more specific roles played in day-to-day life throughout the time that this text has been in preparation (and long before), would require another book to fully enumerate.

Contents

Part III Atlas

Contributors

Jorge R. Barrio, Ph.D.
Distinguished Professor, Department of Molecular and Medical Pharmacology, David Geffen School of Medicine, University of California, Los Angeles, CA

Steven T. DeKosky, M.D.
Professor and Chair, Department of Neurology, University of Pittsburgh, Pittsburgh, PA

Linda M. Ercoli, Ph.D.
Assistant Clinical Professor, Department of Psychiatry and Biobehavioral Sciences, the Semel Institute for Neuroscience and Human Behavior and the Resnick Neuropsychiatric Hospital at the University of California, Los Angeles, CA

Cheri Geist, B.Sc.
Research Associate, Neuronuclear Imaging Section, Department of Molecular and Medical Pharmacology, David Geffen School of Medicine, University of California, Los Angeles, CA

Sung-Cheng Huang, D.Sc.
Professor, Department of Molecular and Medical Pharmacology, David Geffen School of Medicine, University of California, Los Angeles, CA

Vladimir Kepe, Ph.D.
Associate Researcher, Department of Molecular and Medical Pharmacology, David Geffen School of Medicine, University of California, Los Angeles, CA

William E. Klunk, M.D., Ph.D.
Professor, Department of Psychiatry, University of Pittsburgh, Pittsburgh, PA

Victoria Lau, B.Sc.
Research Associate, Neuronuclear Imaging Section, Department of Molecular and Medical Pharmacology, David Geffen School of Medicine, University of California, Los Angeles, CA

Brian J. Lopresti, B.S.
Research Instructor, Department of Radiology, University of Pittsburgh, PET Facility, Pittsburgh, PA

Chester A. Mathis, Ph.D.
Professor, Department of Radiology, University of Pittsburgh, Pittsburgh, PA

Lisa Mosconi, Ph.D.
Assistant Professor, Department of Psychiatry, New York University School of Medicine, New York, NY

Robert D. Nebes, Ph.D.
Professor, Department of Psychiatry, University of Pittsburgh Medical Center, Pittsburgh, PA

Julie C. Price, Ph.D.
Associate Professor, Department of Radiology, University of Pittsburgh, Pittsburgh, PA

Nagichettiar Satyamurthy, Ph.D.
Professor, Department of Molecular and Medical Pharmacology, David Geffen School of Medicine, University of California, Los Angeles, CA

Judith A. Saxton, Ph.D.
Associate Professor, Department of Neurology, University of Pittsburgh, Pittsburgh, PA

John P. Seibyl, M.D.
Senior Scientist, Imaging Division, Institute for Neurodegenerative Disorders, New Haven, CT

Daniel H.S. Silverman, M.D., Ph.D.
Head, Neuronuclear Imaging Section; Associate Chief, Division of Biological Imaging; Associate Professor, Department of Molecular and Medical Pharmacology; Associate Director, UCLA Alzheimer's Disease Center Imaging Core, David Geffen School of Medicine, University of California, Los Angeles, CA

Erin Siu, B.Sc.
Research Associate, Neuronuclear Imaging Section, Department of Molecular and Medical Pharmacology, David Geffen School of Medicine, University of California, Los Angeles, CA

Gary W. Small, M.D.
Professor, Parlow-Solomon Professor on Aging, Department of Psychiatry, David Geffen School of Medicine at University of California Los Angeles, Los Angeles, CA

Nicholas Tsopelas, M.D.
Professor, Department of Psychiatry, Western Psychiatric Institute and Clinic, University of Pittsburgh, Pittsburgh, PA

Part I
Imaging Applications in Current Clinical Practice

Chapter 1
Clinical Evaluation of Dementia and When to Perform PET

Linda M. Ercoli and Gary W. Small

The number and proportion of adults over 65 years is expected to increase rapidly over the next several decades. According to projections from the United States Bureau of the Census,[1] between the years 2000 and 2030, the population aged 65 and over is expected to double from 35 to over 70 million. The largest proportion of older adults will be between the ages of 65 and 74 years, and the largest growth is projected to occur in individuals 85 years and older, increasing from 4.3 to 8.8 million. Because age is the greatest risk factor for dementia, as the population of elderly people increases, so will the number of patients suffering from dementia. Given that early treatment interventions are able to keep patients at higher levels of functioning and future innovative therapies may be able to delay the onset of dementia and slow its progression, it is becoming increasingly important to accurately diagnose dementia as early as possible.

This chapter outlines the basic elements of a clinical diagnostic evaluation for Alzheimer's disease (AD) and other dementias; and also addresses how to identify candidates for a dementia evaluation, discusses the role of neuroimaging in a clinical dementia evaluation, and identifies future directions.

Definition of Dementia

According to the *Diagnostic and Statistical Manual of Mental Disorders,* 4th edition,[2] the essential features of dementia include impaired memory plus impairment in at least one other cognitive domain (e.g., language, executive, and visual-spatial skills), and significant disturbance of work or social functioning or both resulting from cognitive deficits. These features cannot occur exclusively during the course of a delirium, but delirium may occur during the course of dementia. Dementias may also include mood changes, personality alterations, and behavioral disturbances.

Depending on variation in presentation or whether patients present earlier versus later during the course of a dementing disorder, distinguishing between age-related cognitive decline and early dementia, and differentiating among different types of

D.H.S. Silverman (ed.), *PET in the Evaluation of Alzheimer's Disease and Related Disorders*, 3
DOI: 10.1007/978-0-387-76420-7_1, © Springer Science+Business Media, LLC 2009

dementias can be challenging. Diagnostic criteria for various dementing illnesses have been developed to aid in differential diagnosis.[3,4] For instance, dementia of the Alzheimer's type, the most prevalent form of dementia in older adults, is characterized by a gradual onset and progression of symptoms without another identifiable or treatable cause. A definite diagnosis of dementia of the Alzheimer's type can be made only by histopathologic examination of brain tissue, usually postmortem. The National Institute of Neurological and Communicative Disorders and the Alzheimer's Association consensus statement[5] provide criteria and guidelines for the diagnosis of possible and probable AD. Probable AD is similar to progressive dementia of the Alzheimer's type, whereas possible AD includes dementia syndromes with atypical onset, presentation, or progression in which an additional or co-morbid disease (e.g., tumor or cerebral thrombosis) may be implicated but not believed to be the cause of the dementia.

Epidemiology of Dementia and Preclinical Syndromes

Dementia affects approximately 27 million people worldwide, with approximately 5 million new cases annually (one new case every 7 s).[6,7] Although younger persons can suffer from dementia, dementias are most common in older age, and the incidence of dementia doubles every 5 years after age 60. The most common form of dementia is dementia of the Alzheimer's type (or AD), which accounts for approximately 65% of dementias in late life. The prevalence of AD increases with age, afflicting approximately 13% of Americans age 65 and older and up to 50% of those over 85 years. Currently, AD costs the Centers for Medicare and Medicaid Services and U.S. businesses an estimated $148 billion annually.[8,11]

A number of other common forms of dementia have been identified. Vascular dementia (VAD), is estimated to account for approximately 15–20% of dementias[12,13] in the United States and Europe; and up to 50% of dementias in Japan.[14] Dementia with Lewy bodies (DLB) accounts for up to 30% of dementias,[15] and frontotemporal dementia (FTD), a spectrum of disorders that particularly affects persons under 65 years of age, accounts for approximately 5% of dementias[16] although some estimates are higher.[17] Less frequent dementia syndromes include Creutzfeldt-Jakob disease, HIV-associated dementia, neurosyphilis, Parkinson's dementia, normal pressure hydrocephalus, and dementias resulting from exposure to toxic substances (e.g., alcohol, heavy metals, illicit substances), metabolic abnormalities, and psychiatric disorders.

Preclinical dementia syndromes, characterized by milder forms of memory loss and no functional impairment, are prevalent in the general population and have received increasing clinical attention. Their identification is important because early pharmacologic interventions in dementia may delay the onset and slow the progression of AD, extend quality of life, offset medical costs, and delay placement in care facilities.[18,19]

Two common preclinical syndromes include age-associated memory impairment (AAMI)[20] and mild cognitive impairment (MCI).[21,22] AAMI is the mildest form of age-related memory loss. It occurs in persons over 50 years of age and is characterized by self-reported memory complaints, decreased memory performances compared with younger adults (typically defined as 1 standard deviation below young adults on memory tests), but normal memory compared with age peers. The prevalence of AAMI has been estimated at 40% in people 65 years of age or older, and although most cases are benign over the short term, approximately 1% of these individuals develop dementia each year.[20,23] MCI typically involves a more severe loss of memory that is still not associated with functional decline. Persons with MCI show reductions in memory or other cognitive domains compared with age peers. Many persons with MCI show similar cerebral pathology to persons with AD,[24,25] and approximately 15% of persons with MCI develop dementia annually and most often AD.[21,22] The outcome of MCI varies, indicating that it is a heterogeneous disorder. Although eventually most persons with MCI develop AD, some develop other types of dementia, some remain stable, and others revert to normal cognition. Originally, MCI was characterized as an amnestic disorder, but more recently the definition has been expanded to include other cognitive (e.g., amnestic plus other impairments; single or multiple non-memory domains) or etiologic subtypes (e.g., vascular).[22]

Obstacles to Accurate Diagnosis of Dementia

Despite better diagnostic methods and pharmacologic interventions, several obstacles impede the diagnosis of dementia.[26,27] Previous studies indicate that false-negative diagnoses may occur in 50–90% of cases.[28,29] If physicians mistakenly attribute early cognitive decline to normal aging, evaluation and treatment may be delayed until the disease severity and neuronal damage have progressed.

Reduced time that physicians spend with patients is another obstacle to detecting AD. In today's managed care environment, many primary care physicians have limited time to conduct a comprehensive informant interview. Under such circumstances, helpful strategies for obtaining relevant information include enlisting the assistance of nurses or trained staff to interview patients or family on the telephone or at the office before seeing the physician. Questionnaires to collect information on daily function, medications, and family history of dementia can be mailed to the patient or family before the appointment or administered in the waiting room.

Another obstacle to diagnosing dementia is overreliance on and overinterpretation of laboratory findings, particularly CT and MRI results. The diagnosis of dementia usually is a clinical diagnosis. The purpose of laboratory assessment is to identify uncommon treatable causes and common treatable co-morbid conditions.

Similarly, overreliance on typical cutoff scores on mental status or cognitive screening tests, or using such tests for the sole purpose of diagnosis is another obstacle to diagnosing dementia. Highly educated individuals who have suffered cognitive decline may show normal function on cognitive screening tests such as the Mini Mental State Exam (MMSE), whereas persons with low education may appear to have cognitive impairment or dementia when they actually have not declined.[30] Age- and education-corrected normative data are available for some screening tests, such as the MMSE.[31,32] As a rule of thumb, cognitive screening measures are most useful as a quantitative baseline against which to compare future assessments, and not to be used alone for diagnostic purposes. When the diagnosis is unclear, neuropsychological testing may better distinguish between normal aging and dementia, as well as identify deficits that point to a specific diagnosis.

Finally, clinicians often have difficulty distinguishing complaints of the *worried well* (i.e., normal aging) from those of patients who have an underlying brain disorder that results in cognitive decline. Subjective complaints can indicate the presence of mood disorders or early dementia; in any event, they should be taken seriously.[33,34]

Determining When to Conduct a Dementia Evaluation

A variety of symptoms and circumstances may warrant a dementia evaluation. Several of the following issues are worth considering.

Patient or Family Concerns

Any patient or family concerns about cognitive decline or personality, behavioral, or mood changes are indications for a mental status assessment and possibly a dementia evaluation. One recent study showed that collaterals' perceptions, particularly persons who live with or know the patient well, are accurate in reporting a patient's cognitive capabilities.[35]

Functional Impairment

Declines in the ability to conduct higher-level daily activities or patients stopping or reducing the time spent in such activities should prompt a dementia evaluation. Patients with early or mild AD suffer declines in their ability to perform higher-level daily activities such as planning or preparing meals, managing finances or medications, using a telephone, keeping track of appointments, and driving without getting lost. These functional impairments may be the patient's or family's earliest indicators that something is wrong. A dementia evaluation is warranted when patients have dysfunction in higher-level activities but intact basic functions such as eating and maintaining personal hygiene and grooming, because these basic activities often remain normal until later stages of a dementing disease.

Changes in Personality and Behavior

Significant changes in behavior and mood often occur in early dementia.[36] For instance, patients with AD may demonstrate personality changes, irritability, anxiety, apathy, or depression early in the disease process, followed by delusions, hallucinations, aggression, disinhibition, and wandering in middle and late stages. Such behaviors are the most troubling to caregivers, make home management difficult, and frequently lead to family distress and nursing home placement.[37]

Delirium

Delirium is a syndrome of acquired impairment of attention, alertness, and perception[2] that can be the consequence of a general medical condition, such as infection, pharmacologic toxicity, or metabolic disturbance. Delirium is often confused with dementia because both are characterized by global cognitive impairment; however, delirium can be distinguished from dementia by its acute onset, marked fluctuations in cognitive impairment over the course of a day, disruptions in consciousness and attention, and alterations in the sleep cycle. Hallucinations and visual illusions are common. Further complicating the picture, delirium and dementia often co-exist, particularly in a hospital setting; and dementia, a risk factor for delirium, contributes to the higher prevalence of delirium in the elderly.[38,39] Thus, patients with persistent cognitive deficits, even after delirium clears, should undergo a dementia evaluation.

Abrupt Changes in Cognitive, Emotional, or Neurologic Status

Patient presentations or family complaints of an abrupt onset of mood disturbance or change, behavioral changes, changes in sleep/wake cycles, or abrupt cognitive decline should prompt a mental status examination.

Depression

A thorough evaluation should be conducted if patients have gradual or abrupt onset of depression. The distinction between depression and dementia in late life is not always clear, because depression and dementia may be co-morbid, depression may be a prodrome to dementia, or the two may be mistaken for each other, as both involve memory difficulties.[40,41] Noting the level of awareness of cognitive difficulties may be helpful in distinguishing dementia from depression. Demented patients may be aware of cognitive deficits, but they may underestimate their severity and impact on everyday functioning accurately,[42] whereas depressed patients tend to exaggerate memory or cognitive problems. Neuropsychological evaluations also can be helpful in differentiating depression from early dementia.[43,44] Some depressed geriatric patients have a *reversible dementia* syndrome, but such patients require continued monitoring, as nearly 50% develop irreversible dementia within 5 years.[45]

The Basic Dementia Workup

According to most consensus guideline recommendations, the elements of a basic dementia workup include a detailed history, physical and neurologic examinations, basic laboratory tests, and a computed tomography (CT) or magnetic resonance imaging (MRI) scan of the brain.[46] Additional tests—such as diagnostic and laboratory tests, functional neuroimaging and neuropsychological evaluations, speech and speech/language assessment, and genetic testing—are obtained as necessary, pending results of the basic workup.

If time is limited, before meeting with the patient, the physician can send forms and questionnaires for the patient or a collateral to complete to expedite information gathering about the present complaint, current medications and supplements, and family history of dementia. In addition, standardized and validated forms to assess cognitive complaints (e.g., Memory Functioning Questionnaire),[47] and functional activities (e.g., Pfeiffer Functional Activities Questionnaire)[48] also may be included in the packet. Given that patients with cognitive difficulties may not be able to provide accurate information regarding their history, a person who knows the patient well can complete the forms.

During the intake evaluation, the physician conducts the initial history to obtain information about the chief complaint; background information on the onset, course, and progression of deficits or functional impairment; medical and psychiatric history; relevant social history; and to observe patient behavior and assess mood. The physician also conducts a neuropsychiatric screen to formulate diagnostic hypotheses. The initial interview also can serve to establish rapport and a working relationship with the patient.

Chief Complaint and History

The clinician gathers additional information about the patient's chief complaint and medical background. The history includes data about the onset (e.g., abrupt versus insidious and gradual), nature of symptoms, course of the current problems (i.e., fluctuating or progressive), and whether the patient has experienced changes in personality, mood, or daily functioning. It is important to try to construct a timeline of what has changed for the patient and when; therefore, the physician should try to distinguish longstanding difficulties from those of recent onset.

Memory complaints correlate with depression, other psychiatric illnesses, declining physical health, objectively measured memory impairment, or incident dementia,[33,34] and declines in cerebral metabolism.[49] In some persons, memory complaints may be a symptom of an early dementing disorder, especially in persons with cognitive impairment[50] or highly educated persons, who may notice changes before detection with objective tests.[33]

Medical/Psychiatric/Surgical Histories and Review of Systems

Gathering information about previous episodes of memory loss, mood or other psychiatric disorders, and medical conditions and procedures are pertinent to understanding the patient's current presentation. The physician obtains history on basic medical conditions, especially those that may affect cognition, including hypertension, cardiovascular disease, diabetes, head injury with loss of consciousness, sleep apnea, and seizures. Many physical conditions such as cardiac, pulmonary, and kidney dysfunction, toxic or metabolic (e.g., diabetes, thyroid dysfunction) abnormalities, vitamin deficiencies, recent infections including urinary tract infections, seizures, and HIV risk factors can impair mental abilities. Elderly individuals are vulnerable to vascular complications following cerebral hypoperfusion, and the clinician should inquire about related risks, such as congestive heart failure and coronary artery bypass graft or other surgeries under general anesthesia.[51]

Substance Use and Dependence

An accurate history of substance use should include a nonjudgmental inquiry about the amount of alcohol and other substances used, length of use, periods of sobriety, and impact of use on relationships and functioning. Information about substance use is critical because substance abuse or dependence is associated with cognitive difficulties. Recovery of cognitive abilities may be slow in elderly alcohol-abstinent individuals.[52] Smoking history is important, because smoking is a risk factor for cerebrovascular disease.

Medications and Allergies

Review of both prescription and over-the-counter medications is warranted, particularly because some medications, medication interactions, or medication mismanagement may result in or contribute to cognitive dysfunction. Patients with memory difficulties may not properly self-administer medications; therefore, the physician should inquire how patients keep track of medication use (i.e., use of pill organizers) and who administers the medications. Use of natural supplements and herbal remedies has become increasingly common, and the physician should inquire about supplements, which can interact with prescription medications.[53] Also note any history of allergies.

Social, Educational, and Occupational Histories

Assessing educational attainment and performance and occupational history provides additional information about a patient's pre-evaluation level of adjustment and intellectual, occupational, and social functioning. The physician should obtain information regarding marital status or domestic partner, familial and social relationships, and living situation. Such information is useful in determining who may be involved in the patient's care, support, or supervision.

Family History

Physicians should inquire about family history of dementia or psychiatric illnesses, given the genetic contribution to brain aging rates, dementia, and psychiatric disorder risks. For dementia, information about age at onset and specific diagnoses as well as symptoms in family members, if known, is relevant. For psychiatric history, the clinician should ask whether any relatives had psychiatric illnesses such as depression and any treatments received.

Physical Examination

The physical examination includes a basic neurologic examination, which can provide information relevant to the differential diagnosis and the need for examination by a specialist. For instance, in early AD, motor, sensory, and cerebellar portions of the neurologic examination are intact, whereas in vascular or mixed dementia (vascular plus AD) focal motor or sensory signs (excluding fluent aphasia and apraxia) may be present.[54] Parkinsonian rigidity and bradykinesia accompanying dementia onset are suggestive of Lewy body dementia.[55,56]

Laboratory Tests

The American Academy of Neurology[57] currently recommends only vitamin B_{12} and thyroid function for routine laboratory screening. However, additional tests to consider include complete blood count, electrolyte panel, glucose, hepatic and renal function tests, erythrocyte sedimentation rate, arterial blood gas, autoimmune disease screening tests such as antinuclear antibody, toxicology screens, lumbar puncture, electroencephalogram, HIV, heavy metal levels, and a rapid plasma reagin if the history or physical examination is suspicious for any of the conditions for which these tests are indicated.

Mental Status Examination

The mental status evaluation involves observing patients and asking questions to gather information about a patient's behavior and appearance, ambulation and movement, mood and affect, speech, thought processes and content, insight and judgment, and basic cognition.

Observation of patients is an important data-gathering tool that provides clues about cognitive impairment and differential diagnosis. Physicians who meet their patients in the waiting room can note what the patient is doing—engaged in conversation, reading, or staring blankly. Attire and grooming provide clues about difficulty dressing or poor hygiene. Watching patients getting out of chairs provides information about muscle strength or coordination. Gait disturbances, such as limps, broad-based gait, mincing steps, or a leaden tread may be indicative of the presence of an underlying disorder. Physicians should observe for repetitive movements (dyskinesias), tremor, or asymmetries, which can provide information about stroke or other abnormality.

The first element of a mental status test should be the assessment of the patient's level of awareness, because awareness affects the rest of the evaluation. Note if the patient is alert, drowsy, lethargic, sleepy, or in a stupor, or if the patient demonstrates fluctuations in alertness and arousal.

Listening to casual conversation and speech provides information about language functioning and possible focal abnormalities or underlying disorders. The clinician listens to the quality of speech, such as the rhythm, rate, flow, tone, volume, prosody (emotional cadence), and grammatical content, and determines if patients can comprehend. Indicators of language problems include pauses in speech, which may suggest difficulties finding words or slowed information processing; slurred or garbled speech (dysarthria); and mistakes that involve substitutions of incorrect syllables or words (paraphasic errors). Grammatical errors may indicate aphasia. For example, telegraphic speech (i.e., speech that includes noun–verb combinations, but omits articles, prepositions, conjunctions, pronouns, plurals, and past tenses) is an indication of Broca's aphasia. Difficulties following simple commands indicate possible comprehension problems. Difficulties following more complex or lengthy commands can indicate comprehension or memory problems.

Speech provides clues to thought content and thought process. Speech may be linear, goal directed, meaningful, tangential, circumstantial, bizarre, or blocked. Evidence of intrusions or inappropriate responses or content may indicate disinhibition, poor social judgment, or psychosis. Thought content abnormalities include delusions, hallucinations, illusions, ideas of reference, and suicidal and homicidal ideations. In patients with memory problems, recalling events or details of events that never occurred indicates confabulation.

During the interview, assess for symptoms of depressed mood or anxiety. *Mood* refers to a patient's inner state or feelings (i.e., anxious, depressed, sad) or the feeling tone observed by the physician. *Affect* refers to outward expression of emotion, which may include facial expression, tone of voice, body language, and demeanor. The physician may ask how the patient feels, but should also observe affect to determine if it matches the content of the patient's report. The range of emotional expression may be broad, reduced by varying degrees, or labile. Patients may deny, minimize, or not obviously present with depression. Patients also may vary in their willingness to report depression or have reduced awareness or varying expressions of depression because of educational, cultural, generational, or gender-related factors. The clinician should inquire about additional depression symptoms such as changes or disruptions in sleep, appetite, concentration, interest in activities, libido, and energy level; the presence of feelings of guilt, hopelessness, helplessness; and somaticizing. Clinicians should ask about passive thoughts of death (i.e., reports that life is not worth living or patients feeling like they would be better off dead), as well as active suicidal thoughts and about a specific plan or the means to commit suicide in patients with suicidal ideation. The inquiry then concludes with further questions about the presence of other symptoms, such as anxiety, panic, mania, paranoia, hallucinations, homicidal ideation, obsessions, or compulsions. Life transitions, such as retirement, losses (of a loved one, physical mobility, employment, or financial security), moving, personal illness or illness in a family member, or caring for an ill loved one, should alert the clinician to the potential for stress or dysphoria in patients.

The initial evaluation also includes determining whether the patient has sufficient insight into cognitive difficulties and has a sense of how cognitive difficulties affect daily functioning or relationships with others. Some patients present with memory complaints, whereas others minimize them. More severely impaired patients may not be aware of cognitive problems or how cognitive problems impact their judgment [42] or daily function. With cognitively impaired patients, such information is best learned from the family.

Cognitive Screening

Cognitive screenings are brief in-office assessments of cognition that provide information regarding cognitive functioning. Cognitive screening includes using validated screening instruments, such as the MMSE, and brief bedside assessments. Cognitive screenings are usually sensitive to significant cognitive impairment associated with dementia, and in some patients, they can also detect MCI.

Cognitive screening starts with a measure of gross cognition, such as the MMSE,[58] a validated screening tool widely used in the evaluation of memory loss and dementia. The MMSE includes 30 items that assess orientation to time and place, registration of three words, attention, recall of three words, the ability to follow three-step commands, repetition of a phrase, the ability to follow a written command, writing a sentence, and visuospatial ability (figure copying). The exam can be administered in 5–10 min. For the average individual, a score of 23 points or less is consistent with a diagnosis of dementia, scores of 11–20 are generally seen in moderate dementia, and 10 or lower in advanced dementia. Care must be taken in interpreting MMSE scores in persons with either very high or very low levels of education. Patients with higher levels of academic achievement may have high scores on the MMSE (e.g., [27–30]) yet still suffer from dementia, and for patients with fewer than 9 years of education, the typical 23–24 cutoff for dementia may be too stringent and result in a false-positive error.[59] Age and education corrected norms are available.[60,61]

Supplementing the MMSE with additional tests may improve the accuracy of diagnosis[62,63] and provide additional or more extensive information about cognitive function. At the very least, a brief memory and executive function assessment can add to the clinical picture. Additional tests of language and visual-spatial abilities also can be administered, depending on the need for further information or the patient's presentation. A number of resources on mental status testing are available.[64,65]

Assessing delayed recall with a 10-item word list can alert the physician to either MCI or dementia. An example of an easy to administer and validated instrument is the memory test from the Consortium to Establish a Registry for Alzheimer's Disease.[66] The Consortium word list has been administered to numerous patients and cognitively intact controls and is available in several languages. After presenting the word list visually, using cards, three times (in a different order each time), recall and recognition are tested after a 5-min delay. Cognitively intact subjects generally recall six or seven of the words after the delay, patients recalling only three or four of the words may have MCI, and if they also have additional cognitive difficulties and functional impairment, then such a low score would indicate dementia.

Tests of frontal-executive functioning include clock drawing, similarities, sequencing, proverb interpretation, and multiple loops.[64,65] For clock drawing, the patient is instructed to draw a clock with the hands set at 11:10. People with cognitive dysfunction will be stimulus bound (draw the hands at 10 and 11), show impaired planning (crowding numbers or running out of space to put the clock face numbers), neglect (leaving numbers off one side, usually the left, of the clock), or exhibit gross disorganization (inability to draw anything resembling a clock). In hand sequencing, patients are asked to correctly perform a succession of hand movements developed by Luria (the hand is first placed flat, then on one side, and then as a fist, on a flat surface). In addition, patients can be asked to copy a series of figures (triangles, squares, and circles) or multiple loops. Patients with frontal impairment may be unable to alternate at all or more than a few times and instead draw the same figure repetitively (perseveration); patients may experience stimulus or evidence *closing in,* in which they crowd the stimulus figure or sometimes trace over it. Abstraction, another frontal lobe function, can be assessed using proverb interpretation. The patient interprets common proverbs such as, "Don't cry over spilled milk." Concrete answers such as, "The milk spilled so you have to wipe it up," are indications of reduced abstraction ability. On similarities, patients explain how two increasingly disparate items are alike (e.g., ask how a table and a chair are alike). Abstract responses such as "both furniture" indicate better abstraction ability than concrete answers such as "You sit on both." As items become increasingly difficult (e.g., poem–statue), patients with concrete thinking may respond that they are "not alike" or that "a poem describes a statue." Word generation or fluency is another frontal function that can be assessed in the office. The physician can ask the patient to produce as many words as possible (in 1 min) that begin with a particular letter of the alphabet (commonly F, A, and S), excluding proper nouns. Typically, producing fewer than eight F words in 1 min indicates impairment, but cultural and educational factors influence this test and such factors must be considered before determining that fluency is impaired in someone with reduced output. Qualitatively, the physician should also note any perseverations or intrusions of words that do not begin with the specified letter.

For extensive language assessments, patients should be referred to a speech pathologist; but the physician can assess basic elements of language comprehension and production in the office. The MMSE covers simple verbal and written comprehension, production, repetition, and naming. However, impairment may be evident with further testing. For instance, sometimes anomia is evident in a patient after several naming trials or when patients are asked to name low-frequency items. Therefore, physicians can have a set of pictures or objects available to assess naming in greater depth than provided in the MMSE. Similarly, comprehension can be assessed by asking patients to point at objects in the room, first one at a time, and then in serial order, and follow multistage commands. Patients who have difficulty following increasingly lengthy commands may have a memory problem.

When patients have complaints of getting lost in familiar surroundings, the physician can assess visuoconstruction or the ability to copy and produce figures on demand, such as a cross, square, and cube.

The physician can also assess general fund of knowledge with questions such as, "Where is China?" or "Name one (or more) of the presidents after John Kennedy." Asking about news is also helpful in determining recent memory and the patient's understanding of recent events.

In sum, the depth of the mental status examination depends on the need to gather additional data to develop diagnostic hypotheses. Any time that cognition is assessed, the physician needs to keep in mind that performance is influenced by the presence of sensory impairments, age, education, and language proficiency. For a detailed assessment of mental abilities or in cases in which results of the cognitive screening are equivocal, patients should be referred to a clinical neuropsychologist for an evaluation. A speech pathologist should be consulted for in-depth speech and language assessments or when aphasia is noted.

Structural Neuroimaging

Consensus guidelines on the evaluation of dementia recommend routine structural imaging studies to assist in the diagnosis and differential diagnosis of dementia.[46]

Specific indications for structural imaging include MRI scans (or CT if MRI is not available) for cognitive decline or deficits, personality or behavioral change, suspicious historical features, focal neurologic findings, or neurologic indications of stroke, tumor, bleeding, seizure activity, or hydrocephalus.

PET Scans

Including 2-deoxy-2-[^{18}F]fluoro-D-glucose (FDG) positron emission tomography (PET) in a diagnostic workup adds to an understanding of the clinical picture and improves diagnostic accuracy. Physicians as well as family members may erroneously attribute cognitive decline to normal aging,[67–69] especially when patients are in the early stages of a dementing disorder, and estimates of failing to recognize cognitive impairment may range from 40% to 90% of cases.[70–72]

Adding PET to a clinical dementia evaluation can enhance diagnostic sensitivity. In relation to neuropathologic confirmation of the presence or absence of AD, inclusion of PET in a clinical dementia workup increases accuracy for detecting AD compared with clinical workups that do not include PET.[73] Sensitivity pertains to correctly determining the presence of AD, whereas specificity pertains to correctly determining that AD is not present. Previous studies have found that the sensitivity for detecting histopathologically confirmed AD using PET falls in the range of 91.5% ± 3.5%, compared with 66% ± 17% for detecting it on the basis of identifying probable AD in clinical evaluations performed without PET, with comparable specificities for both kinds of workup.[74] If AD is considered to be detected on the basis of clinically identifying either possible or probable AD, sensitivity with and without PET is then comparable, but specificity without PET then falls to a range (55.5% ± 5.5%) that is substantially lower than that achieved when using PET (70% ± 3%). In patients already diagnosed with dementia, a PET scan can clarify the diagnosis, which is relevant to appropriate treatment, for example, in differentiating AD from FTD, because unlike AD, FTD does not respond well to acetylcholinesterase inhibitor treatment.[75]

A major clinical challenge is the early identification of patients who will develop AD or other dementias, which is relevant to earlier treatment intervention and planning for a patient's future needs.[76] Several studies indicate that PET is sensitive to AD-like hypometabolic brain changes in nondemented persons with the apolipoprotein epsilon 4 (APOE-4) genetic risk for AD.[77,78] Results of various investigations indicate that PET predicts cognitive decline in persons with APOE-4,[79] in normal elderly persons,[80] and in persons with mild memory complaints.[81] PET also has been found to predict AD in persons with questionable dementia.[82] Recent studies also support the use of PET to predict the conversion of MCI to dementia[83] or for differentiating stable from progressive amnestic MCI, particularly in combination with memory test performance scores.[84]

Some patients with a normal initial evaluation request a PET study because they are concerned about their personal risk for dementia, such as prior head trauma or a family history of dementia. A negative PET may reassure these *worried well* individuals that they have no evidence of a progressive neurodegenerative dementia. If, however, the scan results are consistent with a progressive neurodegenerative dementia, then patients can consider early treatment intervention strategies to slow progression of cognitive impairment, although this would be considered an off-label use of medication.

Silverman and associates[85–87] developed an algorithm to determine if a PET scan is likely to be useful in diagnosis (Fig. 1.1). According to the algorithm, persons who have cognitive impairment, identified by history and initial cognitive screening, undergo a screening laboratory assessment, pertinent cognitive testing, and, if indicated, structural neuroimaging. If these reveal abnormalities, then the patient is treated and reassessed after treatment is completed. A PET scan is indicated if deficits then persist, or if the initial workup does not reveal an underlying cause. The consequence of not using PET in an evaluation is not only reduced diagnostic sensitivity, but also a possible lost opportunity for early intervention in the case of a missed diagnosis. PET has become increasingly available clinically because of the approval of Medicare funding for PET scanning.

Although PET typically enhances diagnostic sensitivity, errors in specificity can occur despite its use. Persons with DLB, for example, may be mistakenly diagnosed as having AD with or without the use of PET; however, cholinesterase inhibitors commonly used in AD are often beneficial in DLB or mixed dementia.[88–90] Limited research has been conducted on memantine in non-AD dementias, but it appears to be well tolerated in patients with VaD and mixed dementias,[91] and is tolerated in DLB, although some adverse reactions have been reported.[92,93]

Although a diagnosis of AD may be upsetting to the patient and family members, accurate knowledge of diagnosis often reduces anxiety and helps families clarify caregiving tasks. Many patients and family members are relieved when a diagnosis is reached and a treatment plan is enacted, especially after a patient has undergone many inconclusive evaluations and procedures.[73]

Case Study

A case study of a 53-year-old woman who presented to the UCLA Memory Clinic demonstrates the usefulness of PET in a clinical evaluation.[73] The patient began a series of clinical evaluations more than 2 years before coming to the memory clinic. She first presented to her internist with complaints of memory loss and functional impairment at work. She was diagnosed with depression and referred to a neurologist, who saw the patient twice. The neurologist noted that the patient was anxious and "hyperventilated at times," and attributed most symptoms to a psychiatric cause. The neurologist ordered two MRI scans of the brain (with and without contrast) to rule out frontal lobe disease. The noncontrast MRI showed a 1-cm area of abnormal signal in the deep white matter of the right parietal lobe on the T2- but not the T1-weighted image. A subsequent contrast MRI also showed slightly increased signal in that same area. The radiologist interpreted the

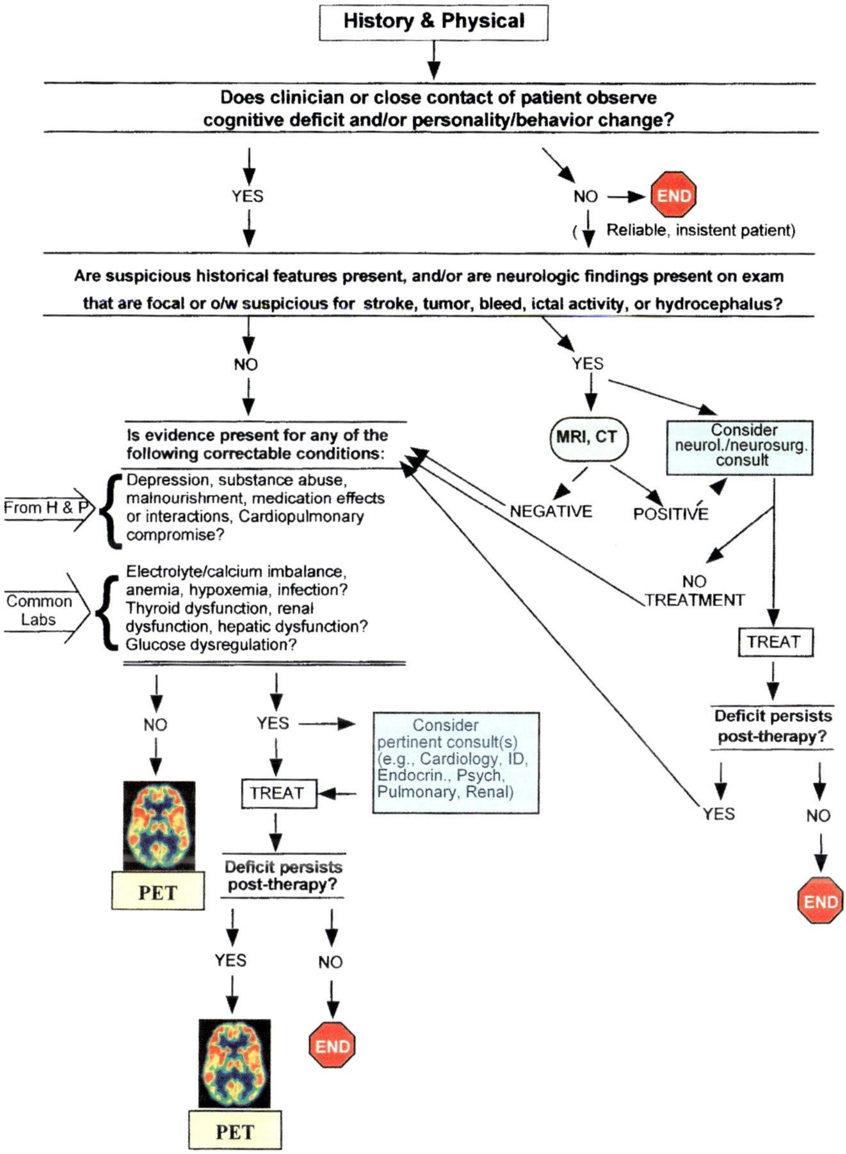

Fig. 1.1 When to get PET. Flow diagram demonstrating diagnostic algorithm for evaluation of geriatric patients with early symptoms of cognitive decline. Cost–benefit analyses have demonstrated that use of this algorithm can provide greater diagnostic accuracy at lower overall financial cost, in the context of the clinical and economic environments of both the United States[85] and continental Europe,[86] than comparable algorithms that fail to employ brain PET scanning in appropriate patients. (Adapted from Silverman et al.[85] with permission.)

finding as being consistent with an ischemic change, and the neurologist's impression was that it was consistent with the patient's history of migraine. The patient saw her internist two more times and was diagnosed with hypothyroidism, depression, and fibromyalgia.

The patient's memory problems persisted, and 8 months later she saw a neuropsychologist. The neuropsychologist noted a significantly reduced performance IQ compared with a normal verbal IQ and determined that the results suggested neurologic difficulties, as well as the possible contributory effects of posttraumatic stress disorder.

The patient still had no conclusive or specific diagnosis after 9 months when she was seen by a geriatric psychiatrist at a University memory clinic. The geriatric psychiatrist performed an intake evaluation, administering an MMSE and reviewing the patient's previous brain imaging studies. The patient was impaired on the MMSE, scoring 18 of 30. An FDG PET scan was performed, and it revealed diffuse, moderately severe cortical hypometabolism, especially affecting the bilateral parietal, left inferior frontal, and temporal cortices and sparing the bilateral sensorimotor and visual cortices. The results were consistent with a neurodegenerative dementia, most likely AD. A follow-up MRI was then obtained, which was still within normal limits. A neuropsychological evaluation performed 1 week after the PET indicated extensive and severe cognitive deficits that could not be explained by the patient's previous diagnoses (i.e., fibromyalgia, attention deficit disorder, depression, posttraumatic stress disorder).

The psychiatrist diagnosed the patient with possible AD on the basis of the PET result, severe cognitive impairment on neuropsychological test results and the unremarkable MRI, and then prescribed an acetylcholinesterase inhibitor. The patient responded well to treatment cognitively, as well as improving in her social functioning. The family also was referred to the Alzheimer's Association, and the patient and her husband were able to proceed with their lives. The patient returned for regular follow-up at the memory clinic every 6–12 months.

Overall, compared with years of conventional evaluations with no specific diagnosis, in contrast, within the course of 1 month after she came to the memory clinic, the patient obtained a PET scan that revealed a pattern consistent with AD, was diagnosed with possible AD, received and subsequently responded to treatment. The patient's young age contributed to the diagnostic delay, as most cases of AD occur after the age of 65. The neurologist suspected FTD, which commonly occurs in persons under 65 years, but the MRI was generally unremarkable. Nevertheless, the sensitivity of PET to early dementia and differentiating AD from FTD underscores the value of PET in a diagnostic workup, particularly after other diagnostic tests yield inconclusive findings.

Neuropsychological Testing

A neuropsychological evaluation consists of administering a battery of standardized tests to assess cognition. Test result interpretation is based on comparing the performance (i.e., test scores) to normative data appropriate to the individual's peer group or cohort (i.e., typically age, education, and when available, gender, and ethnicity). When deficits are noted, their pattern and level of severity can provide information about whether a patient is demented or has MCI and about possible underlying etiologies.

Referral for neuropsychological testing is recommended when the diagnosis is unclear, and the pattern of performance on tests may provide clues regarding differential diagnosis. When the physician or patients or their families want a detailed description of cognition, a neuropsychological evaluation can be useful. Neuropsychological testing is typically more sensitive to detecting mild cognitive deficits than cognitive screening; thus, neuropsychological testing is appropriate when mild deficits are suspected or present when cognitive screening is within normal limits. Neuropsychological testing can be ordered to establish a baseline of cognitive functioning, assess the magnitude and rate of change in patients who have had previous testing, or assess behavioral expressions of treatment response. In addition, neuropsychologists can provide recommendations about compensatory strategies for cognitive impairment, behavioral management, and performance of daily activities.

Neuropsychological testing has limitations. Patients may experience fatigue from testing or anxiety related to testing, and patients without medical insurance may not be able to afford neuropsychological testing. Neuropsychological tests are not direct or perfect measures of everyday life activities;[94] therefore, they may not be optimally sensitive to changes or declines in functional activities in daily life. The sensitivity of neuropsychological testing may be decreased if normative groups are contaminated with cognitively impaired or mildly demented subjects in the older age ranges. Tests that are developed primarily on the majority culture (e.g., predominantly English-speaking white persons) are not appropriate for ethnic minorities, non-native English speakers, or persons with different cultural experiences compared with the majority culture.[95] Neuropsychological testing is sensitive to preclinical cognitive changes.[96,97] However, in persons with normal cognition or high cognitive reserve who can compensate for cognitive difficulties, PET imaging typically is a more powerful early detection tool.[98]

Genetic Testing

Genetic testing may be helpful in identifying mutations in rare families that demonstrate an autosomal dominant inheritance pattern. (Half of relatives develop dementia, often in their fifties or sixties.) Patients with cognitive decline who have a strong family history of early onset dementia are candidates for such tests. In such situations, identifying a rare genetic mutation may inform at-risk relatives of their prognosis.

The possession of the APOE-4 allele is a risk factor for developing AD.[99,100] APOE-4 is a susceptibility gene—it is neither necessary nor sufficient for the development of AD. Knowing its presence may give a patient a conviction of false doom, and its absence may give a false sense of security. Therefore, experts have not recommended APOE assessment as a predictive test in asymptomatic individuals.[101] Recent research has found that many patients who choose to obtain such genetic risk information do not experience adverse psychological effects,[102] although one study reported that persons with knowledge of carrying the APOE-4 genetic risk may alter decisions about purchasing long-term health care insurance.[103]

Making an Initial Diagnosis

After conducting the interview and mental status examination, the physician formulates diagnostic hypotheses. The physician then considers all of the data gathered about the patient's history, functional status, laboratory test results, and physical and mental status examination, and formulates a working diagnosis that provisionally places the patient within one of several broad categories of diagnosis. The first step is to decide whether a patient has evidence of a cognitive deficit.

If the patient's history, MMSE, and other supplemental test results do not suggest cognitive or functional decline, then the patient most likely does not have a cognitive disorder. Patients who have no identifiable memory impairment or patients with AAMI may be reassured that they have normal memory functioning at the time of the evaluation. Because only approximately 1% of persons with AAMI develop dementia annually, the evaluation can be considered a baseline assessment, and they can be monitored with biannual evaluations. If the physician has not obtained a PET scan, then PET in these patients may be helpful in assessing dementia risk, as studies of people with AAMI have indicated that patterns of parietal deficits predict future cognitive decline after several years.[79]

If, however, the MMSE or assessments of delayed recall fall outside of the normal range for age and education, then the patient may have either MCI or dementia. The distinction of MCI versus dementia is often based on functional impairment.[2] If no occupational or social functional impairment exists, and typically only memory is impaired, then the initial impression would be consistent with MCI. Although in the original conception of MCI (i.e., amnestic MCI), memory was the only cognitive domain affected, the definition has been expanded to include other subtypes with mild impairment in other or multiple cognitive domains.[22]

Patients with MCI should be monitored closely. At present, no medications have been approved by the FDA for the treatment of MCI. Some MCI patients may request acetylcholinesterase inhibitor drugs (currently an off-label use), but the results of randomized clinical trials of acetylcholinesterase inhibitors in MCI indicate that efficacy and safety may vary depending on the individual drug and outcome measure assessed.[104–106]

If the patient does have functional impairment (e.g., gets lost while driving in familiar places, forgets to pay bills, cannot manage medications, leaves pots burning on the stove), has evidence of dysfunction in memory and another cognitive domain, and has not had an abrupt change in mental status (suggesting a delirium), then the provisional diagnosis is dementia.

In patients diagnosed with dementia, the next step is differential diagnosis. Differential diagnosis may be challenging, but most cases result from a few pathologies that are identifiable by their clinical courses and neuroimaging findings.

Alzheimer's disease is characterized by insidious onset, early memory loss, language and visuospatial deficits (reflecting the destruction of the temporal and parietal lobes), a progressive course, and lack of early neurologic signs early in the disease course. Cognitive deficits are prominent and become more severe and global as AD progresses. Behavioral and personality changes, including agitation, aggression, and psychosis, often emerge as the disease progresses. Depressed mood often occurs with AD. Brain autopsies of persons with AD indicate an accumulation of the neuropathologic hallmarks of the disease, amyloid neuritic plaques and neurofibrillary tangles. PET patterns reveal hypometabolism in posterior cingulate, parietal, and temporal cortices with frontal involvement as AD progresses.[74]

Vascular Dementia

Often coincident with AD, cerebrovascular damage is the second most common cause of dementia. Numerous types of lesions can cause VaD, including single small but devastating lesions in vital brain regions, or multiple white matter lesions that accumulate over the years because of chronic hypertension. Such heterogeneity produces a varying clinical picture and requires careful consideration of other sources of vascular pathology such as infectious, inflammatory, embolic, and occlusive sources. However, evidence supportive of a diagnosis of VaD[54] includes a close (3-month) temporal relationship between a cerebrovascular event and cognitive decline, neurologic deficits, and evidence of vascular disease on structural neuroimaging (MRI or CT) in the absence of altered level of consciousness. Cognitive deficits are variable depending on the type and location of the cerebral lesion, but executive deficits and psychomotor slowing are common in VaD. PET often demonstrates patchy hypometabolic patterns, both in cortical and subcortical regions, consistent with discrete vascular lesions,[107] but the better spatial resolution of MRI scanning provides a more sensitive measure to detect cerebrovascular disease. As with AD, depression and apathy may be co-morbid with VaD, and first onset of depression in late life is associated with a number of factors, including underlying cerebrovascular disease.[108,109]

Dementia with Lewy Bodies

DLB is another common cause of dementia. Unlike AD, most DLB patients are more likely to be men, and the illness has a shorter course (less than 10 years) than AD. Most cases of DLB occur in persons over 65 years of age. DLB is characterized by a frontal-subcortical cognitive deficit pattern (early and prominent impairment in attention and executive dysfunction, compared with less prominent and later memory impairment), fluctuating level of cognition and alertness, parkinsonism, and visual hallucinations. DLB may be difficult to distinguish from Parkinson's disease, but the parkinsonism in DLB differs from Parkinson's disease by being more often symmetric, with less pronounced tremor (if any). Hallucinations are also more prominent in Parkinson's disease than in DLB. The diagnosis is supported by a history of syncope, falls, confusion, extreme sensitivity to the movement side effects of neuroleptics, delusions, and other types of hallucinations. Single photon emission computed tomography (SPECT) demonstrates hypoperfusion,[110] and PET[111] demonstrates a glucose metabolic pattern similar to AD (parietal, temporal, and frontal deficits), along with occipital hypometabolism.

Frontotemporal Dementia

FTD is a spectrum of disorders characterized by prominent early frontal or temporal dysfunction or both. Depending on the region and hemisphere involved, FTD patients often present first with behavioral syndromes characterized by changes in personality and social functioning, including disinhibition, eccentricity, apathy, emotional blunting, hyperorality, and psychiatric symptoms such as depression and compulsions. Early cognitive symptoms include disturbances in language (reduced output, echolalia, palilalia) and executive dysfunction, and relative sparing of episodic memory and visuospatial functions early on. Patients usually have an earlier average age at onset than AD (the sixth decade on average) and a faster course of progressive deterioration to mutism and profound dementia over approximately a decade. Because behavioral disturbances are prominent early on, psychiatric conditions such as mood and psychotic disorders should be considered in the differential diagnosis. Structural neuroimaging may reveal frontal and temporal (particularly anterior temporal) atrophy. PET and SPECT may show frontotemporal abnormalities with preserved posterior functioning.[112] PET is particularly useful in distinguishing AD from FTD.

Other Dementia Syndromes

Other conditions to be considered in the differential diagnosis include Creutzfeldt-Jakob disease, HIV-associated dementia, neurosyphilis, Parkinson's disease dementia, dementia resulting from exposure to toxic substances (e.g., alcohol, heavy metals, illicit substances), normal pressure hydrocephalus, metabolic abnormalities, and dementias related to psychiatric disorders such as bipolar disorder and schizophrenia. These dementias usually account for a small percentage of cases in typical clinical settings. Should the history, physical examination, or neuroimaging studies suggest one of these less common causes of dementia, further workup and evaluation must be pursued, including possible referral to the appropriate specialist for definitive diagnosis and treatment.

Medical Specialty Resources and Referrals for Patients

Disposition plans vary depending on the diagnosis. For persons with normal cognitive function or AAMI, follow-up assessments every 6 to 12 months or referral back to their primary care or other referring physician may be appropriate. Neuropsychologists can conduct annual evaluations to track cognitive change, if needed.

Patients with AD can be managed and treated successfully by primary care physicians, but patients with more complex presentations or medical histories, with atypical symptoms, or early onset dementia (before 60 years of age) may necessitate referral to specialists. Neurologic consultation is important for patients with parkinsonism, focal neurologic signs, abrupt onset or unusually rapid course or progression, or abnormal neuroimaging findings.

Patients with depression or anxiety require further evaluation and treatment by a specialist. Clinicians can refer patients to geriatric psychiatrists for pharmacologic interventions; or to a geriatric psychiatrist, psychologist, or therapist for psychotherapy (individual and family), behavioral management, management of suicidal behavior, and functional evaluation to make a determination about institutionalization or hospitalization. Neuropsychologists can conduct evaluations to track cognitive change or treatment response. Speech pathologists can provide therapy for patients with aphasia or other language disorders. Social workers can provide counseling or direct patients to helpful community resources. Patients may require referrals to physical therapists, occupational therapists, or recreational specialists for rehabilitation or support in performing basic activities. Day treatment programs offer cognitive and social stimulation for patients, as well as respite for caregivers.

Planning for illness progression and end-of-life issues is important. Patients at risk for dementia or in the early stages of a dementing illness may consult an attorney for making wills, estate planning, or arrangements for end-of-life care or conservatorships. Social workers and other professionals can assist the family in arranging for home healthcare, daycare, or placement in an assisted living center, nursing home, hospice, or rarely a hospital. Medical ethicists or clergy may be consulted for end-of-life issues.

The Future of Neuroimaging in Clinical Evaluations

Innovations in neuroimaging techniques and tracer development hold promise for new clinical applications. Brain imaging will play an important role in the development of surrogate markers that will effectively identify people with mild cognitive decline who are at risk for the development of AD, assist in making the differential diagnosis, and assist in the assessment of drug, anti-amyloid, and other treatment responses.

Imaging of Amyloid Plaques and Neurofibrillary Tangles In Vivo

Evidence from postmortem studies indicates that the accumulation of senile plaques[113] and neurofibrillary tangles,[114] the neuropathologic hallmarks of AD, occurs over the decades before clinical AD diagnosis. The prospect of in vivo visualization of these neuropathologic lesions has driven several groups (e.g., Pittsburgh,[115] UCLA,[116,117] University of Pennsylvania[118]) to search for imaging biomarkers of these pathologies. The early success using ^{18}F-FDDNP[116] to visualize neurofibrillary tangles and senile plaques in AD and research by Klunk et al.[119] on amyloid labeling offer an opportunity to follow the neuropathologic evolution of AD in living subjects. In addition, the ability of ^{18}F-FDDNP to label neurofibrillary tangles suggests that it may be useful in imaging prominent tauopathies, such as FTD, as initial studies have suggested.[120]

Imaging of Neuroreceptor Densities In Vivo

Additional measures of neurodegenerative decline, such as reduced density of medial temporal serotonin receptors as an index of hippocampal pyramidal neuronal loss, might further assist in defining the patterns of dementia and brain aging and augment early detection and disease progression monitoring. ^{18}F-MPPF is a selective molecular imaging probe for 5-HT1A receptors in hippocampus and other brain areas, which permits quantification of 5-HT1A receptor densities in the human brain with PET.[121] Recent research has shown that ^{18}F-MPPF is sensitive to determining the degree of densities of these receptors and can help differentiate between patients with AD, MCI, and normal cognition.[122]

Surrogate Markers for Treatment Response

Neuroimaging shows potential for use as surrogate markers for response to pharmacotherapy. Limited trials have been conducted, but the results indicate that FDG PET is sensitive to differential change and response in regional cerebral metabolism in persons with AD treated with cholinesterase inhibitors compared with placebo.[123,124] Structural MRI is also being examined as a surrogate marker for treatment interventions in AD.[125] Hippocampal atrophy is not specific for AD, but antemortem hippocampal volume has been found to be a marker of pathologic stage[126] and related to hippocampal neurofibrillary tangle burden.[127] In vivo visualization of these brain pathologies will also help develop further understanding of how antiaggregation drugs directly interact with neurofibril aggregates.[128]

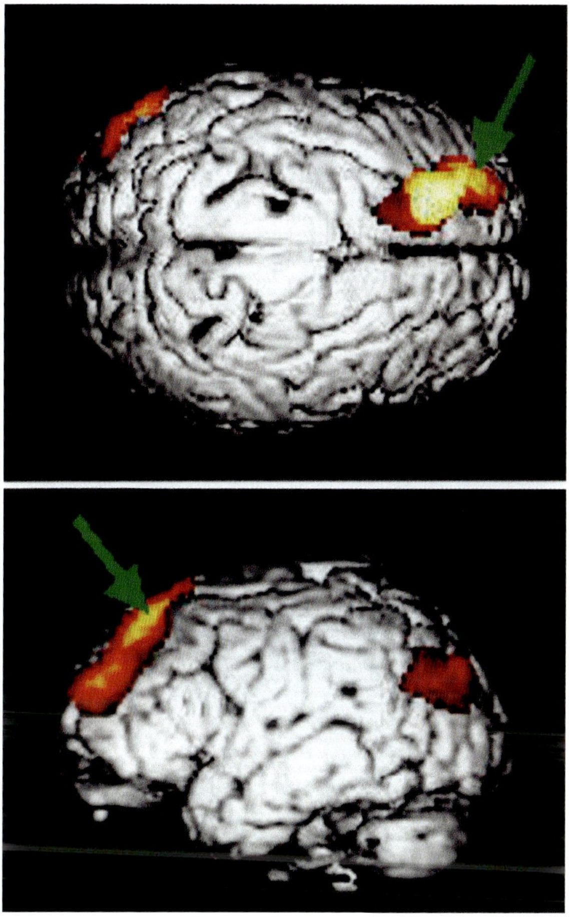

Fig. 1.2 Effects of a healthy lifestyle intervention on resting brain metabolism. The images display a statistical parametric map of FDG-PET data, comparing changes in intervention and control subject groups. Following the intervention comprised of lifestyle instructional information and 2 weeks of implementation at home, a 5% decrease in activity was identified in the left dorsolateral prefrontal cortex of subjects in the intervention group but not the control group. The color scale highlights the location of all cortical voxels in which significantly greater decreases ($P < 0.01$) occurred in the former, involving a stretch of cortex in Brodmann's areas 8, 9, and 10, shown from above the brain (*top*), and from the left lateral viewpoint (*bottom*). The arrows point to the region of peak significance

Surrogate Markers for Response to Preventative Strategies

Finally, neuroimaging may have applications as a surrogate marker for responses to nonpharmacologic preventative strategies, such as lifestyle interventions. Our group conducted a pilot study to determine the effects of a healthy lifestyle intervention, consisting of healthy diet, exercise, and cognitive stimulation, on brain function and other physiologic indexes related to cardiac and brain health.[129] Healthy middle-aged to older volunteers were randomized to a 2-week healthy lifestyle intervention or a control group. The intervention group showed a reduction in frontal lobe activity on PET compared with the control condition, suggestive of more efficient brain functioning or heightened attentional abilities (Fig. 1.2). Currently, larger clinical trials are underway to further assess the role of neuroimaging in assessing the effects of preventative interventions on brain function.

Conclusion

Effective and appropriate treatment of dementia begins with accurate clinical diagnosis. With the advent of pharmacologic and novel medical interventions for the treatment of dementia, early diagnosis is of increasing importance. Neuroimaging can add to clinical evaluations by enhancing sensitivity and specificity and aiding in differential diagnosis. New technologies in neuroimaging will enhance early diagnostic accuracy and serve as biomarkers for treatment response. Although evaluations without neuroimaging are less costly in the short term, appropriate use of neuroimaging in clinical evaluations can save time and cost in the long run. Because FDG PET increases diagnostic sensitivity and specificity of AD, the technique could also improve diagnostic homogeneity in clinical trials of mild-to-moderate AD. Identifying a specific neuroimaging pattern (e.g., parietal and temporal hypometabolism) would result in treating a refined phenotype rather than a clinical syndrome. Through early detection and enhanced diagnostic accuracy, patients can receive treatment that delays dementia onset, slows disease progression, and reduces burdens on society. Patients will be less likely to endure lengthy and multiple costly evaluations.

References

1. US Bureau of the Census. Population projections of the United States by race, sex, age and Hispanic origin: 1995–2050. Current Pop Rep 2000;25–1130.
2. American Psychiatric Association. Diagnostic and Statistical Manual of Mental Disorders, 4th ed. Washington, DC: APA, 1994.
3. Rasmusson DX, Brandt J, Steele C, et al. Accuracy of clinical diagnosis of Alzheimer disease and clinical features of patients with non-Alzheimer neuropathology. Alzheimer Dis Assoc Disord 1996;10:180–188.
4. Larson EB, Edwards JK, O'Meara E, et al. Neuropathologic diagnostic outcomes from a cohort of outpatients with suspected dementia. J Gerontol 1996;51:M313–318.
5. McKhann G, Drachman D, Folstein M, et al. Clinical diagnosis of Alzheimer's disease: report of the NINCDS-ADRDA Work Group under the auspices of Department of Health and Human Services Task Force on Alzheimer's disease. Neurology 1984;34:939–944.
6. Ferri CP, Prince M, Brayne C, et al. Global prevalence of dementia: a Delphi consensus study. Lancet 2005;366:2112–2117.

7. Brookmeyer R, Johnson E, Ziegler G, et al. Forecasting the global burden of Alzheimer's disease. Alzheimers Dement 2007;3:186–91.
8. Jorm AF. The epidemiology of Alzheimer's disease and related disorders. London: Chapman & Hall, 1990.
9. Ritchie K, Kildea D. Is senile dementia "age related" or "aging related?" Evidence from a meta-analysis of dementia prevalence in the oldest old. Lancet 1995;346:931–934.
10. National Institute on Aging. Progress report on Alzheimer's disease 1996. Bethesda: National Institute on Aging; NIH Publication No 96-4137, 1996.
11. Alzheimer's Association. 2008 Alzheimer's Disease Facts and Figures, 2008
12. Brayne C, Gill C, Huppert FA, et al. Incidence of clinically diagnosed subtypes of dementia in an elderly population. Cambridge Project for Later Life. Br J Psychiatr 1995;167:255–262.
13. Hebert R, Brayne C. Epidemiology of vascular dementia. Neuroepidemiology 1995;14:240–257.
14. Ikeda M, Hokoishi K, Maki N, et al. Increased prevalence of vascular dementia in Japan: a community-based epidemiological study. Neurology 2001;57:839–844.
15. Zaccai J, McCracken C, Brayne C. A systematic review of prevalence and incidence studies of dementia with Lewy bodies. Age Ageing 2005;34:561–566.
16. Galariotis V, Bodi N, Janka Z, et al. Frontotemporal dementia—part I. History, prevalence, clinical forms. Ideggyogy Sz 2005;20:164–171.
17. Snowden JS, Neary D, Mann DM. Frontotemporal dementia. Br J Psychiatr 2002;180:140–143.
18. DeKosky S. Early intervention is key to successful management of Alzheimer disease. Alzheimer Dis Assoc Disord 2003;17(Suppl 4):S99–104.
19. Leifer BP. Early diagnosis of Alzheimer's disease: clinical and economic benefits. J Am Geriatr Soc 2003;51(5 Suppl Dementia):S281–288.
20. Crook T, Bartus RT, Ferris SH, et al. Age associated memory impairment: proposed diagnostic criteria and measures of clinical change—report of a National Institute of Mental Health Work Group. Dev Neuropsychol 1986;2:261–276.
21. Petersen RC, Smith GE, Waring SC, et al. Mild cognitive impairment: clinical characterization and outcome. Arch Neurol 1999;56:303–308.
22. Petersen RC. Mild cognitive impairment as a diagnostic entity. J Intern Med 2004;256:183–194.
23. Larrabee GJ, Crook TH. Estimated prevalence of age-associated memory impairment derived from standardized tests of memory function. Int Psychogeriatr 1994;6:95–104.
24. Morris JC, Price AL. Pathologic correlates of nondemented aging, mild cognitive impairment, and early-stage Alzheimer's disease. J Mol Neurosci 2001;17:101–118.
25. Guillozet AL, Weintraub S, Mash DC, et al. Neurofibrillary tangles, amyloid, and memory in aging and mild cognitive impairment. Arch Neurol 2003;60:729–736.
26. Larner AJ. Getting it wrong: the clinical misdiagnosis of Alzheimer's disease. Int J Clin Pract 2004;58:1092–1094.
27. Hoffman RS. Diagnostic errors in the evaluation of behavioral disorders. JAMA 1982;248:964–967.
28. Ross GW, Abbott RD, Petrovich H, et al. Frequency and characteristics of silent dementia among elderly Japanese-American men. The Honolulu-Asia Aging Study. JAMA 1997;277:800–805.
29. Ryan DH. Misdiagnosis in dementia: comparisons of diagnostic error rate and range of hospital investigation according to medical specialty. Int J Geriatr Psychiatr 1994;9:141–147.
30. Tombaugh TN, McIntyre NJ. The mini-mental state examination: a comprehensive review. J Am Geriatr Soc 1992;40:922–935.
31. Crum RM, Anthony JC, Bassett SS, et al. Population-based norms for the Mini-Mental State Examination by age and educational level. JAMA 1993;12:2386–2391.
32. Bleecker ML, Bolla-Wilson K, Kawas C, et al. Age-specific norms for the Mini-Mental State Exam. Neurology 1988;38:1565–1568.
33. Jonker C, Geerlings MI, Schmand B. Are memory complaints predictive for dementia? A review of clinical and population-based studies. Int J Geriatr Psychiatr 2000;15:983–991.
34. Jorm AF, Butterworth P, Anstey KJ, et al. Memory complaints in a community sample aged 60–64 years: associations with cognitive functioning, psychiatric symptoms, medical conditions, APOE genotype, hippocampus and amygdala volumes, and white-matter hyperintensities. Psychol Med 2004;34:1495–1506.

35. Cacchione PZ, Powlishta KK, Grant EA, et al. Accuracy of collateral source reports in very mild to mild dementia of the Alzheimer type. J Am Geriatr Soc 2003;51:819–823.
36. Mega MS, Cummings JL, Fiorello T, et al. The spectrum of behavioral changes in Alzheimer's disease. Neurology 1996;46:130–135.
37. Stern Y, Alpert M, Brandt J, et al. Utility of extrapyramidal signs and psychosis as predictors of cognitive and functional decline, nursing home admission and death in Alzheimer's disease. Prospective analysis from the Predictors Study. Neurology 1994;44:2300–2307.
38. Lerner AJ, Hedera P, Koss E, et al. Delirium in Alzheimer disease. Alzheim Dis Assoc Disord 1997;11:16–20.
39. Francis J, Kapoor WN. Prognosis after hospital discharge of older medical patients with delirium. J Am Geriatr Soc 1992;40:601–606.
40. Devanand DP, Sano M, Tang MX, et al. Depressed mood and the incidence of Alzheimer's disease in the elderly living in the community. Arch Gen Psychiatr 1996;53:175–182.
41. Reifler BV. Diagnosing Alzheimer's disease in the presence of mixed cognitive and affective symptoms. Int Psychogeriatr 1997;9(Suppl 1):59–64.
42. Derouesne C, Thibault S, Lagha-Pierucci S, et al. Decreased awareness of cognitive deficits in patients with mild dementia of the Alzheimer type. Int J Geriatr Psychiatr 1999;14:1019–1030.
43. desRosiers G, Hodges JR, Berrios G. The neuropsychological differentiation of patients with very mild Alzheimer's disease and/or major depression. J Am Geriatr Soc 1995;43:1256–1263.
44. Visser PJ, Verhey FR, Ponds RW, et al. Distinction between preclinical Alzheimer's disease and depression. J Am Geriatr Soc 2000;48:479–484.
45. Alexopoulos GS, Meyers BS, Young RC, et al. The course of geriatric depression with "reversible dementia": a controlled study. Am J Psychiatr 1993;150:1693–1699.
46. Knopman DS, DeKosky ST, Cummings JL, et al. Practice parameter: diagnosis of dementia (an evidence-based review). Report of the Quality Standards Subcommittee of the American Academy of Neurology. Neurology 2001;56:1143–1153.
47. Gilewski MJ, Zelinski EM, Schaie KW. The Memory Functioning Questionnaire for assessment of memory complaints in adulthood and old age. Psychol Aging 1990;5:482–490.
48. Pfeffer RI, Kurosaki TT, Harrah CH Jr, et al. Measurement of functional activities in older adults in the community. J Gerontol 1982;37:323–329.
49. Ercoli LM, Siddarth P, Huang S-C, et al. Perceived loss of memory ability and cerebral metabolic decline in persons with the apolipoprotein e-4 genetic risk for Alzheimer's disease. Arch Gen Psychiatr 2006;63:442–448.
50. Schmand B, Jonker C, Hooijer C, et al. Subjective memory complaints may announce dementia. Neurology 1996;46:121–125.
51. Roman GC. Brain hypoperfusion: a critical factor in vascular dementia. Neurol Res 2004;26:454–458.
52. Munro CA, Saxton J, Butters MA. The neuropsychological consequences of abstinence among older alcoholics: a cross-sectional study. Alcohol Clin Exp Res 2000;24:1510–1516.
53. Delgoda R, Westlake AC. Herbal interactions involving cytochrome p450 enzymes: a mini review. Toxicol Rev 2004;23:239–249.
54. Roman GC, Tatemichi TK, Erkinjuntti T, et al. Vascular dementia: diagnostic criteria for research studies. Report of the NINDS-AIREN International Workshop. Neurology 1993;43:250–260.
55. McKeith IG, Perry EK, Perry RH. Report of the second dementia with Lewy body international workshop: diagnosis and treatment. Consortium on Dementia with Lewy Bodies. Neurology 1999;22:902–905.
56. McKeith LG, Galasko D, Kosaka K, et al. Consensus guidelines for the clinical and pathologic diagnosis of dementia with Lewy bodies (DLB): report of the Consortium on DLB international workshop. Neurology 1996;47:1113–1124.
57. Practice parameter for diagnosis and evaluation of dementia (summary statement). Report of the Quality Standards Subcommittee of the American Academy of Neurology. Neurology 1994;44:2203–2206.
58. Folstein MF, Folstein SE, McHugh PR. "Mini-Mental State." A practical method for grading the cognitive state of patients for the clinician. J Psychiatr Res 1975;12:189–198.

59. Brayne C, Calloway P. The association of education and socioeconomic status with the Mini Mental State Examination and the clinical diagnosis of dementia in elderly people. Age Aging 1990;19:91–96.
60. Bleecker ML, Bolla-Wilson K, Kawas C, et al. Age-specific norms for the Mini-Mental State Exam. Neurology 1988;38:1565–1568.
61. Crum RM, Anthony JC, Bassett SS, et al. Population-based norms for the Mini-Mental State Examination by age and educational level. JAMA 1993;269:2386–2391.
62. Galasko D, Klauber MR, Hofstetter CR, et al. The Mini-Mental State Examination in the early diagnosis of Alzheimer's disease. Arch Neurol 1990;47:49–52.
63. Commenges D, Gagnon M, Letenneur L, et al. Improving screening for dementia in the elderly using, Mini-Mental State Examination subscores, Benton's Visual Retention Test, and Isaacs' Set Test. Epidemiology 1992;3:185–188.
64. Strub RL, Black FW. The Mental Status Examination in Neurology, 2nd ed. Philadelphia: F. A. David, 1986.
65. Coffey CD, Cummings JL (eds). The American Psychiatric Press Textbook of Geriatric Neuropsychiatry. Washington, DC: American Psychiatric Press, 2000.
66. Morris JC, Mohs RC, Rogers H, et al. Consortium to establish a registry for Alzheimer's disease (CERAD) clinical and neuropsychological assessment of Alzheimer's disease. Psychopharm Bull 1988;24:641–652.
67. Mant A, Eyland EA, Pond DC, et al. Recognition of dementia in general practice: comparison of general practitioners' opinions with assessments using the Mini-Mental State Examination and Blessed dementia rating scale. Fam Pract 1988;5:184–188.
68. McCartney JR, Palmateer LM. Assessment of cognitive deficit in geriatric patients: a study of physician behavior. J Am Geriatr Soc 1985;33:467–471.
69. Ross GW, Abbott RD, Petrovitch H, et al. Frequency and characteristics of silent dementia among elderly Japanese-American men: the Honolulu-Asia Aging Study. JAMA 1997;277:800–805.
70. Ryan DH. Misdiagnosis in dementia: comparisons of diagnostic error rate and range of hospital investigation according to medical specialty. Int J Geriatr Psychiatr 1994;9:141–147.
71. Watson LC, Lewis CL, Fillenbaum GG. Asking family about memory loss. Is it helpful? J Gen Intern Med 2005;20:28–32.
72. Chodosh J, Petitti DB, Elliott M, et al. Physician recognition of cognitive impairment: evaluating the need for improvement. J Am Geriatr Soc 2004;52:1051–1059.
73. Silverman DH, Small GW. Prompt identification of Alzheimer's disease with brain PET imaging of a woman with multiple previous diagnoses of other neuropsychiatric conditions. Am J Psychiatr 2002;159:1482–1488.
74. Silverman DH. Brain F-18-FDG PET in the diagnosis of neurodegenerative dementias: comparison with perfusion SPECT and with clinical evaluations lacking nuclear imaging. J Nucl Med 2004;45:594–607.
75. Chow TW. Treatment approaches to symptoms associated with frontotemporal degeneration. Curr Psychiatry Rep 2005;7:376–380.
76. Chang CY, Silverman DH. Accuracy of early diagnosis and its impact on the management and course of Alzheimer's disease. Expert Rev Mol Diagn 2004;4:63–69.
77. Reiman EM, Caselli RJ, Yun LS, et al. Preclinical evidence of Alzheimer's disease in persons homozygous for the epsilon 4 allele for apolipoprotein E [see comments]. N Engl J Med 1996;334:752–758.
78. Small GW, Mazziotta JC, Collins MT, et al. Apolipoprotein E type 4 allele and cerebral glucose metabolism in relatives at risk for familial Alzheimer disease. JAMA 1995;273:942–947.
79. Small GW, Ercoli LM, Silverman DH, et al. Cerebral metabolic and cognitive decline in persons at genetic risk for Alzheimer's disease. Proc Natl Acad Sci USA 2000;97:6037–6042.
80. de LeonMJ, Convit A, Wolf OT, et al. Prediction of cognitive decline in normal elderly subjects with 2-[(18)F]fluoro-2-deoxy-D-glucose/poitron-emission tomography (FDG/PET).Proc Natl Acad Sci USA 2001;98:10966–10971.
81. Small GW, La Rue A, Komo S, et al. Predictors of cognitive change in middle-aged and older adults with memory loss. Am J Psychiatr 1995;152:1757–1764.

82. Kuhl DE, Small GW, Riege WH, et al. Cerebral metabolic patterns before diagnosis of probable Alzheimer's disease. J Cereb Blood Flow Metab 1987;7(Suppl 1):S406.
83. Chetelat G, Desgranges B, de la Sayette V, et al. Mild cognitive impairment: can FDG-PET predict who is to rapidly convert to Alzheimer's disease? Neurology 2003;60:1374–1377.
84. Anchisi D, Borroni B, Franceschi M, et al. Heterogeneity of brain glucose metabolism in mild cognitive impairment and clinical progression to Alzheimer disease. Arch Neurol 2005;62:1728–1733.
85. Silverman DH, Gambhir SS, Huang HW, et al. Evaluating early dementia with and without assessment of regional cerebral metabolism by PET: a comparison of predicted costs and benefits. J Nucl Med 2002;43:253–266.
86. Moulin-Romsee G, Maes A, Silverman D, et al. Cost-effectiveness of F-18-fluorodeoxyglucose positron emission tomography in the assessment of early dementia from a Belgian and European perspective. Eur J Neurol 2005;12:254–263.
87. Silverman DH, Small GW, Chang CY, et al. Positron emission tomography in evaluation of dementia: regional brain metabolism and long-term outcome. JAMA 2001;286:2120–2127.
88. Malouf R, Birks J. Donepezil for vascular cognitive impairment. Cochrane Database Syst Rev 2004;1:CD004395.
89. McKeith I, Del Ser T, Spano P, et al. Efficacy of rivastigmine in dementia with Lewy bodies: a randomised, double-blind, placebo-controlled international study. Lancet 2000;356:2031–2036.
90. Roman GC, Wilkinson DG, Doody RS, et al. Donepezil in vascular dementia: combined analysis of two large-scale clinical trials. Dement Geriatr Cogn Disord 2005;20:338–344.
91. Memantine for dementia. Cochrane Database Syst Rev 2005;20:CD003154.
92. Sabbagh MN, Hake AM, Ahmed S, et al. The use of memantine in dementia with Lewy bodies. J Alzheimers Dis 2005;7:285–289.
93. Ridha BH, Josephs KA, Rossor MN. Delusions and hallucinations in dementia with Lewy bodies: worsening with memantine. Neurology 2005;65(3):481–482.
94. Chaytor N, Schmitter-Edgecombe M. The ecological validity of neuropsychological tests: a review of the literature on everyday cognitive skills. Neuropsychol Rev 2003;13:181–197.
95. Teng EL, Manly JJ. Neuropsychological testing: helpful or harmful? Alzheimer Dis Assoc Disord 2005;19:267–271.
96. Saxton J, Lopez OL, Ratcliff G, et al. Preclinical Alzheimer disease: neuropsychological test performance 1.5 to 8 years prior to onset. Neurology 2004;63:2341–2347.
97. Tierney MC, Yao C, Kiss A, et al. Neuropsychological tests accurately predict incident Alzheimer disease after 5 and 10 years. Neurology 2005;64:1853–1859.
98. Mortimer JA, Borenstein AR, Gosche KM, et al. Very early detection of Alzheimer neuropathology and the role of brain reserve in modifying its clinical expression. J Geriatr Psychiatry Neurol 2005;18:218–223.
99. Saunders AM, Strittmatter WJ, Schmechel D, et al. Association of apolipoprotein E allele E4 with late-onset familial and sporadic Alzheimer's disease. Neurology 1993;43:1467–1472.
100. Corder EH, Saunders AM, Strittmatter WJ, et al. Gene dose of apolipoprotein E type 4 allele and the risk of Alzheimer's disease in late onset families. Science 1993;261:921–923.
101. Pitner JK, Bachman DL. A synopsis of the practice parameters on dementia from the American Academy of Neurology on the diagnosis of dementia. Consult Pharm 2004;19:52–63.
102. Roberts JS, Cupples LA, Relkin NR, et al. Genetic risk assessment for adult children of people with Alzheimer's disease: the Risk Evaluation and Education for Alzheimer's Disease (REVEAL) study. J Geriatr Psychiatry Neurol 2005;18:250–255.
103. Zick CD, Mathews CJ, Roberts JS, et al. Genetic testing for Alzheimer's disease and its impact on insurance purchasing behavior. Health Aff (Millwood) 2005;24:483–490.
104. Loy C, Schneider L. Galantamine for Alzheimer's disease and mild cognitive impairment. Cochrane Database Syst Rev 2006;25:CD001747.
105. Petersen RC, Thomas RG, Grundman M, et al. Vitamin E and donepezil for the treatment of mild cognitive impairment. N Engl J Med 2005;352:2379–2388.
106. Salloway S, Ferris S, Kluger A, et al. Donepezil 401 Study Group. Efficacy of donepezil in mild cognitive impairment: a randomized placebo-controlled trial. Neurology 2004;63(4):651–657.

107. Mielke R, Heiss WD. Positron emission tomography for diagnosis of Alzheimer's disease and vascular dementia. J Neural Transm Suppl 1998;53:237–250.
108. Alexopoulos GS. Vascular disease, depression, and dementia. J Am Geriatr Soc. 2003;51:1178–1180.
109. Camus V, Kraehenbuhl H, Preisig M, et al. Geriatric depression and vascular diseases: what are the links? J Affect Disord 2004;81:1–16.
110. Lobotesis K, Fenwick JD, Phipps A, et al. Occipital hypoperfusion on SPECT in dementia with Lewy bodies but not AD. Neurology 200113;56:643–649.
111. Minoshima S, Foster NL, Sima AA, et al. Alzheimer's disease versus dementia with Lewy bodies: cerebral metabolic distinction with autopsy confirmation. Ann Neurol 2001;50:358–365.
112. Duara R, Barker W, Luis CA. Frontotemporal dementia and Alzheimer's disease: differential diagnosis. Dement Geriatr Cogn Disord 1999;10(Suppl 1):37–42.
113. Braak H, Braak E. Neuropathological staging of Alzheimer-related changes. Acta Neuropathol 1991;82:239–259.
114. Price JL, Morris JC. Tangles and plaques in nondemented aging and "preclinical" Alzheimer's disease. Ann Neurol 1999;45:358–368.
115. Klunk WE, Wang Y, Huang GF, et al. The binding of 2-(4′-ethylaminophenyl)benzothiazole to postmortem brain homogenates is dominated by the amyloid component. J Neurosci 2003;23:2086–2092.
116. Shoghi-Jadid K, Small GW, Agdeppa ED, et al. Localization of neurofibrillary tangles and beta-amyloid plaques in the brains of living patients with Alzheimer's disease. Am J Geriatr Psychiatry 2002;10:24–35.
117. Small GW, Kepe V, Ercoli L, et al. Positron emission tomography scanning of cerebral amyloid and tau deposits in mild cognitive impairment. N Engl J Med 2006;355:2652–2663.
118. Kung HF, Kung MP, Zhuang ZP, et al. Iodinated tracers for imaging amyloid plaques in the brain. Mol Imaging Biol 2003;5:418–426.
119. Klunk WE, Engler H, Nordberg A, et al. Imaging brain amyloid in Alzheimer's disease with Pittsburgh Compound-B. Ann Neurol 2004;55:306–319.
120. Small GW, Kepe V, Huang S-C, et al. *In vivo* brain imaging of tau aggregation in frontal temporal dementia using [F-18]FDDNP positron emission tomography. 9th International Conference on Alzheimer's Disease and Related Disorders, 2004.
121. Passchier J, van Waarde A, Vaalburg W, Willemsen ATM. On the quantitation of [^{18}F]MPPF binding to 5-HT1A receptors in the human brain. J Nucl Med 2001:42;1025–1031.
122. Kepe V, Barrio JR, Huang SC, et al. Serotonin 1A receptors in the living brain of Alzheimer's disease patients. Proc Natl Acad Sci USA 2006;103:702–707.
123. Potkin SG, Anand R, Fleming K, et al. Brain metabolic and clinical effects of rivastigmine in Alzheimer's disease. Int J Neuropsychopharmacol 2001;4:223–30.
124. Mega MS, Cummings JL, Masterman DM, et al. Cognitive and metabolic responses to metrifonate therapy in Alzheimer's disease. Neuropsychiatr Neuropsychol Behav Neurol 2001;14:63–68.
125. Fox NC, Black RS, Gilman S, et al. Effects of Abeta immunization (AN1792) on MRI measures of cerebral volume in Alzheimer disease. Neurology 2005;64:1563–1572.
126. Jack CR Jr, Dickson DW, Parisi JE et al. Antemortem MRI findings correlate with hippocampal neuropathology in normal aging and dementia. Neurology 2002;58:750–757.
127. Silbert LC, Quinn JF, Moore MM, et al. Changes in premorbid brain volume predict Alzheimer's disease pathology. Neurology 2003;61: 487–492.
128. Agdeppa ED, Kepe V, Petric A, et al. *In vitro* detection of (S)-naproxen and ibuprofen binding to plaques in the Alzheimer's brain using the positron emission tomography molecular imaging probe 2-(1-{6-[(2-[^{18}F]fluoroethyl)(methyl)amino]-2-aphthyl}ethylidene)malononitrile. Neuroscience 2003;117:723–730.
129. Small GW, Silverman DHS, Siddarth P, Ercoli LM, Miller KJ, Wright BC, Bookheimer SY, Barrio JR, Phelps ME. Effects of a 14-day healthy aging lifestyle program on cognition and brain function. Am J Geriatr Psychiatr 2006;14:538–545.

Chapter 2
Clinical Interpretation of Brain PET Scans: Performing Visual Assessments, Providing Quantifying Data, and Generating Integrated Reports

Daniel H.S. Silverman

Visual assessment of brain FDG PET data represents a fundamental skill, independent of the particular clinical indication toward which it is being applied. In our imaging facility, we routinely employ a systematic approach for evaluating regional metabolism throughout the brain. In addition, beginning in 2004, software tools approved by the Food and Drug Administration for quantifying relative regional activity became available to assist with that evaluation. This chapter first describes key aspects of a skilled visual assessment, and then examines methods of regional quantification that are practical in typical clinical environments, and, finally, illustrates an approach toward scan interpretation that integrates the visual and quantifying information present in clinical PET scans.

Visual Assessment

Systematic visual examination of a clinical brain PET scan involves a number of key elements that are important to include in every assessment, at least implicitly, and if abnormalities are identified, then certainly explicitly mentioned in the interpretive report. These elements can generally be considered in five sequential steps, as outlined here.

Step 1: Optimizing Technical Quality

An important initial step in examining any imaging study is to assess its technical quality. This is done implicitly and, assuming that technical quality is adequate, this part of the assessment will not usually enter into the language of the clinical report. Considerations with respect to technical quality include filtering at a level that is not so rough (small full width at half maximum) as to leave the images too noisy, nor so smooth (large full width at half maximum) as to degrade the resolution to the point of not being able to make out small areas of variation in metabolism; displaying the images at sufficient zoom to allow them to be adequately seen, but

D.H.S. Silverman (ed.), *PET in the Evaluation of Alzheimer's Disease and Related Disorders*,
DOI: 10.1007/978-0-387-76420-7_2, © Springer Science+Business Media, LLC 2009

still all included side by side in presenting a splash view of slices on the screen from one end of the brain to the other (e.g., superior to inferior planes, in the transaxial orientation), so that relative levels of metabolism throughout the brain can be readily compared; assessing the blood glucose level of the patient at the time of tracer administration (levels that are too high compete for FDG transport across the blood–brain barrier, as well as across the membrane of cells in the brain, reducing the statistical count quality of the image); and placing the patient's brain symmetrically with respect to the plane of the ring of detectors, so that the ability to assess symmetry in the brain will not be compromised or complicated by tilt. Parameters for filtering smoothness and zoom usually need only be established at the outset for each type of instrument at each imaging facility, and as these are in part a matter of subjective taste of the interpreters, should be initially determined empirically. Images of a representative brain or phantom can be reconstructed by the technologists with a variety of zoom sizes and using filters over a range of full width at half maximum. In contrast, blood glucose levels and symmetry of placement will need to be considered for each acquired study.

For neuropsychiatric indications, patients should fast for at least 4 h before a FDG PET study, as with whole body studies done for oncologic indications; regimens for managing antidiabetic medications and food intake in diabetic patients can also be carried out in the same way as for whole body oncology studies. We do a *finger-stick* assessment of each patient before administration of FDG. A blood glucose level below 150 mg/dL (8.3 mmol/L) is desirable. It is recommended to have a policy in place such that if the level is much in excess of this (e.g., 180 or 200 mg/dL) that the interpreting physician be notified. Depending on the situation of the patient (e.g., distance of residence, schedule flexibility) and of the imaging facility (e.g., whether a physician is on site, and tightness of camera schedule), several options are possible. It may be decided to send the patient home and reschedule the study for a different day and different time of day; or, it may be decided to wait 1–2 h and re-check the blood glucose level to see if it has decreased to an acceptable level; or regular insulin may be administered intravenously according to a sliding scale, blood glucose re-checked in 20–30 min, and FDG administered at that time if its level has fallen appreciably (if not, another dose of insulin followed by another 20–30 min wait can be tried). If this latter approach is used, it is important to wait for at least 20 min after each insulin administration before giving FDG, in order to avoid driving the radiotracer into peripheral tissues and thus defeat the purpose of diminishing competition with blood glucose for uptake into the brain[1].

On the other hand, for neuro-oncologic indications, the instruction to the patient to fast before the PET scan may be omitted entirely; in fact, the patient should be advised to come to a morning study after having had a good breakfast, or to an afternoon study following a good lunch. This is apparently due to uptake of glucose into normal brain tissue becoming saturated at lower concentrations than is the case for the uptake of glucose into the higher-grade brain tumors for which FDG PET is obtained, and so the target-to-background contrast of tumor relative to normal brain tissue is actually enhanced by the presence of an elevated blood glucose level.

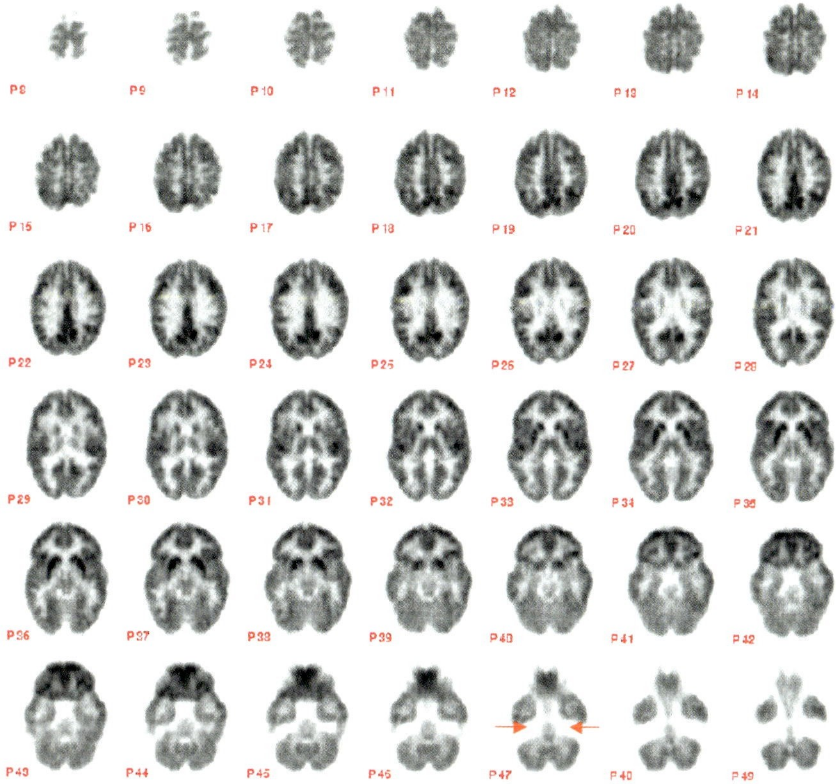

Fig. 2.1 Normal FDG PET brain scan of a healthy middle-aged adult

The PET scan (Fig. 2.1) should be inspected to ensure symmetric presentation. This can be done readily on transaxial views with respect to in-plane rotation by simply looking for tilt of the long axis of the brain away from the vertical, and with respect to out-of-plane rotation by examining structures below where most of the brain tissue lies, such as the photopenia representing the petrous ridges of the skull (Fig. 2.1, *arrows*), ensuring that they are symmetric in appearance (thus avoiding problems relating to asymmetry of the brain tissue itself). If visual inspection reveals asymmetric placement, the technologist responsible for processing the image can be asked to re-orient the brain image symmetrically, making the job of interpretation much more straightforward. This is particularly worthwhile since most facilities now obtain brain images by three-dimensional (3D) acquisition, providing resolution that is more nearly isotropic for all dimensions of the brain data. We would also recommend that the processing technologists be trained to automatically inspect the reconstructed images for asymmetry in the manner described previously, and as a matter of routine re-slice the brain volume to produce the most symmetric presentation, in advance of providing the images to the workstations where they will be interpreted.

Steps 2 and 3: Global Assessments

If it has not already been done, this is the time to set the color scale and its intensity thresholds to optimize the pixel display and to do so in a way that is reproducible from scan to scan. For this purpose, we recommend always beginning with a linear scale, such as the inverse linear grayscale; one knows that if a brain region has twice as much radioactivity associated with it, then it will be twice as dark in this black-on-white image. In the brain, FDG reflects the energy-expensive process of synaptic activity, and synapses are concentrated in the gray matter structures of the brain. Once the color scale has been selected, it is thus important to take maximal diagnostic advantage of the scale by spreading out most of its gradations over the gray matter intensities of the brain image. To do this, the lower intensity threshold can be raised until just before cortex appears affected, usually when approximately 90% of the scalp activity has been pushed into the background range of the scale (i.e., white, in the case of the inverse grayscale); the upper intensity threshold can then be adjusted until approximately 10% of the brain appears in the upper range of the scale (i.e., black, in the case of the inverse grayscale). In this way, the entire gray range of the color scale will be spread over 90% of the range of gray matter level metabolism of the brain. A problem in using color scales such as *rainbow* scales and other nonlinear display scales for the initial diagnostic assessment is that the way that the image appears to the interpreter becomes highly susceptible to precisely where the upper and lower intensity thresholds have been set. Therefore, it is recommended that those other scales be used, if at all, only after the interpreter has examined the brain scan using the more reproducible display offered by the linear scale as detailed previously.

Once technical quality has been taken care of, the next step in examining a brain PET scan is to assess the gross structure of the patient's brain. We emphasize *gross* structure, because fine structural details should of course be assessed using structural imaging modalities (CT or MR) that provide the highest spatial resolution. It is nevertheless worth taking note at this stage of structural features of the scan such as areas of missing or deformed tissue that may represent moderate-sized cerebrovascular insults; asymmetry secondary to mass effects; relative expansion of the white matter/ventricular space suggestive of hydrocephalus; posttraumatic, postsurgical, or other disease-related changes; or extra tissue that may represent tumor. Most routinely, however, what will be assessed at this stage is the degree of any atrophy that is present, which can then be qualitatively rated as *slight, mild, moderate,* or *severe.* Generalized atrophy can be assessed at the level of the lateral ventricles by examining the interhemispheric fissure (Fig. 2.2, *arrows in leftmost image of second row*) and at the level of the third ventricle by examining the separation between the left and right sides of the thalamus (Fig. 2.2, *arrow in middle image, third row*). In young healthy subjects, before the onset of atrophy, left and right cerebral hemispheres, as well as left and right thalami, will be in close apposition to each other. To the extent that widening is seen at both levels, those findings are consistent with generalized atrophy. Evident sulcal widening within each hemisphere should also be mentioned. In describing the atrophy apparent on functional images secondary to age-related change, we use the qualitative terms *slight, mild,* and *moderate* to indicate the degree

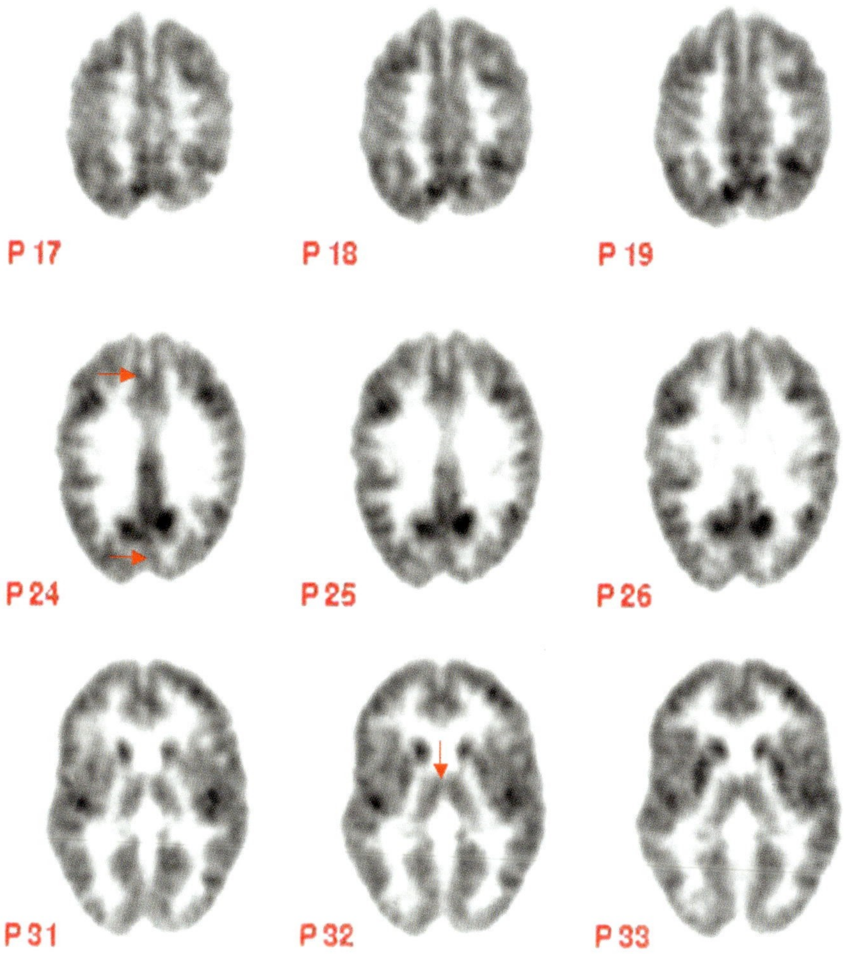

Fig. 2.2 Structural examination of brain PET scan

of atrophy typically seen in scans of patients in their forties to sixties, sixties to seventies, and seventies to eighties respectively, and use *severe* to indicate a degree of atrophy generally seen only under pathologic circumstances, whereas the descriptor itself is used independently of the age of the particular patient being evaluated. For example, it might be stated in describing the scan of a 50-year-old subject that there is moderate widening of the interhemispheric fissure and interthalamic distance, consistent with a degree of generalized atrophy that is greater than typical for a patient of this age; precisely the same description would be given if the scan belonged to an 80 year old, except for omission of the words *greater than*.

One reason that the description of global structural changes is necessary relates to the third step in our systematic approach, an assessment of the level of global metabolism of the cerebral cortex (Fig. 2.3). This is because we can have altered metabolism

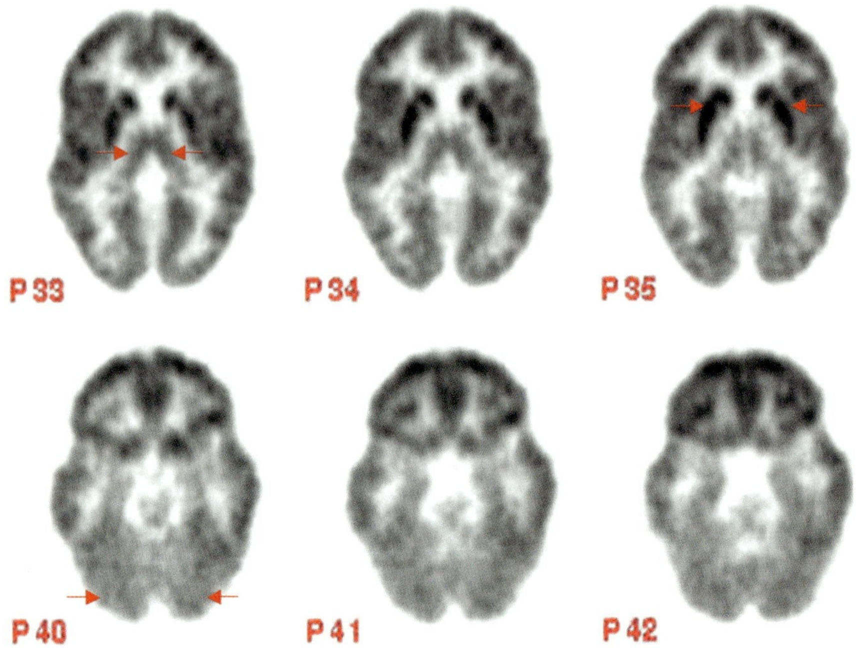

Fig. 2.3 Assessment of global metabolism in brain PET scan. See text for details

in two different ways. For example, *hypometabolism* can be present in an absolute sense, meaning that there would be (if one were to measure it semi-invasively) fewer milligrams of glucose being used per minute per 100 g of gray matter, or *hypometabolism* can be present in which there is less glucose being used because there is less gray matter remaining. Thus, it is important to have an idea of how much brain tissue is present in order to know how much metabolism it is fair to expect.

In assessing global cortical metabolism, it is critically important to use internal reference structures, so as not to be misled by anomalies of the way in which the brain is displayed. A couple rules of thumb can be especially useful in assessing the global level of cortical metabolism. First, in a healthy person in the absence of significant atrophy, the putamen and caudate nuclei of the basal ganglia (Fig. 2.3, *arrows in rightmost image, first row*) should have a level of metabolism approximately 9%–15% higher than frontal and parietal cortex, whereas the cerebellar cortex (Fig. 2.3, *arrows in leftmost image, second row*) should have a level of metabolism at least 10% lower than frontal and parietal cortex. This means that average cortex should have a level of metabolism (or darkness, on the inverse linear grayscale, shown in Fig. 2.3) falling approximately midway between that of the cerebellum and basal ganglia. Second, in a healthy person in the absence of significant atrophy, the thalamus (Fig. 2.3, *arrows in leftmost image, first row*) should have a level of metabolism approximately isometabolic with the frontal and parietal cortex. To the extent that the average cortical metabolic level is seen to fall closer to the cerebellar level than the basal ganglia level of metabolism, and correspondingly below the level of thalamic metabolism, that would be consistent with global cortical hypometabolism. When this pattern is seen, the first thing to check is whether it can be accounted for by a similar level of global cortical atrophy, as often occurs in older patients. (Also see comments below on effects of normal aging on cerebellar metabolism, which can further contribute to this pattern.) If so, combining this with the global structural assessment of the prior step, it is appropriate to state something such as, "a moderate degree of generalized atrophy typical for age, with atrophy-associated global cortical hypometabolism, is seen." Other common causes of global cortical hypometabolism include central nervous system depressants such as those used as muscle relaxants, anxiolytics, hypnotics, and for sedation, as well as falling asleep during the FDG uptake period.

If, conversely, basal ganglia and thalamic levels of metabolism appear to fall below the level of general cortical metabolism, one should strongly suspect that image reconstruction was performed without adequate attenuation correction. Inadequate attenuation correction causes the deeper structures of the brain to appear washed out because of the greater degree of attenuation occurring as the photons emitted from the more central structures pass through more surrounding tissue, before they are able to reach the scanner detectors. In this case, the scan should be reconstructed with proper attenuation correction before interpretation is rendered. If the problem has stemmed from a failed transmission scan, the study often can still be salvaged by applying a calculated attenuation correction algorithm, taking advantage of the relatively regular ellipsoid shape of the brain.

Steps 4 and 5: Focal Assessments

The final steps of our systematic examination of brain PET are to evaluate for focal cortical and focal noncortical abnormalities. These steps tend to be, understandably, the most difficult to master, as the brain is composed of dozens of distinct structural and functional regions, each comprising its own characteristic levels of metabolism.[2–5] Thus, it is necessary to develop through experience a strong sense of what the normal range of appearance should be for each region, to recognize when an individual region falls outside of that range, and finally, to arrive at a differential diagnosis that accounts for the constellation of any abnormalities noted.

In carrying out the fourth step, identifying focal cortical abnormalities, it is important to distinguish areas of true hypometabolism from areas of apparent hypometabolism caused by tissue loss and partial volume effects. This is done by concomitantly being attuned to the structural details of the brain (e.g., where the gyri are thicker and where they are thinning, where the sulci are widened by atrophic changes) and also where metabolism in adjacent tissue has been diminished by other processes. Visual assessments of cortical metabolism should be made only while mentally accounting for such changes. As an example of a common interpretive error, the superior aspects of parietal cortex may appear to be diminished in intensity in older patients, leading to the description of biparietal hypometabolism, and possibly the misinterpretation of the scan as revealing early Alzheimer's disease. Isolated superior biparietal hypometabolism should in fact never be interpreted as representing Alzheimer's disease, which characteristically affects inferior parietal cortex before more superior cortex is affected. What this pattern most often reflects is the atrophy of normal aging, in which sulcal widening affecting the external face of the cortical ribbon leads to a partial volume effect apparent in the most superior transaxial planes, which can be readily confirmed by examining the corresponding sagittal views.

Once structural considerations are taken into account, the next issue facing the interpreter is to know the relative levels of metabolism to expect among different regions of the cortex. The most important characteristic features of cortical metabolism as reflected in the FDG PET images are summarized here. First, metabolism in the *temporal cortex* is visibly lower than cortical metabolism in the frontal, parietal, and occipital lobes in the brains of healthy adults of all ages. Moreover, it is normal for anterior temporal metabolism to be lower than posterior temporal metabolism. Because of partial volume effects with surrounding white matter levels of metabolism, it is also normal for medial temporal cortical metabolism to appear lower than lateral temporal metabolism.

Second, it is normal for the *cingulate cortex* (the medially lying cortex seen immediately above the white matter of the corpus callosum on sagittal planes viewed near midline, as well as in the most inferior transaxial planes sliced along the canthomeatal line to demonstrate a continuous strip of cortex stretching anteriorly to posteriorly; Fig. 2.4) to demonstrate visibly higher metabolism in the posterior cingulate than in the anterior cingulate cortex and than average cortex of the frontal, parietal, and of course temporal lobes. The posterior cingulate cortex has, in fact, the highest level of metabolism of any non-sensory/motor-activated part of the cerebral cortex and can be 20%–40% more metabolic than average cortex found in the other regions of young healthy brains. The cingulate cortex is a part of the brain that tends to atrophy faster than average cortex, however, so that the gradient of posterior cingulate to frontoparietotemporal cortex becomes less apparent with age. Nevertheless, it should maintain an appearance of intensity more similar to basal ganglia than to

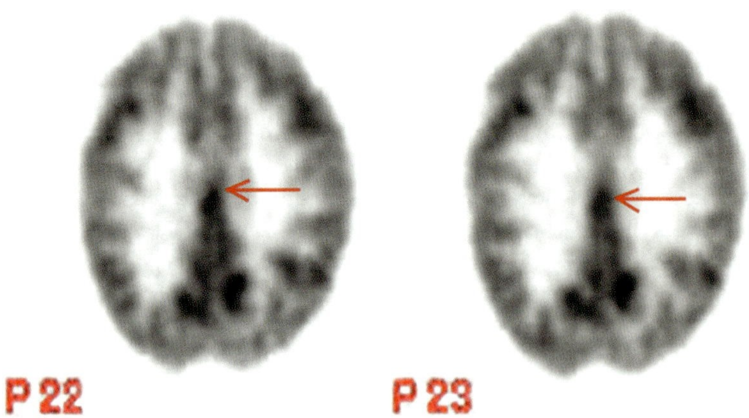

Fig. 2.4 Examination of metabolism of posterior cingulate cortex

average cortex in healthy subjects. Assessment of this cortical region takes on special importance in the context of a dementia evaluation, because the posterior cingulate cortex happens to also be the region of the brain in which metabolism declines most significantly in the earliest stages of Alzheimer's disease.[6]

Third, heterogeneity resulting from variable *sensory activation* can be expected. Thus, in a PET scan acquired after FDG uptake has proceeded with eyes open (as we recommend), it is normal for metabolism in the occipital lobe to appear greater than metabolism in other lobes of the brain. Likewise, if the patient's attention was attracted asymmetrically to either the left or right visual field during the uptake period, asymmetric occipital metabolism may be seen. For similar reasons, metabolism in sensorimotor cortex, and in the superior temporal lobe corresponding to auditory cortex, is often seen to be mildly elevated above the level of metabolism found in surrounding cortex.

Fourth, apart from the sensorimotor region, metabolism along the *lateral aspect of the frontal and parietal lobes,* after accounting for gyral thickness and sulcal width, should be fairly homogeneous in the brains of adults in the middle-age range. As for focal noncortical abnormalities, we have already reviewed what relative levels of metabolism to expect for cerebellum, thalamus, and basal ganglia structures. At this point, any asymmetries in metabolism of those structures from left to right, or nonuniformities in metabolism of those regions from anterior to posterior, should be noted. In looking for those abnormalities, it is important to examine the parts of each structure in the planes in which they are most robust, to avoid partial volume effects caused by activity in these relatively thin structures being averaged with the relatively low level activity above and below them. One should bear in mind, for example, that the plane in which the right caudate nucleus head of the basal ganglia appears most robust may differ from the plane in which the right lentiform nucleus of the basal ganglia is best appreciated, or that the plane in which a structure is best seen on one side of the brain may be slightly offset from the plane in which its contralateral counterpart is best seen.

Lastly, with respect to *effects of healthy aging* on cortical metabolism (Fig. 2.5), because the metabolism of the prefrontal region, particularly the most medial and anterior portions of the frontal lobe (Fig. 2.5, *arrows in left image of bottom row*), typically declines faster than metabolism of average cortex, it is normal for prefrontal metabolism to be slightly greater than parietal metabolism in young people, and slightly lower than parietal metabolism in older adults. Otherwise, the pattern of metabolism seen throughout the cortex in healthy brains remains relatively stable throughout adulthood. Finally, it should be noted that the metabolism of the cerebellum tends to increase during normal aging. This is seen visually not only as a relative effect caused by global hypometabolism of the cortex, but also reflects an actual increased rate of glucose utilization by the cerebellum in absolute terms in elderly subjects.[3]

Quantification

Several issues need to be considered with respect to quantifying brain PET studies in the context of rendering clinical interpretations. For example, is it necessary to quantify the scans or is visual interpretation adequate? When is it most helpful to

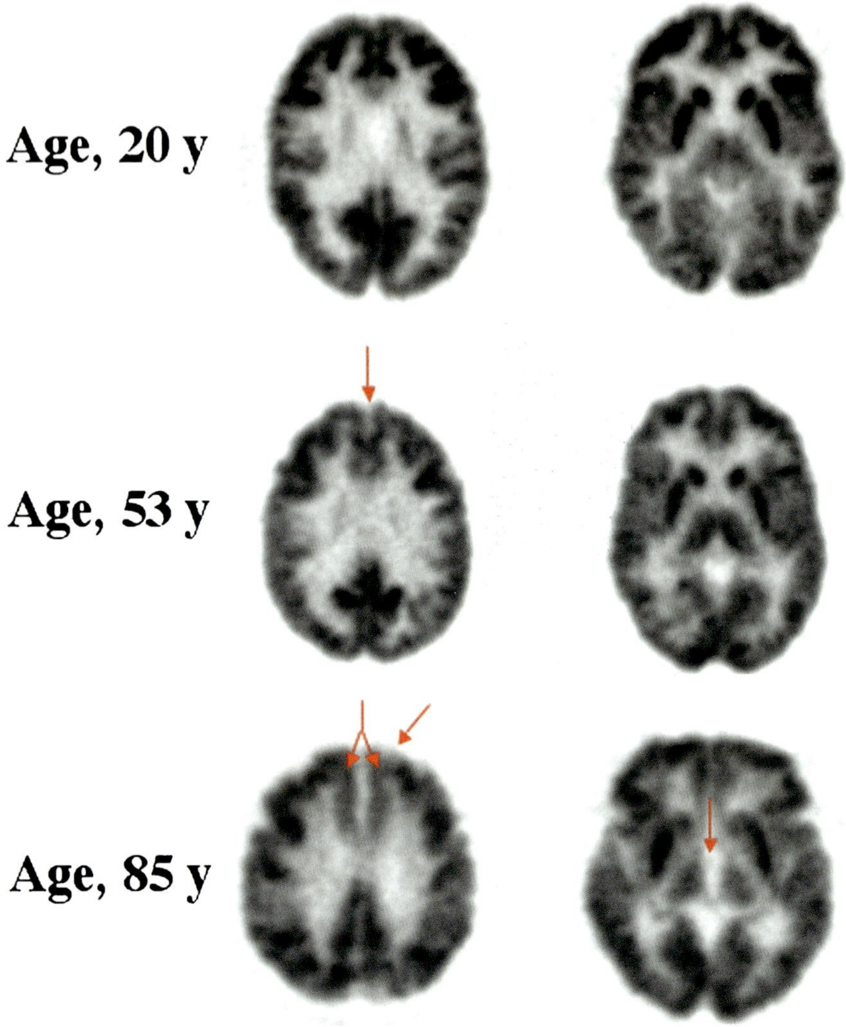

Fig. 2.5 Structural and metabolic patterns in FDG PET scans associated with age in healthy adults

perform quantification? What strategies may be employed to obtain quantifying data, and what software packages are available for implementing those strategies?

With respect to whether quantification of brain PET is necessary, the answer is clearly no, in the sense that it has been seen that substantial diagnostic and prognostic accuracies with regard to dementing disorders are achievable through visual interpretation alone[7-10] when performed by experienced readers of brain PET scans. Nevertheless it may be helpful in several ways to have quantitative information available. For example, for readers without a lot of experience in reading brain PET who are faced with the task of rendering an occasional interpretation (a common occurrence, given the traditionally relatively low volume of neurologic PET scans relative to oncologic PET scans in many clinical environments), it may be useful for increasing their interpretive confidence and accuracy. We recently assessed this type of utility in a systematic examination of the readings of brain PET scans by five physicians in our nuclear medicine residency program; with use of an FDA-approved commercially available software tool dedicated to brain PET quantification, the physicians interpreted scans correctly 8%–13% more often (based on the criterion standard of long-term clinical follow-up), relative to relying on their visual analyses alone. The information can also be used to provide even expert readers with quantitative context (e.g., "Lateral temporal metabolism appears asymmetric, with left-sided activity measuring 15% lower than on the right.") or statistical support (e.g., "Activity in posterior cingulate cortex falls 3.5 standard deviations below the normal mean for this region."), to supplement their interpretations with findings they visually have noted, as well as to perhaps draw their attention to imaging findings that may have been overlooked initially.

Of course, quantification is essential for the purpose of addressing questions that are intrinsically quantitative, not only questions about groups of subjects (e.g., "In healthy human brain tissue, how much more metabolically active is the posterior cingulate than the anterior cingulate cortex?" or "Which patients have more severe hypometabolism in posterior cingulate cortex—Alzheimer or frontotemporal dementia patients?"), but also quantitative questions in an individual patient relative to a normal group ("How hypometabolic is the posterior cingulate cortex in this patient, who clinically appears to have mild AD?") or statistical questions ("Is the observed degree of hypometabolism in the inferior parietal cortex statistically significant for that brain region?").

Another useful role for quantification of brain PET images is in defining the degree of change over time between two or more scans obtained for the same patient. For example, neurodegenerative dementing processes are associated with inexorable decline of the metabolism of involved brain regions. The metabolic decline precedes and parallels symptomatic decline. Thus, if a patient's memory measurably worsens over 1 or 2 years and that deterioration is a result of incipient Alzheimer's disease, it can then be expected that metabolism of posterior cortical regions will have declined during that interval. In the absence of a pathologic process, on the other hand, regional cerebral metabolism tends to be more quantitatively stable than neuropsychological performance (the latter being more prone to day-to-day, and even hour-to-hour, variability related to factors such as motivation, alertness, practice effects, and so forth). Thus, a significant decline in regional metabolism can be expected to provide a more sensitive (better signal-to-noise ratio because of smaller test variance) and more specific (based on characteristic patterns of regional cerebral involvement, coupled with being less prone to influence from nondisease processes) indicator of the presence of Alzheimer's and other neurodegenerative disease processes, than changes in neuropsychological test scores of individual patients. In patients with initially borderline abnormal scans who have regional hypometabolism suggesting the presence of an incipient disease process, quantifiable interval decline in the quantitatively borderline regions adds assurance to the diagnosis that the initial scan suggests, even if those changes remain very mild.

Once the decision to quantify brain PET data has been made, the next issues to be addressed involve choosing an appropriate strategy for obtaining quantifying data and selecting a software package among several now available with which to implement that strategy. The quantifying approaches that are in clinical use generally fall into either of two categories: (1) those based on measuring activity in a neuroanatomically or functionally defined region of interest (ROI) of the brain, and (2) those based on measurements of activity in individual image pixels or their 3D counterpart, *voxels*.

ROIs that are manually defined by an operator with appropriate neuroanatomic training on images containing pertinent anatomic landmarks provide a gold standard of regional activity. As might be expected, however, such an approach requires a level of neuroanatomic expertise and is sufficiently time- and labor-intensive that it is not considered to be practical to implement for routine clinical interpretations of brain PET images. An exception is when there is a well-defined focus (or small number of foci) to be measured (e.g., an area of suspected tumor growth), around which ROIs can be easily defined. In the evaluation of dementia, in contrast, numerous regions in need of quantification exist, but they are not easy to define (dorsolateral prefrontal cortex, inferior parietal lobule, posterior cingulate cortex, angular and marginal gyri, sensorimotor cortex, and so forth).

During the last decade, a number of innovative investigators developed voxel- or pixel-based approaches designed to reduce the time and labor involved in the manual ROI method, such as the statistical parametric mapping approach initially developed by Friston and colleagues in the United Kingdom, as implemented in several versions of SPM software, and the three-dimensional stereotactic surface projection (3D SSP) method developed by Minoshima and his colleagues in the United States as implemented in NeuroStat and, more recently, other versions of 3D SSP-based software. These methods, which can sample thousands of pixel/voxel units denoted by their location in an image derived from warping the patient's individual scan into some form of template space, lend themselves to relatively automated output of quantitative or statistical units and then referred to locations in the original patient's brain image, which they are meant to represent. This allows for a rapid sampling of the brain volume, without neuroanatomic expertise needed for the quantification process itself. Of course, to analyze the output, the reader must possess an appropriate level of neuroanatomic expertise and must generally also assume that the individual pixel/voxel units have been assigned locations that correspond closely with the neuroanatomic sites in the patient's brain, before the image-warping process, from which the measured activity was derived.

The standardized region of interest (SROI) approach combines elements of both the manual ROI and pixel/voxel-based approaches. Anatomically and functionally defined regions are defined on a brain template, thereby essentially encoding the neurologic expertise of the developers into the program. Hundreds of these SROIs can be predefined and then applied to an individual patient's brain, which has undergone elastic transformation to the template space (or, alternatively, the template-defined SROIs may be warped to the patient's brain scan), so that the end-user can obtain an automated determination of the levels of activity measured in all brain regions in a matter of seconds, rather than the many hours it would require to obtain comparable information by the manual ROI method.

In the United States, the FDA approves medical imaging software to be marketed for clinical applications under its purview to regulate medical devices. The first software product dedicated to the quantification of brain PET scans to receive approval from the FDA was released in 2004, and it employs the SROI approach described previously. The essential features and algorithms underlying that software were originally developed by the author and his colleagues at the University of California, Los Angeles (UCLA) to facilitate research focused on measuring the utility of brain PET applied to diagnostic and prognostic assessments of patients undergoing clinical evaluation for cognitive impairment. The University of California subsequently licensed marketing and development rights to Syntermed, Inc. (Atlanta, GA), which distributes the software package under the name NeuroQ. Other FDA-approved products that have been commercially released at the time of this writing include Scenium (Siemens AG, New York, NY) and MIMneuro (MIMvista Corp., Cleveland, OH). These products differ from each other, not only with respect to the visual appearance of their displays and the display features offered, but in more substantive ways as well, including the underlying algorithms used for quantification, the tradeoffs made in versatility versus dedicated application to clinical brain PET interpretation, the degree to which straightforward quality control by the user versus presentation of the output following an opaque *black box* quantification process is enabled, the options provided for normalizing the PET data, and the readiness with which the findings evident in the visual display can be related to the numeric results of analysis, as might be given in a clinical report. Although we use a wide variety of software applications for analysis of brain PET scans applied to a diverse range of our research activities at UCLA (including packages not approved by the FDA, such as SPM), the product we use for automated quantification of brain PET to assist with rendering our clinical interpretations continues to be NeuroQ. For this reason, it has been employed, and its output illustrated, in many of the cases described in this book; this is a direct reflection of the actual working practices of the authors and should not be interpreted as implying its superiority over other products that are available for quantifying brain PET scans.

Clinical Reports

Once a patient's scan has been analyzed qualitatively and quantitatively, the remaining task faced by the examiner is to prepare a clinical report that describes the pertinent findings and integrates them to logically support a prognostic or diagnostic conclusion, addressing the clinical question for the which patient is being evaluated. If the approach for systematic examination of the brain PET scans described in this chapter is followed, it lends itself readily to direct translation of that process into a written report. Findings can be sequentially listed as technical comments (when necessary, to qualify an interpretation), global structural and metabolic assessments, focal cortical observations, focal noncortical observations, and (when performed) quantitative and statistical measures, all in a standard three- or four-item format. We discourage listing quantifying measures that are not pertinent to the visual observations; this minimizes the risk of being distracted from the interpretation by numeric artifacts and avoids losing the reader of the report in a sea of numbers. By the time patients are symptomatic for whatever it is that has led to their referral, any neuropathologic processes underlying their symptoms that have metabolic consequences generally will have had an impact on brain function that is visually observable (or, as Bob Dylan put it, "You don't need a weatherman to know which way the wind blows"—although it may be of interest to supplement that qualitative determination with a statement about how fast it is blowing.) To make all this more concrete, consider the case of a 73-year-old woman who underwent brain FDG PET for evaluation of mild cognitive changes, whose scan demonstrates mild hypometabolism that covers areas that are highly characteristic of incipient Alzheimer's disease (Fig. 2.6, *left*). As we follow along the lateral contour from the frontal cortex (*top half of image*) to parietotemporal cortex (*bottom half of image*) seen in that plane, metabolism is seen to mildly decline bilaterally and is slightly lower on the right side of the brain (*left side of image*). The right parietotemporal cluster of regions was found to fall more than three standard deviations below normal. Also in that leftmost image, the posterior cingulate cortex is seen to display a similar level of metabolism, even though this region normally should be considerably more metabolically active than average cortex. A systematic examination of the remainder of the patient's scan led to the following report of findings and overall conclusion.

Findings

1. The gross structure of the brain demonstrates mild widening of the interhemispheric fissure and interthalamic space, consistent with mild generalized cerebral atrophy.
2. The pattern of FDG metabolism in this scan shows mild but extensive bilateral parietal (somewhat worse on right) and posterior cingulate cortical hypometabolism and mild bilateral temporal cortical hypometabolism. The occipital metabolism is less prominent than is typically seen in an eyes-open study.
3. Basal ganglia metabolism is robust, and the activity of the thalamus and brainstem is unremarkable. The cerebellar cortex shows mild crossed cerebellar diaschisis with the left-sided metabolism slightly lower than right.
4. SROI analysis quantifies the posterior cingulate and parietotemporal cortical metabolism as falling approximately 2–3 standard deviations below normal mean, and temporal regions as ranging from approximately 1–5 standard deviations below normal mean, all as normalized to pons.

Conclusion

The conclusion is posterior-predominant mild cortical hypometabolism, particularly affecting parietal, temporal, and posterior cingulate cortex, as described previously. This pattern is most commonly seen in the context of Alzheimer's-like changes occurring in the patient's brain.

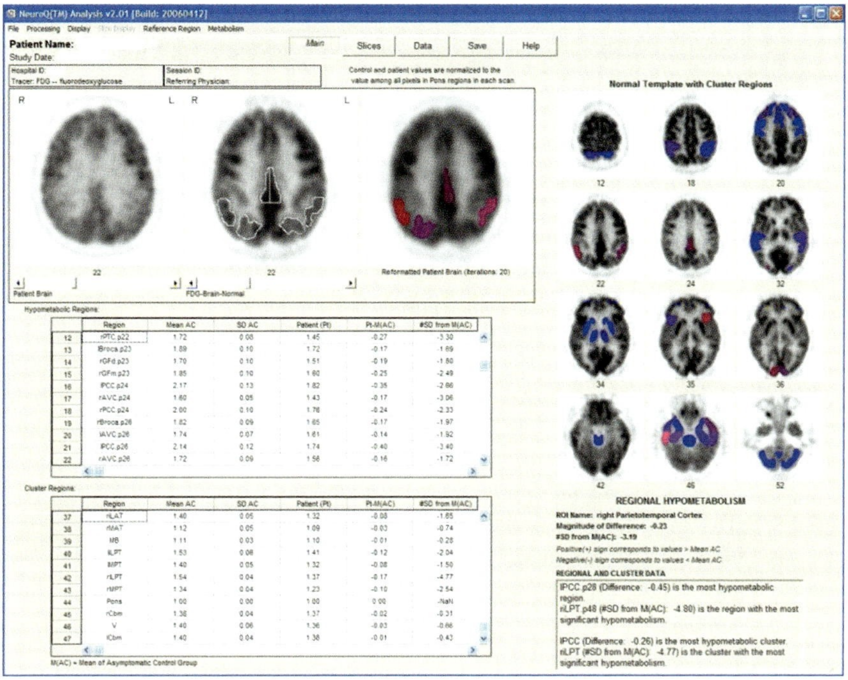

Fig. 2.6 Results of quantification of a brain PET scan, using a standardized region of interest (SROI) approach. Among the three larger images on the left side of the window, the *leftmost image* shows an axial plane from the patients' original PET scan, the *center image* shows the corresponding plane from the normal template on which are outlined SROI contours sampling posterior cortical regions in white, and the *rightmost image* demonstrates that plane from the patient's scan after being transformed into template space, with those areas sampled by the SROIs that are hypometabolic (as defined by falling in the lowest 5% of a normal distribution) displayed in color. On the *right side of the window,* 12 axial planes from the template are shown extending from superior to inferior levels for anatomic reference, with the superimposed color scale corresponding to the results of quantification of the patient's brain data. In that two-dimensional scale, areas that are bright blue are normal, areas that are bright red are the most abnormal in both magnitude and in terms of statistical significance of the abnormality relative to a normal database, and intermediate shades represent areas of abnormality that may be statistically significant, but by a lesser magnitude. (Courtesy of NeuroQ, Syntermed, Inc., Atlanta, GA.)

The first three items in the Findings section are based on visual analysis of the patient's scan, examined in the order detailed in the first section of this chapter. The fourth item in the Findings section described results of scan quantification that are pertinent to that visual analysis and the diagnostic assessment that is about to be presented. As articulated in the Conclusion, note that in the absence of clinical dementia, regardless of how characteristic the scan findings are, a diagnosis of Alzheimer's disease per se cannot be reached, given that a key criterion for having that disease is the presence of dementia. Nevertheless, the presence of the biochemical processes that will eventually lead to that diagnosis is indicated by the pattern of metabolism, as conveyed in the final sentence of the report. Similarly, although not a part of this patient's current clinical picture, if it can be confirmed that the patient had eyes open during the FDG uptake period, the decrease in occipital metabolism could reflect early changes associated with cortical deposition of Lewy bodies.

Summary

Regardless of what other tools are brought to bear on the process, the clinical interpretation of brain PET scans must be built on the foundation of a skilled visual assessment of the pattern of radiotracer uptake. That assessment involves examining at least five aspects of the study, as detailed in this chapter: (1) technical quality, (2) structural integrity of the brain, (3) global metabolism, particularly of the cortex, (4) focal cortical metabolism, and (5) focal noncortical metabolism (most often including basal ganglia, thalamus, cerebellum, and brainstem). In the past few years, software tools have become available to assist with this analysis, which can be used to lend quantitative and statistical support to interpretations suggested by the observed uptake patterns. Applying the acquired skills and tools in this way to FDG PET scans obtained of patients undergoing scanning for dementia-related conditions, qualitative and quantitative findings may be fluidly integrated into final written reports that contribute to the diagnostic evaluation as described in the next chapter.

References

1. Buchert R, Santer R, Brenner W, et al. Computer simulations suggest that acute correction of hyperglycemia with an insulin bolus protocol might be useful in brain FDG PET. Nuklearmedizin 2009:(in press).
2. Minoshima S, Frey KA, Burdette JH, et al. Interpretation of metabolic abnormalities in Alzheimer's disease using three-dimensional stereotactic surface projections (3D-SSP) and normal database. J Nucl Med 1995;36:237P.
3. Moeller JR, Ishikawa T, Dhawan V, et al. The metabolic topography of normal aging. J Cereb Blood Flow Metab 1996;16:385–398.
4. Ishii K, Sakamoto S, Sasaki M, et al. Cerebral glucose metabolism in patients with frontotemporal dementia. J Nucl Med 1998;39:1875–1878.
5. Silverman DHS, Alavi A. PET imaging in the assessment of normal and impaired cognitive function. Radiol Clin North Am 2005;43:67–77.
6. Minoshima S, Giordani B, Berent S, et al. Metabolic reduction in the posterior cingulate cortex in very early AD. Ann Neurol 1997;42:85–94.
7. Silverman DHS. Brain F-18-FDG PET in the diagnosis of neurodegenerative dementias: comparison with perfusion SPECT and with clinical evaluations lacking nuclear imaging. J Nucl Med 2004;45:594–607.
8. Silverman DHS, Small GW, Chang CY et al. Positron emission tomography in evaluation of dementia: regional brain metabolism and longterm outcome. JAMA 2001;286:2120–2127.
9. Silverman DH, Truong CT, Kim SK, et al. Prognostic value of regional cerebral metabolism in patients undergoing dementia evaluation: comparison to a quantifying parameter of subsequent cognitive performance and to prognostic assessment without PET. Mol Genet Metab 2003;80:350–355.
10. Silverman DH, Mosconi L, Ercoli L, et al. Positron emission tomography scans obtained for the evaluation of cognitive dysfunction. Semin Nucl Med 2008;38:251–61.

Chapter 3
FDG PET in the Evaluation of Mild Cognitive Impairment and Early Dementia

Lisa Mosconi and Daniel H.S. Silverman

Alzheimer's disease (AD) is the most common form of dementia in mid- to late life and one of the most serious health problems in the industrialized world. The elderly are the fastest growing part of the population, and increases in life expectancy will inevitably lead to a further increase in the prevalence of AD. Moreover, age-associated cognitive impairments affect 10 times as many individuals.[1] The risk of developing AD doubles approximately every 5 years between the ages of 65 and 85 years, and as the baby boomer generation ages, it is estimated that in 30 years 15 to 20 million elderly nationwide may have some cognitive disability.[1,2] The demographics of aging thus suggest a great need to diagnose AD accurately and distinguish it specifically from the many other possible causes of cognitive impairment. As strategies to delay disease progression and possibly prevent or offset the onset of AD are under development,[3] it is extremely important to recognize individuals at high risk for developing AD who may particularly benefit from early therapeutic interventions.

Remarkable progress has been made in the understanding of the cascade of molecular events leading to AD. In the last decade, genetic abnormalities have been identified, new pathophysiologic mechanisms discovered, therapeutic agents approved, and diagnostic tests developed. Nonetheless, fundamental questions remain unanswered and the lack of specific biological markers hinders the management of AD. With the development of specific and effective prevention treatments, improved early detection of AD will be increasingly critical for medical care.

The definitive diagnosis of AD is based on the postmortem observation of specific pathologic lesions: intracellular neurofibrillary tangles (NFT) and β-amyloid deposition in the form of extracellular senile plaques and blood vessel deposits, synapse dysfunction, and loss.[4–6] AD pathology translates to functional and structural brain damage, mainly involving the brain regions in which the concentration of cell loss is the greatest in AD (see Morrison and Hof for review).[7] Invariably, in AD major circuits are structurally disrupted through synapse loss and neuronal death, and selective vulnerability exists with respect to which neurons die and which are resistant to neurodegeneration. The pyramidal cells in the entorhinal cortex and the CA1 and subiculum regions of the hippocampus and the perforant path that connects

D.H.S. Silverman (ed.), *PET in the Evaluation of Alzheimer's Disease and Related Disorders*,
DOI: 10.1007/978-0-387-76420-7_3,

the hippocampus to the neocortex are particularly vulnerable to degeneration, whereas primary sensory and motor areas show minimal neuronal loss.[7]

Several studies have shown that the progression of AD pathology in the brain can be staged and the pathologic changes associated with the cognitive decline characteristic of AD develop many years before the clinical manifestations of the disease become apparent using standard approaches to assessment.[8–11] When a brain contains few NFT, they are concentrated in limbic and paralimbic structures, such as the medial temporal lobes (MTL, i.e., hippocampus, transentorhinal and entorhinal cortices, and parahippocampal gyrus), the amygdala, and the nucleus basalis of Meynert. These parts of the brain play a critical role in the neural control of memory function. This initial *low limbic* stage of NFT distribution provides an anatomic substrate for the relatively common memory impairments associated with aging. In the next *high limbic* stage of NFT density, NFT become more numerous in the limbic regions and begin to cluster in the adjacent inferior temporal and fusiform gyri and in the connected orbitofrontal regions, insula, and temporal poles. This stage is associated with mild cognitive impairment (MCI), forgetfulness, and preclinical AD.[9] Finally, NFT spread to the parietotemporal and prefrontal association cortices that are involved in the neural control of perception, attention, and language.[8,9] The corresponding *low* and *high neocortical* stages are associated with mild and then severe dementia.

Compared with NFT, neuritic plaques show significant interindividual variations of distribution. There does not seem to be as close a relationship between the regional amyloid deposition and the pattern of neuropsychological deficits, and the correlation between plaque density and dementia is relatively poor (see Mesulam for review).[12] β-Amyloid depositions often show initial predilection for the neocortex and are found in the MTL at later stages of disease.[13–15] It has been suggested that some form of soluble, circulating amyloid may be more detrimental in the early AD stages than its fibrillar form.[16]

Both NFTs and plaques are often found in the brain of nondemented elderly individuals,[6] which makes the definition of boundaries between normal aging and the early stages of AD particularly problematic. Conversely, neuropathologic studies indicate that extensive synapse loss (i.e., loss of connections between neurons) is found in AD, although not in aging. Severe synapse loss is found in AD brains, with reductions ranging from 30% to 90%.[6,17] Synaptic abnormalities are seen as the proximate cause of dementia in AD and provide a better correlate of the pattern and severity of cognitive impairment than amyloid plaques or NFTs.[18] By contrast, synapse and neuronal loss occur to a modest degree in the aging brain. With increasing age, brain changes are noted on macroscopic and microscopic evaluations. Following the attainment of a maximum weight around 18 years of age, the size and weight of the human brain gradually decreases over the adult life span,[7] and by age 80 years, it is estimated that the brain has lost on average 15% of its original adult weight, which translates to very mild generalized cerebral atrophy and ventricular enlargement.[19]

Longitudinal in vivo imaging studies have begun to provide a bridge between clinical- and neuropathology-based staging models. As our ability to detect brain changes related to AD improves, so does our ability to detect patients at increased risk for AD by using neuroimaging. Neuroimaging techniques offer the opportunity to track AD-related brain changes in vivo, which is critical for creating an early diagnostic capacity. Substantial neuronal loss results in structural brain changes that can be visualized as gross atrophy by using magnetic resonance imaging (MRI). Recent MRI studies in AD patients have shown that cortical atrophy occurs in defined sequences as the disease progresses, substantiating the pattern of NFT accumulation observed in cross-section at autopsy.[20] Most MRI studies have shown that severe hippocampal atrophy is consistently found in mild AD patients,[21–26] whereas volume reductions in the cortical regions become apparent in moderate to severe AD.[23,25–27] Evidence suggests that the volume loss detected on MRI is related to both the extent of NFT pathology and to the magnitude of neuronal loss.[28,29] As neuronal degeneration and the formation of insoluble amyloid deposits and neuritic tangles gradually progress, AD pathology is known to have the general effect of disrupting axonal transport and inducing widespread metabolic declines. Several studies have shown that synaptic and dendritic loss precedes frank neuronal loss, with accompanying astrogliosis and hyperphosphorylation of tau,[30] and is most prominent in limbic and then cortical regions corresponding to the clinical deficits.[8,18,30] As the metabolic declines are a direct consequence of dysfunction and loss at the synapse (a principal site for energy substrate utilization), the detection of abnormalities in brain function may be particularly useful in the early detection of AD.

The molecular bases of brain metabolism and its variation over the life span are well understood and characterized. In the average adult human, the brain represents approximately 2% of the body weight, and nonetheless accounts for approximately 20% of the oxygen and calories consumed by the body.[31] This constant metabolic activity largely consists of the oxidation of glucose to carbon dioxide and water, resulting in the production of adenosine triphosphate, the energy carrier in the living cells. Therefore, glucose is the common path for the bioenergetics of nearly all neurochemical processes. Relatively recent studies have shown that most brain energy is used to sustain postsynaptic currents and action potentials, which account for 85% of the total energy consumption, rather than activity in presynaptic terminals and glial cells.[32] Among other imaging modalities, PET imaging using 2-[^{18}F] fluoro-2-deoxy-D-glucose (FDG) as the tracer has the unique ability to provide quantitative estimates of the local cerebral metabolic rate of glucose consumption (micromoles per minute per gram of tissue) as derived from emission data and arterial blood samples mathematically analyzed by means of kinetic models. The metabolic signal detected with FDG PET, as an index of neuronal integrity, is mainly associated with glutamate signaling in the brain,[33] as greater than 80% of the brain's neurons are excitatory and 90% of those synapses are glutamatergic.[32–35]

In healthy aging, metabolic rates are relatively stable over time, with most subjects showing whole brain metabolic variability of less than 10%.[36] By contrast, AD patients present with severe reductions in the rate of brain glucose consumption and higher regional and whole brain variability,[37] which reflect decreased synaptic functioning and density.[35,38] The metabolic reduction in AD cannot be accounted for by a rate limitation in glucose delivery or abnormal coupling between oxidation and phosphorylation, as phosphorus metabolites levels are usually within the normal range in mild to severe AD patients.[39]

During the three decades in which FDG PET imaging has been applied to the study of AD, several important thematic contributions emerged. Primary among them has been the detection of the metabolic signature in AD relative to normal elderly controls, followed by the differential diagnosis of AD from other neurodegenerative diseases, and finally longitudinal imaging measures of disease progression. The focus of the early FDG PET studies in AD was to identify general evidence for brain damage that was specifically associated with AD and with the severity of the clinical symptoms. Compared with age-matched healthy normal control subjects, AD patients show regional metabolic reductions involving the parietotemporal and posterior cingulate cortices, and the frontal areas in more advanced disease, in comparison with the relatively spared primary motor and visual areas, cerebellum, thalamus, and basal ganglia nuclei.[37] These findings have been accumulating since the early 1980s, and this pattern of hypometabolism is now largely accepted as a reliable in vivo hallmark of AD, because of its accuracy in distinguishing AD from normal aging as well as from other diseases that affect the brain regionally and globally. FDG PET metabolic measures correlate with longitudinal progression and clinical worsening of disease[40–42] and are sensitive to pharmacologic treatments in dementia.[43,44]

Several events transformed the functional imaging field during the last 15 years. With increasing technical improvements, early SPECT and PET cameras have been replaced by modern multiheaded SPECT gamma cameras and PET equipment with higher spatial resolution, which increased our ability to measure accurately brain metabolism in small brain structures. Since the late 1990s with improvements in the spatial resolution of FDG PET systems and MRI-PET coregistration, reports of hippocampal metabolic abnormalities in AD and MCI also appeared[45–51] (Fig. 3.1) along with neo cortical hypometabolism. A newer generation of PET scanners is now equipped with up to 120,000 lutetium oxyorthosilicate scintillating crystals, yielding a spatial resolution of 2.2 mm.[52] Moreover, modern equipment and software allow reformatting of the PET images in any spatial orientation and coregistration to any other imaging modalities, as well as the implementation of accurate protocols for performing atrophy correction. In order to clarify the brain changes implicated in the disease onset, it is important

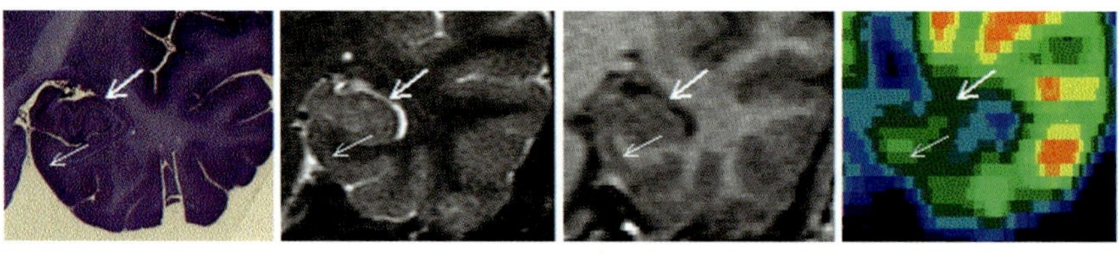

Fig. 3.1 The hippocampal formation: from postmortem to in vivo imaging. *From left to right:* Coronal histologic sections and in vivo coregistered T2- and T1-weighted magnetic resonance imaging (MRI) and FDG PET scans of a patient with mild cognitive impairment (MCI) (female, age 75 at MRI/PET, age 84 at death), showing normal hippocampal (*thick arrow*) and entorhinal cortex (*thin arrow*) volumes on MRI and reduced FDG uptake on PET

to determine the extent to which hypometabolism measured with FDG PET is related to the effects of brain atrophy.[53,54] The presence of brain atrophy artificially lowers the FDG PET measures because of the partial volume effects of cerebrospinal fluid and white matter, and the resulting metabolic measures reflect the combined effects of hypometabolism and atrophy. Although non–atrophy-corrected metabolic measures may be diagnostically useful as they reflect the presence of an underlying neurodegenerative process, measures of brain metabolism per unit brain volume (i.e., as obtained with atrophy correction) allow addressing questions about the biological mechanisms involved in AD by providing a better estimate of the extent of metabolic impairment per unit tissue.

Preclinical Detection of Alzheimer's Disease

Along with technical improvements leading to the new generation of high-resolution PET scanners, advances in the clinical and neuropsychological characterization of AD have led to the conceptualization of a predementia stage, referred to by many as MCI. MCI is seen as a transitional stage between normal aging and dementia including but not exclusive to the AD type.[55] Despite a lack of uniformity of accepted clinical criteria, several imaging studies have investigated this heterogeneous prodromal AD condition, particularly in MCI patients with severe memory impairments (i.e., *amnestic* MCI), who are at especially high risk for declining to AD, with an estimated conversion rate of over 10% per year.[55] Predicting clinical progression by using qualitative measures on clinical scales is particularly challenging for patients presenting in the early stages of disease. There is evidence that PET examinations have higher predictive value than the clinical measures in identifying the presence of a progressive neurodegenerative disease.[56,57] As ample data suggest that reduced brain metabolism may predispose normal individuals to cognitive decline, the use of FDG PET in the clinical diagnostic workup is of great interest.

Scientific progress in different fields, including the discovery of gene mutations and susceptibility genes for AD, the production of transgenic mice to further clarify disease mechanisms and screen candidate treatments, and the recent development of treatments such as amyloid β-peptide immunization,[58] have raised the hope of developing prevention treatments for AD. However, given the low incidence and slow progression of normal elderly to AD (1%–3%/year),[2] using traditional clinical endpoints to test the efficacy of such treatments would require very large samples, long follow-up, and great expense to follow cognitively normal persons treated with a candidate primary prevention therapy to assess impact on development of AD dementia.[59]

Increasing evidence suggests that FDG PET imaging can be used to expedite the process by detecting brain abnormalities in individuals who might be at risk for AD but who have not yet developed symptoms. The knowledge of established risk factors for AD has enabled investigators to develop enrichment strategies for longitudinal imaging studies to reduce the sample sizes and study duration. Some studies used statistical power analyses to test the feasibility of using brain glucose metabolism as an outcome measure in long-term treatment studies of AD in comparison with cognitive test scores.[42,60] It was estimated that to detect a 33% treatment response with 80% power in a typical 1-year, double-blind, placebo-controlled treatment study, a cognitive study using the Mini Mental State Examination would require 224 AD patients per group, whereas as few as 36 patients per group would be needed for an FDG PET study.[42]

Several alternative approaches have been undertaken for the investigation of preclinical AD with FDG PET. One approach involves examining individuals from families with early onset AD (FAD). FAD is characterized by autosomal dominant inheritance and a specific age at onset for a given pedigree (see Tanzi and Bertram for review).[61] Although penetrance is not complete, study of at risk, presymptomatic individuals close to the expected age at onset provides information about preclinical AD-related brain changes. However, these rare genetic mutations account for less than 5% of AD cases in the general population,[61] and the natural history of the more common late-onset sporadic AD may be different than that of FAD. One approach to reduce the sample sizes and follow-up intervals in sporadic AD involves monitoring MCI patients, particularly of the amnestic type, who are more likely to develop AD in the near future.[55,62] In an effort to further anticipate the early detection of AD, recent studies have focused on normal elderly at genetic risk for AD, as determined by their being carriers of known susceptibility genes for late life AD such as the apolipoprotein E E4 allele.[63] Finally, other studies have monitored normal elderly individuals to the onset of MCI. The main findings obtained with the different approaches to the early detection of AD are reviewed in what follows.

Familial Early-Onset Alzheimer's Disease

Autosomal dominant mutations have been identified in three genes, i.e., amyloid precursor protein (APP) and presenilin (PS-) 1 and 2 genes, which determine early-onset FAD. Most imaging studies in FAD cases carrying these mutations were performed with MRI. Serial MRI examinations in affected and at risk FAD members of a British pedigree with mutations in the APP and PS-1 genes reported that the onset of dementia is accompanied by progressive MTL and whole brain atrophy.[64–66] A few FDG PET studies in FAD have been performed that examined the same British FAD patients.[67,68] These cross-sectional FDG PET examinations showed parietotemporal, posterior cingulate, and frontal cortical hypometabolism in most FAD cases, which also showed mild atrophy in the same regions.[67,68] Longitudinal FDG PET studies in FAD would be of interest to compare hypometabolism with atrophy as preclinical markers of incipient dementia and to assess whether the rate of metabolic reductions also increases close to conversion. However, evidence shows that familial and sporadic AD patients present with comparable brain pathology at autopsy,[12] although FAD patients typically develop dementia at 40–50 years of age, consistent with a faster and more aggressive progression of brain damage than in sporadic AD.

Mild Cognitive Impairment

Amnestic MCI is seen as a transitional state between healthy aging and dementia, during which individuals are able to perform usual activities of daily living but suffer isolated memory difficulties exceeding those expected on the basis of normal aging, which makes these individuals at higher risk for developing future AD.[55,62] However, not all MCI patients develop AD, as subjects may remain stable over time, revert to a normal state, or progress to another dementia.[62] As the clinical diagnosis per se is often uncertain in MCI and clinical assessment requires multiple examinations and laboratory tests over time, PET evaluations are increasingly used to support the clinical diagnosis at the early stages of AD.

Despite some commonalities, different clinicians in different countries have used variable criteria for diagnosing prodromal AD. Several subcategories exist, including amnestic MCI, MCI single non-memory domain, MCI multiple domains, cognitive impairment no dementia, questionable AD, and minimal AD, among others.[62] These variable clinical inclusion criteria translated to variable imaging findings, generally showing mild and heterogenous brain damage. A newer designation, Mild Decline in Cognition (MDC), is distinguished from those labels by virtue of not defining "impairment" relative to some reference database used to compare patients to "normals," but rather by comparing patients' cognitive abilities to their own prior performance levels, and documenting that decline has occurred.56 This is especially valuable in the context of elucidating neurodegenerative disease processes, using brain imaging parameters that are measurably affected well in advance of patients falling below some normal reference range defining "impairment," as they suffer from the early stages of a trajectory of inexorable decline.

As the extent of brain hypo metabolism highly correlates with dementia severity, in keeping with their clinical presentation, MCI patients usually present on PET with mild global and regional hypometabolism (Fig. 3.2). FDG PET examinations revealed that MCI patients show a pattern of brain hypometabolism that is topographically consistent with that observed in clinical AD. However, some studies did not observe the same distribution of cortical metabolic deficits in MCI,[69–73] particularly in the case of very mildly affected subjects,[48,50] whereas other studies have reported cortical metabolic deficits in the parietotemporal and posterior cingulate cortex in MCI patients of the amnestic type and in those close to converting to AD.[49,68,74–79] FDG PET studies that have examined the MTL in MCI reported evidence for metabolic reductions, irrespective of the severity and type of cognitive impairment.[46–51] MTL hypometabolism in MCI can be identified on visual inspection of the PET scans (Fig. 3.3), and the inclusion of qualitative evaluations of the MTL along with the traditionally inspected cortical regions can improve the accuracy of the PET diagnosis in distinguishing MCI from normal aging and AD.[51]

Studies that used quantitative measures have shown significant absolute reductions of glucose metabolic rates in MCI patients relative to controls. These reductions are milder than in AD and affect the MTL (7%–17%),[47–51] lateral temporal (8%),[47] and posterior cingulate cortices (23%).[49] More severe metabolic reductions within the same regions and extending to the parietotemporal and frontal regions were found

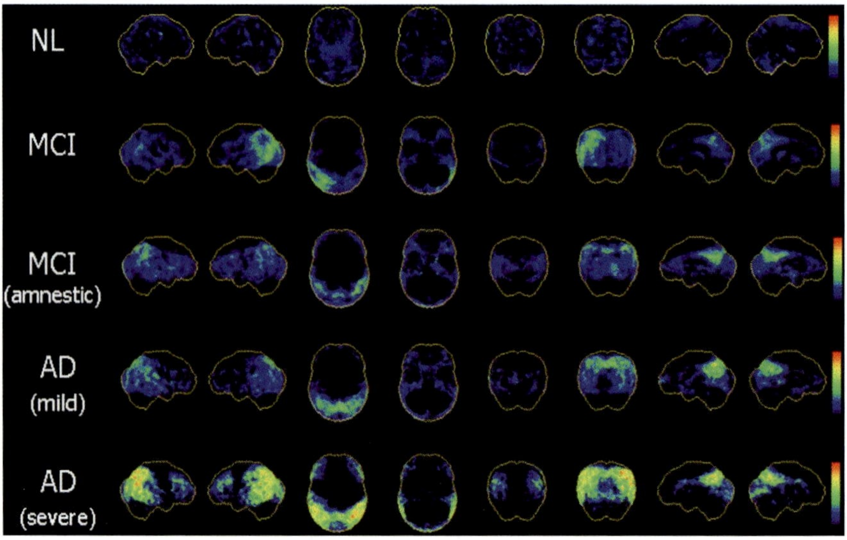

Fig. 3.2 FDG PET findings correlate with the severity of cognitive impairment. Brain regions showing reduced metabolism are displayed as Z-score maps as derived from 3D stereotactic surface projection analysis.[74] Color coding represents statistical significance (Z score) of regional metabolic reductions in comparison with a database of healthy normal subjects (50% women, aged 50–80 years). Z-score maps are displayed in the right and left lateral, top and bottom, anterior and posterior, left and right medial views of a reference standardized brain. No regions of hypointensity are found for a representative normal (NL) subject. Metabolic reductions are found for the nonamnestic mild cognitive impairment (MCI), amnestic MCI, mild Alzheimer's disease (AD), and severe AD patients, who present with gradually more severe hypometabolism in the lateral association and posterior cingulate cortices ($P < 0.001$), with relative sparing of the primary sensorimotor (lateral and medial views) and occipital cortex (medial views)

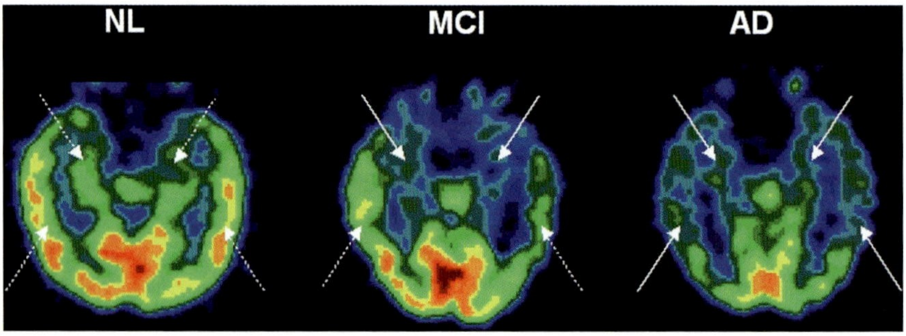

Fig. 3.3 Cortical and medial temporal lobes (MTL) FDG uptake in normal (NL), mild cognitive impairment (MCI), and Alzheimer's disease (AD) subjects. FDG PET axial scans of a normal subject (male, age 66 years, 16 years education, MMSE = 30), an MCI patient (female, age 67 years, 14 years education, MMSE = 30), and an AD patient (male, age 66 years, 14 years education, MMSE = 23) are displayed in the hippocampal plane, showing normal (*dashed arrow*) cortical and MTL FDG uptake in NL aging, questionable cortical uptake and reduced (*solid line*) MTL uptake in MCI, and reduced cortical and MTL uptake in AD

in AD patients.[48–51] Overall, these data are consistent with pathology studies suggesting a progression from the early involvement of the MTL (associated with memory loss and clear but minimal functional deficits) to diagnosable AD with both MTL and cortical involvement, and substantiate the clinical conceptualization of MCI as a transitional stage between normal aging and dementia.

A growing body of longitudinal FDG PET studies has been carried out to examine the predictive value of cerebral metabolic measures in the decline from MCI to AD. The major findings are summarized in Table 3.1. All longitudinal FDG PET studies in MCI were consistent in demonstrating metabolic changes associated with incipient AD that share the same topography of the characteristic AD PET pattern, i.e., reduced parietotemporal and posterior cingulate cortex metabolism, and are detectable several years before clinical diagnosis.[74–77,80–83] The metabolic reductions at the MCI stage are more pronounced in those MCI patients who eventually developed AD as compared with those who remained stable and predict AD with accuracies ranging from 75% to 100%.[75–77,81–83] Interestingly, these results were obtained using a variety of image analysis techniques, from the traditional manual regions of interest approach to most recent automated voxel-based analysis.[74,84] With any method, PET metabolic measures proved sensitive predictors of future

Table 3.1 Prediction of decline from mild cognitive impairment (MCI) to Alzheimer's disease using FDG PET

Reference	Subjects: decliners/ nondecliners	Follow-up (years)	Major findings	Predictive accuracy
Minoshima et al. (1997)[74]	8/23	2	Reduced parietotemporal and posterior cingulate cortex MRglc	Not reported
Herholz et al. (1999)[75]	19/52	2	Reduced cortical MRglc	78%
Arnaiz et al. (2001)[76]	9/20	3	Reduced parietotemporal cortex MRglc	75%
Chetelat et al. (2003)[77]	7/17	1.5	Reduced parietotemporal and posterior cingulate cortex MRglc	94%–100%
Drzezga et al. (2003)[80]	8/22	1	Reduced parietotemporal, posterior cingulate, and/or frontal cortex MRglc	Not reported
Mosconi et al. (2003)[81]	8/37	1	Reduced parietal cortex MRglc	89%
Drzezga et al. (2005)[82]	12/18	1.4	Reduced parietotemporal, posterior cingulate, and/or frontal cortex MRglc	90%
Anchisi et al. (2005)[83]	14/67	1	Reduced parietotemporal and posterior cingulate cortex MRglc	92%

MRglc, metabolic rate for glucose.

AD. Moreover, evidence exists that the metabolic reductions in the declining MCI patients are progressive, indicating that PET measures are both predictors and correlates of decline to AD.[80]

A relatively recent study examined the individual predictive value of the PET diagnosis for the decline from MCI to AD.[82] By using automated techniques to facilitate the PET diagnosis, this study examined the baseline PET scans of 30 MCI patients for the presence of a pattern of hypometabolism indicative of a progressive neurodegenerative disease, by statistical comparison of each patient to an age-matched reference database of normal controls.[85] Decline to AD was observed in 12 of 30 (40%) of the MCI patients over an interval of 1.5 years. The PET diagnosis correctly predicted decline to AD, with 92% sensitivity and 89% specificity, yielding a positive predictive value of 85% and a negative predictive value of 94%.[82]

Although MCI patients have less severe cognitive symptoms than in AD, the observation that they often present with advanced pathology[6] and the fact that they decline within 1–3 years of the first examination indicate that findings in MCI are not strictly *preclinical,* and studies that follow normal subjects until the onset of cognitive impairment will be important for examining the earliest AD stages.

Apolipoprotein E Genotype and the Risk for Alzheimer's Disease

FDG PET studies have examined the effects of established genetic risk factors for sporadic AD, such as the apolipoprotein E E4 allele,[63] on brain metabolism in nondemented individuals. As compared with the noncarriers, asymptomatic normal individual carriers of the E4 genotype show reduced metabolism in the same regions as clinically affected AD patients.[60,86–89] These mild but definite metabolic reductions were found prior to the onset of cognitive symptoms and brain atrophy.[86,89] There is evidence in middle-aged E4 carriers that the metabolic reductions are progressive and correlate with reductions in cognitive performance.[60,86] Moreover, as such hypometabolism was observed in 20- to 40-year-old subjects, these metabolic reductions are considered the earliest brain abnormalities yet found in living persons at risk for AD.[89] It remains uncertain whether the brain abnormalities detected are due to early pathologic changes of AD.

From Normal Aging to Cognitive Impairment

FDG PET has also been used to study the decline from normal to MCI.[47] The aim of this longitudinal FDG PET study was to follow normal elderly subjects long enough to identify metabolic harbingers of future clinical decline to MCI. This study showed that reduced baseline metabolic levels in the entorhinal cortex, which is part of the hippocampal formation, predict an MCI diagnosis 3 years later.[47] At baseline, when all subjects were normal, entorhinal cortex metabolism was reduced 18% in those subjects who declined to MCI relative to those who did not decline at the follow-up. The baseline metabolic reduction predicted decline to MCI with 83% sensitivity and 85% specificity. No cortical regions showed preclinical effects. Moreover, progressive metabolic reductions in the entorhinal cortex and in the left lateral temporal lobe paralleled the onset of MCI, which is of interest, as an ideal biomarker for AD severity must correlate with disease progression. These effects remained significant after correcting the metabolic values for the partial volume effects of cerebrospinal fluid from the MRI-coregistered PET scans. Atrophy correction had the effect of increasing regional metabolism in both the declining (10%–21%) and the nondeclining groups (5%–15%), with the greatest adjustment seen in the entorhinal cortex. After correcting for atrophy, the decliners still showed 11% reduced entorhinal cortex metabolism as compared with the nondecliners, and the predictive accuracy was almost as high, at 80%.[47] This result suggests that the early brain metabolic reductions in AD are relatively independent of the partial volume effects of the increasing cerebrospinal fluid pool, which is consistent with previous PET report of significant metabolic reductions in MCI and AD after atrophy correction.[47,48,50,54,90]

As many MCI patients do not develop AD, it remains to be established whether the observed metabolic reductions are related to future AD. These findings are consistent with MRI studies in normal subjects showing that MTL volume reductions correlate with the decline from normal to MCI[91–93] and also predict future dementia.[94]

Comparing SPECT and PET

SPECT has historically been a more widely available functional brain imaging modality and more commonly used imaging resource for the evaluation of dementia. Most clinical and research studies employing SPECT for the diagnosis of dementia are perfusion based. Although specific radiopharmaceuticals and instrumentation differ from those used in PET, the principles of interpretation, as well as the underlying neurobiological processes, are similar. PET scans typically provide better spatial resolution, however, and the magnitude of hypometabolism seen with FDG PET is generally greater than the amplitude of hypoperfusion seen with SPECT.[95–97] It should further be kept in mind that the generally parallel relationship between the cortical metabolism, which is usually measured with PET and the perfusion measured with SPECT, can break down in the presence of certain disorders, such as cerebrovascular disease.

As might be expected, studies of AD using SPECT have yielded results similar to those using PET, but generally demonstrate less sensitivity and decreased overall accuracy. Higher diagnostic accuracy achieved with PET has been documented in side-by-side studies done contemporaneously, the most powerful experimental design for making such comparisons. These include studies of AD patients with mild symptoms[98] and studies with *high-resolution* SPECT scanners,[99,100] and those investigations show that PET is approximately 15% to 20% more accurate than SPECT.

Some investigators have found that the accuracy of SPECT studies may be improved through use of quantifying software to assist in interpretation.[101] Even so, when the ability of PET and SPECT to identify abnormalities in patients with suspected AD using such software-based techniques have been compared side by side, differences persist. For example, to assess the number of abnormal voxels relative to an age-matched control group for each technique using statistical parametric mapping,[75] the best correspondence was in parietotemporal and posterior cingulate cortices (ratio = 0.90); nevertheless, tracer uptake reductions were significantly more pronounced with PET than with SPECT. Researchers also measured the correlation between clinical severity of impairment and the number of abnormal voxels, which was somewhat better for PET than for SPECT. A higher sensitivity of PET may be especially relevant when identifying disease in its earliest stages in order to target patients for therapy while irreversible neurodegeneration is limited.

Future Implications

Although a cure for AD does not exist, symptomatic treatment has been proved to slow the decline of cognitive and functional abilities, especially in earlier stages. Emerging therapies targeting presumed pathogenic mechanisms are in development. Disease-modifying therapies would be most important to initiate during the earliest phases of the disease, making it especially important to have an early clinical diagnosis of AD, when treatments could potentially arrest the degenerative process at a time when damage to brain tissue is minimized.

As our understanding of the biology of dementia processes advances, it will also become possible to better select treatments for patients suffering from early stages of dementia. Currently, categorizations such as MCI, cognitive impairment with no dementia, and age-associated or age-consistent memory impairment are not uniformly applied across investigative groups or clinical centers, and, more importantly, groups of patients defined by such clinically based categories encompass individuals with several different biological forms and stages of disease. The opportunity to establish categories reflecting more directly the underlying biology of the disease process by using approaches involving pertinent neuroimaging methods is now at hand and can be expected to play an increasing role in defining diagnoses, both for the purpose of selecting appropriate subjects for research trials and for assessing patients for clinical diagnosis and treatment.

Conclusion

In summary, metabolic imaging can be successfully used for the early detection of the effects of AD on the brain, even in the earlier stages of disease when clinical symptoms are not fully expressed and the regional brain damage may be limited.

References

1. Brookmeyer R, Gray S, Kawas C. Projections of Alzheimer's disease in the United States and the public health impact of delaying disease onset. Am J Public Health 1998;88:1337–1342.
2. Petersen RC, Smith GE, Waring SC, et al. Mild cognitive impairment: clinical characterization and outcome. Arch Neurol 1999;56:303–308.
3. Scarpini E, Scheltens P, Feldman H. Treatment of Alzheimer's disease: current status and new perspectives. Lancet Neurol 2003;2:539–547.
4. Ball MJ, Hachinski V, Fox A, et al. A new definition of Alzheimer's disease: a hippocampal dementia. Lancet 1985;1:14–16.
5. Manolio TA, Kronmal RA, Burke GL, et al. Magnetic resonance abnormalities and cardiovascular disease in older adults. The Cardiovascular Health Study. Stroke 1994;25:318–327.
6. Price JL, Morris JC. Tangles and plaques in nondemented aging and "preclinical" Alzheimer's disease. Ann Neurol 1999;45:358–368.
7. Morrison JH, Hof PR. Life and death of neurons in the aging brain. Science 1997;278:412–419.
8. Braak H, Braak E. Development of Alzheimer-related neurofibrillary changes in the neocortex inversely recapitulates cortical myelogenesis. Acta Neuropathol 1996;92:197–201.
9. Delacourte A, David JP, Sergeant N, et al. The biochemical pathway of neurofibrillary degeneration in aging and Alzheimer's disease. Neurology 1999;52:1158–1165.
10. Morris JC, Storandt M, McKeel DW, et al. Cerebral amyloid deposition and diffuse plaques in "normal" aging: evidence for presymptomatic and very mild Alzheimer's disease. Neurology 1996;46:707–719.
11. Braak H, Braak E. Neuropathological staging of Alzheimer-related changes. Acta Neuropathol 1991;82:239–259.
12. Mesulam MM. Neuroplasticity failure in Alzheimer's disease: bridging the gap between plaques and tangles. Neuron 1999;24:521–529.
13. Arriagada PV, Marzloff K, Hyman BT. Distribution of Alzheimer-type pathologic changes in nondemented elderly individuals matches the pattern in Alzheimer's disease. Neurology 1992;42:1681–1688.
14. Giannakopoulos P, Hof PR, Mottier S, et al. Neuropathological changes in the cerebral cortex of 1258 cases from a geriatric hospital: retrospective clinicopathological evaluation of a 10-year autopsy population. Acta Neuropathol 1994;87:456–468.
15. Ulrich J. Alzheimer changes in nondemented patients younger than sixty-five: possible early stages of Alzheimer's disease and senile dementia of Alzheimer type. Ann Neurol 1985;17:273–277.
16. Lambert MP, Barlow AK, Chromy BA, et al. Diffusible, nonfibrillar ligands derived from Abeta1-42 are potent central nervous system neurotoxins. Proc Natl Acad Sci USA 1998;95:6448–6453.
17. Gomez-Isla T, Hollister R, West H, et al. Neuronal loss correlates with but exceeds neurofibrillary tangles in Alzheimer's disease. Ann Neurol 1997;41:17–24.
18. Terry RD, Masliah E, Salmon DP, et al. Physical basis of cognitive alterations in Alzheimer's disease: synapse loss is the major correlate of cognitive impairment. Ann Neurol 1991;30:572–580.
19. Jernigan TL, Archibald SL, Berhow MT, et al. Cerebral structure on MRI, Part I: Localization of age-related changes. Biol Psychiatry 1991;29:55–67.
20. Thompson PM, Hayashi KM, de Zubicaray GI, et al. Dynamics of gray matter loss in Alzheimer's disease. J Neurosci 2003;23:994–1005.
21. Kesslak JP, Nalcioglu O, Cotman CW. Quantification of magnetic resonance scans for hippocampal and parahippocampal atrophy in Alzheimer's disease. Neurology 1991;41:51–54.
22. Jack CRJr, Petersen RC, O'Brien PC, et al. MR-based hippocampal volumetry in the diagnosis of Alzheimer's disease. Neurology 1992;42:183–188.
23. Killiany RJ, Moss MB, Albert MS, et al. Temporal lobe regions on magnetic resonance imaging identify patients with early Alzheimer's disease. Arch Neurol 1993;50:949–954.

24. Convit A, de Leon MJ, Tarshish C, et al. Hippocampal volume losses in minimally impaired elderly. Lancet 1995;345:266.
25. de Toledo-Morrell L, Sullivan MP, Morrell F, et al. Alzheimer's disease: in vivo detection of differential vulnerability of brain regions. Neurobiol Aging 1997;18:463–468.
26. Jack CRJr, Petersen RC, Xu YC, et al. Medial temporal atrophy on MRI in normal aging and very mild Alzheimer's disease. Neurology 1997;49:786–794.
27. Convit A, de Leon MJ, Tarshish C, et al. Specific hippocampal volume reductions in individuals at risk for Alzheimer's disease. Neurobiol Aging 1997;18:131–138.
28. Bobinski M, Wegiel J, Tarnawski M, et al. Relationships between regional neuronal loss and neurofibrillary changes in the hippocampal formation and duration and severity of Alzheimer disease. J Neuropath Exp Neurol 1997;56:414–420.
29. Bobinski M, de Leon MJ, Wegiel J, et al. The histological validation of post mortem magnetic resonance imaging-determined hippocampal volume in Alzheimer's disease. Neuroscience 2000;95:721–725.
30. Saura CA, Choi S, Beglopoulos V, et al. Loss of presenilin function in the adult brain causes memory and synaptic plasticity impairments and age-dependent neurodegeneration. Neuron 2004;42:23–36.
31. Clark DD, Sokoloff L. Circulation and energy metabolism of the brain. In: Siegel GJ, Agranoff BW, Albers RW, et-al., eds, Basic Neurochemistry. Molecular, Cellular and Medical Aspects. Philadelphia: Lippincott-Raven, 1999:637–670.
32. Attwell D, Iadecola C. The neural basis of functional brain imaging signals. Trends Neurosci 2002;25:621–625.
33. Magistretti PJ, Pellerin L, Rothman DL, et al. Energy on demand. Science 1999 ;283:496–497.
34. Fonnum F. Glutamate: a neurotransmitter in mammalian brain. J Neurochem 1984;42:1–11.
35. Herholz K. PET studies in dementia. Ann Nucl Med 2003;17:79–89.
36. Bartlett EJ, Barouche F, Brodie JD, et al. Stability of resting deoxyglucose metabolic values in PET studies of schizophrenia. Psych Res Neuroimaging 1991;40:11–20.
37. Mazziotta JC, Phelps ME. Positron emission tomography studies of the brain. In: Phelps ME, Mazziotta JC, Schelbert H, eds, Positron Emission Tomography and Autoradiography: Principles and Applications for the Brain and Heart. New York: Raven, 1986:493–579.
38. Mielke R, Kessler J, Szelies B, et al. Normal and pathological aging—findings of positron-emission-tomography. J Neural Transm 1998;105:821–837.
39. Murphy DGM, Bottomley PA, Salerno JA, et al. An in vivo study of phosphorus and glucose metabolism in Alzheimer's disease using magnetic resonance spectroscopy and PET. Arch Gen Psychiatry 1993;50:341–349.
40. Smith GS, de Leon MJ, George AE, et al. Topography of cross-sectional and longitudinal glucose metabolic deficits in Alzheimer's disease: pathophysiologic implications. Arch Neurol 1992;49:1142–1150.
41. Jagust WJ, Friedland RP, Budinger TF, et al. Longitudinal studies of regional cerebral metabolism in Alzheimer's disease. Neurology 1988;38:909–912.
42. Alexander GE, Chen K, Pietrini P, et al. Longitudinal PET evaluation of cerebral metabolic decline in dementia: a potential outcome measure in Alzheimer's disease treatment studies. Am J Psychiatry 2002;159:738–745.
43. Nordberg A, Lilja A, Lindqvist H, et al. Tacrine restores cholinergic nicotinic receptors and glucose metabolism in Alzheimer patients as visualised by PET. Neurobiol Aging 1992;13:747–758.
44. Tuszynski MH, Thal L, Pay M, et al. A phase 1 clinical trial of nerve growth factor gene therapy for Alzheimer disease. Nat Med 2005;11:551–555.
45. de Leon MJ, McRae T, Rusinek H, et al. Cortisol reduces hippocampal glucose metabolism in normal elderly but not in Alzheimer's disease. J Clin Endocrinol Metab 1997;82:3251–3259.
46. Ouchi Y, Nobezawa S, Okada H, et al. Altered glucose metabolism in the hippocampal head in memory impairment. Neurology 1998;51:136–142.

47. de Leon MJ, Convit A, Wolf OT, et al. Prediction of cognitive decline in normal elderly subjects with 2-[18F]fluoro-2-deoxy-D-glucose/positron-emission tomography (FDG/PET). Proc Natl Acad Sci USA 2001;98:10966–10971.
48. De Santi S, de Leon MJ, Rusinek H, et al. Hippocampal formation glucose metabolism and volume losses in MCI and AD. Neurobiol Aging 2001;22:529–539.
49. Nestor PJ, Fryer TD, Smielewski P, et al. Limbic hypometabolism in Alzheimer's disease and mild cognitive impairment. Ann Neurol 2003;54:343–351.
50. Mosconi L, Tsui WH, De Santi S, et al. Reduced hippocampal metabolism in mild cognitive impairment and Alzheimer's disease: automated FDG-PET image analysis. Neurology 2005;64:1860–1867.
51. Mosconi L, De Santi S, Li Y, et al. Visual rating of medial temporal lobe metabolism in mild cognitive impairment and Alzheimer's disease using FDG-PET. Eur J Nucl Med 2006;33:210–221.
52. Heiss W-D, Habedank B, Klein JC, et al. Metabolic rates in small brain nuclei determined by high-resolution PET. J Nucl Med 2004;45:1811–1815.
53. Meltzer CC, Zubieta JK, Brandt J, et al. Regional hypometabolism in Alzheimer's disease as measured by positron emission tomography after correction for effects of partial volume averaging. Neurology 1996;47:454–461.
54. Ibanez V, Pietrini P, Alexander GE, et al. Regional glucose metabolic abnormalities are not the result of atrophy in Alzheimer's disease. Neurology 1999;50:1585–1593.
55. Petersen RC, Doody R, Kurz A, et al. Current concepts in mild cognitive impairment. Arch Neurol 2001;58:1985–1992.
56. Silverman DH, Mosconi L, Ercoli L, et al. Positron emission tomography scans obtained for the evaluation of cognitive dysfunction. Semin Nucl Med 2008;38:251–61
57. Silverman DHS, Truong CT, Kim SK, et al. Prognostic value of regional cerebral metabolism in patients undergoing dementia evaluation: comparison to a quantifying parameter of subsequent cognitive performance and to prognostic assessment without PET. Mol Genet Metab 2003;80:350–355.
58. Schenk D, Barbour R, Dunn W, et al. Immunization with amyloid-beta attenuates Alzheimer-disease-like pathology in the PDAPP mouse. Nature 1999;400:173–177.
59. Silverman DHS, Gambhir SS, Huang HW, et al. Evaluating early dementia with and without assessment of regional cerebral metabolism by PET: a comparison of predicted costs and benefits. J Nucl Med 2002;43:253–266.
60. Reiman EM, Caselli RJ, Chen K, et al. Declining brain activity in cognitively normal apolipoprotein E epsilon 4 heterozygotes: a foundation for using positron emission tomography to efficiently test treatments to prevent Alzheimer's disease. Proc Natl Acad Sci USA 2001;98:3334–3339.
61. Tanzi R, Bertram L. New frontiers in Alzheimer's disease genetics. Neuron 2001;32:181–184.
62. Petersen RC, Stevens JC, Ganguli M, et al. Practice parameter: early detection of dementia: mild cognitive impairment (an evidence-based review). Report of the Quality Standards Subcommittee of the American Academy of Neurology. Neurology 2001;56:1133–1142.
63. Corder EH, Saunders AM, Strittmatter WJ, et al. Gene dose of apolipoprotein E type 4 allele and the risk of Alzheimer's disease in late onset families. Science 1993;261:921–923.
64. Fox NC, Warrington EK, Rossor MN. Serial magnetic resonance imaging of cerebral atrophy in preclinical Alzheimer's disease. Lancet 1999;353:2125.
65. Fox NC, Crum WR, Scahill RI, et al. Imaging of onset and progression of Alzheimer's disease with voxel-compression mapping of serial magnetic resonance images. Lancet 2001;358:201–205.
66. Scahill RI, Schott JM, Stevens JM, et al. Mapping the evolution of regional atrophy in Alzheimer's disease: unbiased analysis of fluid-registered serial MRI. Proc Natl Acad Sci USA 2002;99:4703–4707.
67. Kennedy AM, Newman SK, Frackowiak RS, et al. Chromosome 14 linked familial Alzheimer's disease. A clinico-pathological study of a single pedigree. Brain 1995;118:185–205.

68. Kennedy AM, Frackowiak RSJ, Newman SK, et al. Deficits in cerebral glucose metabolism demonstrated by positron emission tomography in individuals at risk of familial Alzheimer's disease. Neurosci Lett 1995;186:17–20.
69. Jagust WJ. Functional imaging in dementia: an overview. J Clin Psychiatry 1994;55(Suppl):5–11.
70. Reed BR, Jagust WJ, Seab JP, et al. Memory and regional cerebral blood flow in mildly symptomatic Alzheimer's disease. Neurology 1989;39:1537–1539.
71. Powers WJ, Perlmutter JS, Videen TO, et al. Blinded clinical evaluation of positron emission tomography for diagnosis of probable Alzheimer's disease. Neurology 1992;42:765–770.
72. Small GW, Okonek A, Mandelkern MA, et al. Age-associated memory loss: initial neuropsychological and cerebral metabolic findings of a longitudinal study. Int Psychogeriat 1994;6:23–44.
73. McKelvey R, Bergman H, Stern J, et al. Lack of prognostic significance of SPECT abnormalities in non-demented elderly subjects with memory loss. Can J Neurol Sci 1999;26:23–28.
74. Minoshima S, Giordani B, Berent S, et al. Metabolic reduction in the posterior cingulate cortex in very early Alzheimer's disease. Ann Neurol 1997;42:85–94.
75. Herholz K, Nordberg A, Salmon E, et al. Impairment of neocortical metabolism predicts progression in Alzheimer's disease. Dementia Geriatr Cog Dis 1999;10:494–504.
76. Arnaiz E, Jelic V, Almkvist O, et al. Impaired cerebral glucose metabolism and cognitive functioning predict deterioration in mild cognitive impairment. NeuroReport 2001;12:851–855.
77. Chetelat G, Desgranges B, De La Sayette V, et-al.Mild cognitive impairment: can FDG-PET predict who is to rapidly convert to Alzheimer's disease. Neurology 2003;60:1374–1377.
78. Cohen G. Age differences in memory for texts: production deficiency or processing limitations? In: Light L, Burke D, eds, Language, Memory and Aging. New York: Cambridge University Press, 1990:171–190.
79. Berent S, Giordani B, Foster N, et al. Neuropsychological function and cerebral glucose utilization in isolated memory impairment and Alzheimer's disease. J Psychiatry Res 1999;33:7–16.
80. Drzezga A, Lautenschlager N, Siebner H, et al. Cerebral metabolic changes accompanying conversion of mild cognitive impairment into Alzheimer's disease: a PET follow-up study. Eur J Nucl Med Mol Imag 2003;30:1104–1113.
81. Mosconi L, Sorbi S, Nacmias B, et al. Brain metabolic differences between sporadic and familial Alzheimer's disease. Neurology 2003;61:1138–1140.
82. Drzezga A, Grimmer T, Riemenschneider M, et al. Prediction of individual outcome in MCI by means of genetic assessment and 18F-FDG PET. J Nucl Med 2005;46:1625–1632.
83. Anchisi D, Borroni B, Franceschi M, et al. Heterogeneity of brain glucose metabolism in mild cognitive impairment and clinical progression to Alzheimer disease. Arch Neurol 2005;62:1728–1733.
84. Friston KJ, Holmes AP, Worsley KJ, et al. Statistical parametric maps in functional imaging: a general linear approach. Hum Brain Mapp 1995;2:189–210.
85. Minoshima S, Frey KA, Koeppe RA, et al. A diagnostic approach in Alzheimer's disease using three-dimensional stereotactic surface projections of fluorine-18-FDG PET. J Nucl Med 1995;36:1238–1248.
86. Small GW, Mazziotta JC, Collins MT, et al. Apolipoprotein E type 4 allele and cerebral glucose metabolism in relatives at risk for familial Alzheimer disease. JAMA 1995;273:942–947.
87. Reiman EM, Caselli RJ, Yun LS, et al. Preclinical evidence of Alzheimer's disease in persons homozygous for the E4 allele for apolipoprotein E. N Engl J Med 1996;334:752–758.
88. Small GW, Ercoli LM, Silverman DHS, et al. Cerebral metabolic and cognitive decline in persons at genetic risk for Alzheimer's disease. Proc Natl Acad Sci USA 2000;97:6037–6042.
89. Reiman EM, Chen K, Alexander GE, et al. Functional brain abnormalities in young adults at genetic risk for late-onset Alzheimer's dementia. Proc Natl Acad Sci USA 2004;101:284–289.

90. Meltzer CC, Leal JP, Mayberg HS, et al. Correction of PET data for partial volume effects in human cerebral cortex by MR imaging. J Comput Assist Tomogr 1990;14:561–570.
91. Jack CR, Peterson RC, Xu Y, et al. Rates of hippocampal atrophy correlate with change in clinical status in aging and AD. Neurology 2000;55:484–489.
92. Rusinek H, De Santi S, Frid D, et al. Regional brain atrophy rate predicts future cognitive decline: 6-year longitudinal MR imaging study of normal aging. Radiology 2003;229:691–696.
93. Jack CRJr, Shiung MM, Gunter JL, et al. Comparison of different MRI brain atrophy rate measures with clinical disease progression in AD. Neurology 2004;62:591–600.
94. den Heijer T, Geerlings MI, Hoebeek FE, et al. Use of hippocampal and amygdalar volumes on magnetic resonance imaging to predict dementia in cognitively intact elderly people. Arch Gen Psychiatry 2006;63:57–62.
95. Hoffman JM, Hanson MW, Welsh KA, et al. Interpretation variability of 18FDG-positron emission tomography studies in dementia. Invest Radiol 1996;31:316–322.
96. Masterman DL, Mendez MF, Fairbanks LA, et al. Sensitivity, specificity, and positive predictive value of technetium 99-HMPAO SPECT in discriminating Alzheimer's disease from other dementias. J Geriatr Psychiatry Neurol 1997;10:15–21.
97. Van Heertum RL, Tikofsky RS, Ruben AB. Dementia. In: Van Heertum RL, Tikofsky RS, eds, Functional Cerebral SPECT and PET Imaging, 3rd ed. New York: Lippincott Williams & Wilkins, 2000:127–188.
98. Mielke R, Heiss WD. Positron emission tomography for diagnosis of Alzheimer's disease and vascular dementia. J Neural Transm Suppl 1998;53:237–250.
99. Messa C, Perani D, Lucignani G, et al. High-resolution technetium-99m-HMPAO SPECT in patients with probable Alzheimer's disease: comparison with fluorine-18-FDG PET. J Nucl Med 1994;35:210–216.
100. Mielke R, Pietrzyk U, Jacobs A, et al. HMPAO SPECT and FDG PET in Alzheimer's disease and vascular dementia: comparison of perfusion and metabolic pattern. Eur J Nucl Med 1994;21:1052–1060.
101. Imabayashi E, Matsuda H, Asada T, et al. Superiority of 3-dimensional stereotactic surface projection analysis over visual inspection in discrimination of patients with very early Alzheimer's disease from controls using brain perfusion SPECT. J Nucl Med 2004;45:1450–1457

Chapter 4
PET and SPECT in the Evaluation of Patients with Central Motor Disorders

John P. Seibyl

Clinical Classification and Pathophysiology of Movement Disorders

In the nearly 200 years since the first modern clinical description of the spectrum of bradykinesia, tremor, and gait disturbance by James Parkinson, tremendous progress has been made in the understanding and clinical management of movement disorders.[1] In particular, the discovery of the pathologic changes occurring in the brain in patients with these disorders directly led to the development of effective symptomatic treatments and set the current focus on the next generation of therapeutics designed to interrupt the progression of disease. Neuroimaging methods, especially positron emission tomography (PET) and single photon emission tomography (SPECT), have now assumed an important role in the refinement in understanding of differential diagnosis and clinical course by providing disease-relevant biomarkers that complement other clinical measures. Nonetheless, as scintigraphic methods are still early in the routine application to the diagnosis and management of Parkinson's disease (PD) and related disorders, intense interest and some controversy remains as to their ultimate clinical application.

The development of PET and SPECT imaging in movement disorders has been accelerated by the early descriptions of the loss of dopamine neurons having cell bodies in the substantia nigra.[2] This elucidation of a key pathophysiologic feature of PD provided the impetus for rational therapies aimed at dopamine replacement and neuroimaging agents.[3] Moreover, with the development of radiopharmaceuticals that label specific dopaminergic targets in patients in vivo comes further refinement of our understanding of the pathophysiology with regard to differential diagnosis, and by extension, better informed strategies for the use of current therapeutics. Insofar as PET and SPECT imaging agents provide a biomarker of the disease process, imaging information complementary with clinical information serves a role in the assessment of the next generation of drugs for movement disorders. This chapter describes the development and application of PET and SPECT radiopharmaceuticals to the key questions in movement disorders, with a description of current clinical and research applications.

D.H.S. Silverman (ed.), *PET in the Evaluation of Alzheimer's Disease and Related Disorders*,
DOI: 10.1007/978-0-387-76420-7_4,

Movement disorders comprise a spectrum of diseases with many common features but significant differences with regard to etiology, clinical course, and treatment. Movement disorders may be generally divided into four major categories (Table 4.1); primary or idiopathic parkinsonism, secondary parkinsonism, Parkinson's plus syndromes, and hereditary neurodegenerative disorders.

Classification schemas are primarily based on clinical features of the movement disorder, and less commonly on pathophysiology, genetics, and etiology, if known. Idiopathic parkinsonism (PD) comprises approximately 80% of movement disorders and may be divided into the preponderant sporadic type or less common familial variant.[4] Typically, PD onset is gradual, with a slowly insidious development and progression of symptoms. Most patients present with unilateral symptoms; often upper extremity tremor or bradykinesia that becomes bilateral over time. Gait disturbance may manifest early, although postural instability and freezing are later features of the illness. A significant minority of patients may develop dementia later in their course. Similarly, autonomic dysfunction may be noted in early disease, but is typically seen in more advanced PD. The rate of progression of

Table 4.1 Major classification of movement disorders

Primary Parkinson's disease
Sporadic
Familial
Parkinson's plus syndromes
Multiple system atrophy
Shy-Drager syndrome
Olivopontocerebellar atrophy
Striatonigral degeneration
Progressive supranuclear palsy
Corticobasal degeneration
Secondary Parkinson's disease
Vascular
Drug induced
Infectious
Metabolic
Toxin induced
Structural/tumor
Psychogenic
Traumatic
Hydrocephalus
Other disorders with altered motor function
Dementia with Lewy bodies
Alzheimer's dementia
Huntington's disease
Wilson's disease
Lubag (Filipino X-linked dystonia)
Machado-Joseph disease
Pick's disease
Hallervorden-Spatz syndrome

symptoms is highly variable both between patients and also within an individual patient's illness course, with some clinical studies suggesting that PD patients progress fastest in the early stages of disease.[5,6]

Early in the disease course idiopathic PD may be difficult to distinguish from Parkinson's plus syndromes and other processes. The latter disorders are less common than PD, but exhibit significant overlap of clinical symptoms. Some clinical features that help distinguish among these disorders, to varying degrees of success, include age of onset, the presence and type of tremor, gaze palsies, early onset of postural instability and dysautonomias, timing of dementia, presence of ataxia, hallucinations, apraxia, symmetry of onset, acuteness of onset, and response to dopaminergic therapies (Table 4.2). Perhaps the most effective tool in the clinician's diagnostic armamentarium is time; for most patients the development and progression of symptoms results in a clearer clinical diagnosis.

Compared with other neurodegenerative disorders, symptomatic treatment of PD is effective, although with several important caveats.[7,8] The stalwarts of PD treatment are the dopamine replacement strategies. Levodopa (L-dopa) in combination with carbidopa to inhibit peripheral drug metabolism has been the mainstay of PD treatment for several decades.[9,10] L-Dopa is incorporated in presynaptic dopamine cells as converted by tyrosine hydroxylase into dopamine. L-Dopa dose must be increased over time as the drug becomes less potent. Many patients develop rapid cycling between severe bradykinesia and dyskinetic movements, reflecting trough and peak levels of L-dopa in brain. Slow-release versions of L-dopa have been developed to accommodate the short half-life of the drug and produce longer response duration. Nonetheless, the occurrence of motor side effects such as dyskinesia and other non-motor effects such as hallucinations and paranoid ideation continues to plague treatment with what is still considered the most potent symptomatic treatment of PD.[11]

In this regard, the increasing use of dopamine agonists represents the second main pillar of dopamine-replacement approaches to PD treatment. These agents have been shown to result in less drug-related dyskinesia than L-dopa, although

Table 4.2 Clinical features of common movement disorders

Symptom	Idiopathic Parkinson's disease	Multiple system atrophy	Progressive supranuclear palsy
Tremor	In some	Atypical tremor	No
Symmetric symptom onset	Unusual	Yes	Yes
Postural instability	Late feature	Yes	Yes
Motor freezing	Late feature	—	—
Dementia	Late feature in some	—	—
Dysautonomias	Sometimes	Yes	No
Olfaction	Diminished	?	?
Response to L-dopa	Good	Minimal early on	Minimal early on
Gaze palsy	No	No	Yes
Clinical progression	Slow, variable	Rapid	Rapid

they are more expensive. Large clinical trials, including the CALM-PD study and the REAL-PET study in PD patients, have evaluated the effects of treatment with L-dopa combined with the dopamine agonists pramipexole (CALM-PD) and ropinirole (REAL-PET). The combinations demonstrate significantly less wearing off, motor fluctuations, and dyskinesias than occur with L-dopa alone.[12–14] Patients are frequently tried on combinations of dopaminergic replacement treatments to help prolong the effect of the drug and minimize side effects.[15,16] Many movement disorder specialists advocate waiting as long as possible before the initiation of treatment, understanding the chronic nature of symptomatic therapy and the high likelihood of developing a treatment complication.

In addition to L-dopa/carbidopa and the dopamine agonists, a number of other therapeutic options are available. Anticholinergic drugs are used based on the neurochemical interplay of dopaminergic and cholinergic neuronal systems and the fact that cholinergic function is affected to a lesser degree than dopamine neuronal function in PD. These agents are generally second-line therapy, especially in patients with tremor-predominant symptoms. Catechol-*O*-methyltransferase inhibitors are another class of drugs used as adjuvant treatment of PD. These drugs are thought to enhance the amount of L-dopa taken into the brain and are speculated to prolong the effect of dopamine in the dopamine synapse. Selegiline is another frequently prescribed medication for PD patients, thought to be an antioxidant with possible neuroprotective effects, although this mechanism remains unproved in the clinic (Table 4.3). Deep brain stimulation, involving an electrode implantation into the subthalamic nucleus or internal segment of the globus pallidus, is an increasingly common symptomatic treatment for advanced PD patients. Although the exact mechanism is unknown, deep brain stimulation improves many of the cardinal symptoms of PD as well as reduces medication-provoked dyskinesias.[17,18]

Table 4.3 Common symptomatic treatments for Parkinson's disease

Drug	Purported Mechanism	Examples
L-Dopa/carbidopa	Precursor of dopamine	Carbidopa-levodopa
Dopamine agonists	Stimulate postsynaptic receptors	Pramipexole, ropinirole, pergolide, cabergoline, bromocriptine
Catechol-*O*-methyltransferase inhibitor	Enhances uptake of L-Dopa	Tolcapone, entacapone
Anticholinergics	Blocks opposing acetylcholine neurons	Benztropine, trihexyphenidyl
Other		
Amantadine	Enhanced dopamine release, delayed reuptake	Amantadine
Selegiline	Antioxidant, mild symptomatic effects, irreversible MAO-B inhibitor	L-deprenyl
MAO-B inhibitors	Prevents metabolism of dopamine	Rasagiline

Over the last several years, therapeutic approaches to PD have expanded beyond aiming for symptomatic treatment to modifying the disease course. These new disease-modifying approaches are represented by treatments to either restore lost dopamine cell functions via cell transplantation or use of neural growth factors or neuroprotective therapies aimed at slowing down the inexorable loss of neuronal function. Neuroprotective treatments derive from an improved understanding of the mechanisms of cell death pathways (apoptosis) and potential ways to interrupt these processes (Fig. 4.1), whereas neurorestorative approaches are based on the advancement of tissue transplant methods, identification and improvement in the brain delivery of neurotrophic factors, and the possibility of gene therapies for enhancing the viability of brain neurons or encouraging neuronal proliferation and interconnection. All of these treatments remain experimental without current use in PD or other movement disorders based on well-controlled clinical trials[19–28] (Table 4.4).

Nonetheless, the prospect of successful development of these new approaches in the future alters the clinical management of movement disorder patients. The possibility of a disease-modifying therapy puts heightened emphasis on determining an early

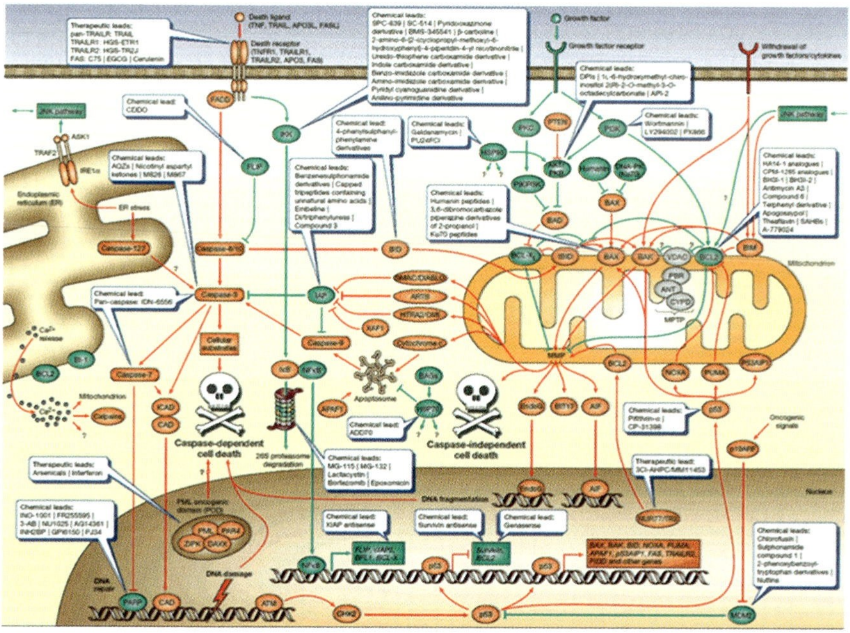

Fig. 4.1 Schematic diagram indicating the rich complexity of cellular mechanisms involved in apoptosis. Elaboration of the biochemical schema of programmed cell death provides potential targets for neuroprotective interventions in degenerative diseases such as Alzheimer's and Parkinson's in which apoptotic pathways may be implicated in the initiation or maintenance of neuronal loss. (Reprinted from Reed and Huang[112] with permission. Copyright ©2006 Macmillan Magazines Ltd.)

Table 4.4 Drugs and mechanisms purporting to affect neurodegeneration

Targets pathways	Drugs/interventions
Antioxidants	Co-Q10, dopamine agonists
Mitochondrial drugs	Co-Q10
Growth factors	Glial cell-derived neurotrophic factor (GDNF), immunophilin ligands
Glutamatergic agents	Receptor modulators
Adenosine agent	A2A antagonists
Inflammation	Nonsteroidal antiinflammatory
Caspase inhibitors	Mixed lineage kinase (MLK) inhibitors
Apoptosis	Propargylamines, dopamine agonists
Other	Cell replacement, stem cell
	Gene therapies
	Deep brain stimulation

and accurate diagnosis to permit earlier intervention. This mandate even extends to the presymptomatic patient, as it is understood that some significant portion of neurons have degenerated before the manifestation of clinical symptoms in PD. Hence the requirement of effective salvage of remaining functional neurons based on the identification of at-risk patients becomes paramount. Given the difficulty in accurate diagnosis in the early course of movement disorders, the strategy of creating algorithms for enriching the at-risk population and subsequent confirmation of diagnosis is an area of intense clinical focus. Ideally, an easily administered, relatively inexpensive screening test, such as a proteomic assay, olfactory testing, or other method with high sensitivity, could be used to identify individuals for either treatment directly or more specific evaluation, including a neuroimaging evaluation. These algorithms are currently under clinical evaluation, but the role of neuroimaging measures with PET or SPECT may prove critical.[29]

Imaging Targets and Properties of Imaging Probes for Movement Disorders

Similar to the discovery of drugs such as L-dopa, the development of radiopharmaceuticals for PD imaging flows directly from an understanding of the pathophysiology in the PD brain. Since the first descriptions of postmortem PD brain indicating the reduction of pigmented neurons in the substantia nigra and elucidation of the nigral–striatal dopamine pathway and its implication in motor dysfunction, the development of imaging markers of the dopamine synapse was an early objective of PET and SPECT researchers.[30–34] Interest has been focused on imaging biomarkers directed at the presynaptic dopamine nerve terminals, with specific targets including dopamine synthesis (^{18}F-FDOPA PET), the dopamine transporter (DAT, multiple PET and SPECT agents), or vesicular transporter (^{11}C VMAT2 PET) (Fig. 4.2).

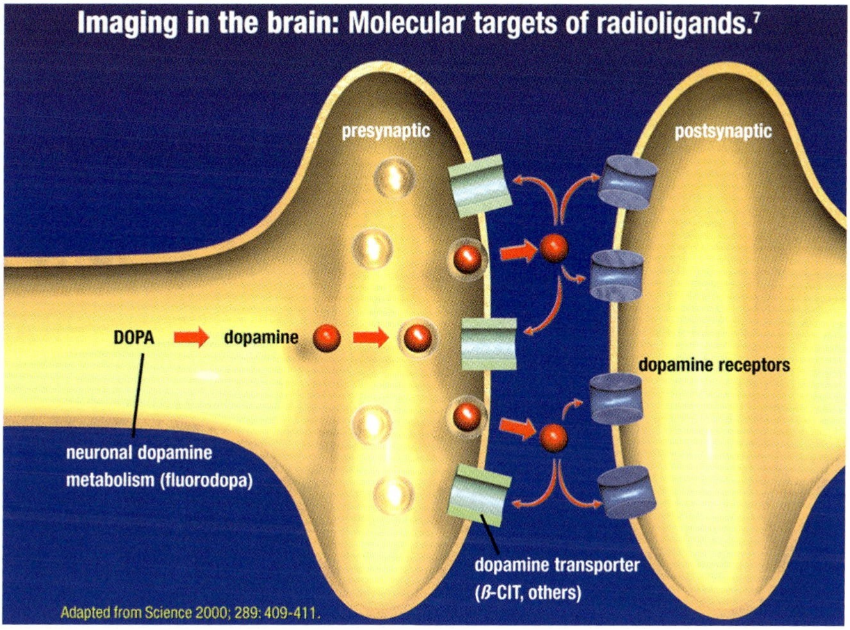

Fig. 4.2 Dopamine neuronal synapse indicating the targets of common presynaptic imaging markers in Parkinson's disease. Radiopharmaceuticals provide a putative measure of neuronal integrity by binding to sites on the presynaptic dopamine neuron, with highest density in the striatum. Hence these imaging agents can provide a quantitative measure of disease. (From Marek and Seibyl[113] with permission.)

^{18}F-FDOPA is taken up into dopamine neurons and converted to ^{18}F-dopamine by aromatic amino acid decarboxylase, where it remains trapped in the cell. Following release into the synapse, dopamine is taken back up into the presynaptic neuron through the DAT, a membrane-bound protein that is the site of action of drugs such as cocaine. A number of analogs of cocaine have been synthesized as radioligands for DAT, including ^{11}C WIN 35,428, ^{18}F β-CFT, and ^{11}C RTI-32 for PET; and ^{123}I β-CIT, ^{123}I FP-CIT, ^{123}I Altropane, and ^{99m}Tc-TRODAT-1 for SPECT.[35–42] Similar to cocaine, many of the analogs exhibit nanomolar binding affinity for the serotonin transporter (SERT) as well as DAT. Imaging studies suggest that over 95% of the signal in the striatum is DAT-related because administration of SERT-selective agents does not produce displacement of activity in the striatum in either preclinical or human studies.[43] Another presynaptic dopamine neuron target, the monoamine transporter VMAT2, is located intracellularly on vesicles rather than on the presynaptic terminal cell membrane. This transporter repackages dopamine and other monoamines into vesicles within the presynaptic terminal. The PET radiopharmaceutical ^{11}C DTBZ binds to VMAT2, and although the transporter is not specific for dopamine, it is estimated that 95% of VMAT2 is associated with dopamine terminals in the striatum.[44] Preclinical studies suggest that this transporter is not subject to regulatory effects of DAT, although controlled within-subject human studies with imaging agents for DAT have yet to confirm this.[45]

All these presynaptic markers demonstrate high uptake in the striatum, an area representing the terminal projections of nigral dopaminergic neurons. Postmortem evaluations of PD brain demonstrate reductions in all these targets with more involvement in the putamen relative to the caudate. Hence for all the presynaptic imaging markers of dopaminergic integrity there is a highly specific pattern of loss of uptake in the striatum with asymmetry consistent with pathologic findings at postmortem as well as a clinical phenomenology (e.g., left versus right asymmetry of symptoms corresponds with greatest reduction of radiotracer uptake occurring on the side of the brain contralateral to symptoms).

The largest patient experience with presynaptic imaging markers of dopaminergic neuronal function in PD is with ^{18}F-FDOPA PET, a marker of dopamine neuronal metabolism, and ^{123}I dopamine transporter (DAT) agents FP-CIT and β-CIT SPECT, and to a lesser extent ^{11}C VMAT2, ^{99m}Tc TRODAT, and ^{123}I Altropane (Fig. 4.3).[30,46,47] Despite these agents targeting different aspects of presynaptic dopamine function, studies in PD patients show remarkable similarity between these radiopharmaceuticals. For example, in newly diagnosed hemi-Parkinson's patients who present with unilateral symptoms, all these radiopharmaceuticals demonstrate reduced uptake in the striatum on the side contralateral to the symptoms as expected, but also show smaller changes on the ipsilateral side to motor symptoms. These patients almost invariably develop bilateral motor symptoms, while maintaining a functional differential between

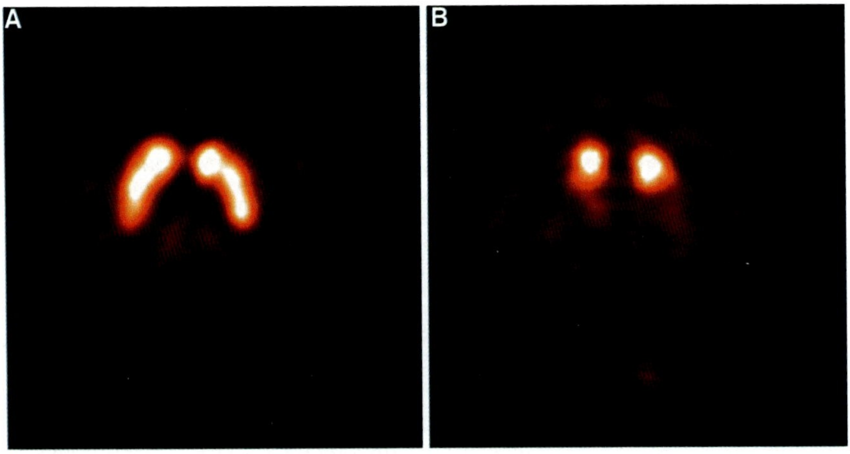

Fig. 4.3 Transaxial image in a healthy control (*A*) and idiopathic Parkinson's patient (*B*) following injection and imaging with the dopamine transporter imaging agent ^{123}I β-CIT. As analogues of cocaine, the dopamine transporter agents demonstrate high uptake in the striatum, where dopaminergic nigrostriatal projections normally show high density. This moderately affected patient demonstrates qualitative loss of uptake with relatively greater involvement in the posterior aspect of the striatum (putamen) relative to the caudate

the side contralateral to initial symptom presentation and the ipsilateral side. Investigators have taken this to suggest that imaging with presynaptic markers of dopaminergic function is sensitive to changes occurring in the brain even before symptom formation.[48] Such observations fuel speculation that imaging provides highly specific and complementary information to clinical evaluation. The latter assessments include tools such as the Unified Parkinson's Disease Rating Scales (UPDRS), which represents the integrated effects of neuronal cell loss and CNS compensatory mechanisms as well as any symptomatic drugs present at the time of assessment. Further, cross-sectional studies in all the presynaptic dopamine system imaging markers show good correlation with clinical Hoehn-Yahr stage or symptom rating such as the total UPDRS and UPDRS motor subscores.[49] Finally, all these imaging markers have been evaluated in longitudinal clinical studies of disease progression and disease monitoring following a disease-modifying intervention. Again, these radiopharmaceuticals are remarkably consistent in the demonstration of striatal signal loss of approximately 4%–11% per year, although with significant variability among PD patients, similar to the variability in the clinical assessment of symptom progression.[50–54]

Although these data provide some theoretical support for development of imaging techniques to assess at-risk patients, the fact that longitudinal studies in progressing PD patients demonstrate a discrepancy between clinical and imaging measures of disease progression (summarized later in this chapter) has led to speculation about the factors that might influence the presynaptic dopamine imaging markers. Do quantitative methods using these markers reflect the density of terminals, or are there regulatory effects on enzymes or transporters on terminals such that imaging measures are not reflective of neuronal cell number? How do dopaminergic medications affect imaging biomarkers? Interest in these issues has been fueled by reports in large-scale PD patient trials in which clinical and imaging findings provide different possible interpretations and point to the need for a new series of clinical imaging trials to address the application of measures of dopaminergic function in PD studies.[12,14,55]

To this end, recent studies with ^{18}F-FDOPA PET focus on extrastriatal targets in movement disorder patients. Is it possible to image not just the terminal extent of nigrostriatal cells, but also the cell bodies located in the substantia nigra? Ito and others have suggested that voxel-wise parametric analyses of ^{18}F-FDOPA PET can delineate signal reduction on the nigra as well as striatal regions.[56]

Hence the use of PET and SPECT agents for interrogating the presynaptic dopamine system depends on the nature of the clinical or research question posed. If the goal is to produce high-quality images for visual or qualitative evaluation of the pattern and extent of striatal signal loss for the purposes of describing a dopaminergic deficit (usually in the context of diagnostic assessment), then all the agents mentioned are useful. If the purpose of the scan is to measure an incremental signal loss in a patient to assess the rate of change of the imaging signal, then a quantitative or semi-quantitative outcome measure is required. Visual analysis of the images is not an adequate means for detecting the relative signal change. The changes on the serial scans are extremely subtle in PD, which progresses inexorably, but slowly. The prerequisite for quantitation in this setting produces many challenges as factors unrelated to the density of binding sites affect the quantitative signal. These include the pharmacokinetics of the radiotracer, signal-to-noise characteristics, and methods of image

Table 4.5 Factors affecting measurement of striatal binding ratios

Neuronal degeneration
Age
Allelic variants of dopamine transporter
Pharmacokinetic factors of the radiopharmaceutical, metabolism, protein binding of parent compound
Patient hydration
Drugs competing with the radioligand for binding at the target site
Patient cooperation, ability to remain motionless
Equipment: Resolution and sensitivity of selected camera, collimator
Performance drifts in cameras over time
Photon flux, counts in image
Reconstruction/filtration
Size and placement of regions of interest

analysis. For example, region of interest analyses of striatal binding ratios in DAT images in a subject will be influenced by such parameters as the timing of the scan postinjection; the size of the striatal regions of interest; reconstruction, filtration, and attenuation correction algorithms; technical factors such as motion; in addition to clinical factors, including the age of the subject, genotype (variant allelic polymorphisms exist for DAT), state of hydration, and so forth (Table 4.5). Ultimately, it is useful to have an imaging outcome measure that is linearly related to a physiologic parameter, such as density of binding sites (B_{max}).[42] For some agents, the washout from the target site is so slow that kinetic modeling theory would predict a simple ratio of the striatal uptake to the background region that is linearly related to B_{max}, the density of dopamine transporter binding sites.

Imaging Assessments for Differential Diagnosis of Movement Disorders

The diagnosis of PD and related disorders is based on clinical evaluation. The most widely accepted clinical definition of PD requires the presence of two of three cardinal motor signs (tremor, rigidity, and bradykinesia) and a response to L-dopa.[57] At the onset of disease, accurate diagnosis is challenging because of the subtlety and nonspecificity of symptoms. The diagnoses most commonly mistaken for PD include vascular parkinsonism, essential tremor, drug-induced parkinsonism, and Alzheimer's disease (Fig. 4.4). Studies suggest that almost one third of patients are incorrectly diagnosed with PD by primary care physicians initially. Even among movement disorder specialists, the rate of misdiagnosis of PD is reported to be 10% to 12%.[58,59]

Other recent studies provide suggestive evidence that movement disorder experts misdiagnose PD early in its course when recruiting subjects for early PD clinical trials. For example, in the REAL-PET study, comparing ropinirole and L-dopa as initial treatments in untreated patients, 11% (21 of 193) of enrolled subjects had

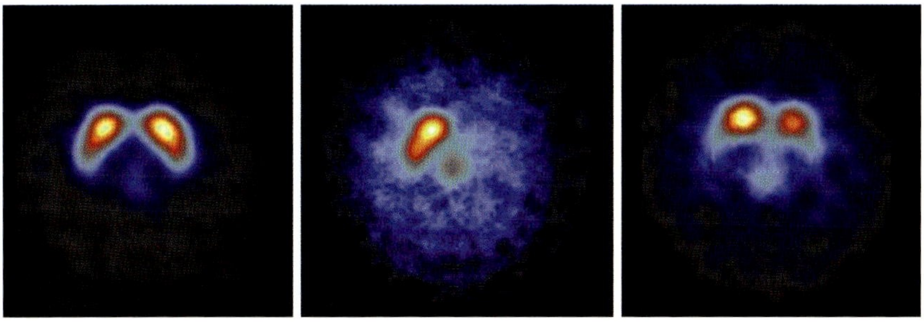

Fig. 4.4 Transaxial dopamine transporter (DAT) SPECT images in a healthy control (*left*), a patient with a history of arteriovenous malformation and mild bradykinesia (*center*), and a mild-to-moderate idiopathic Parkinson's patient (*right*). Vascular processes may result in PD symptoms, but a very different pattern of striatal signal loss than the typical PD patient shown with left–right asymmetry of uptake and greater putaminal involvement

scans without reduction in ^{18}F-dopa striatal uptake at baseline and 2 years later.[14] Understanding that current diagnostic gold standards are currently clinical measures, studies that recruit the earliest PD patients with regard to disease onset consistently demonstrate the greatest percentage of ^{18}F-FDOPA or ^{123}I β-CIT normal scans.[11] Full characterization of these scans without evidence of dopaminergic deficits (SWEDD) is ongoing, but highly suggestive that at least a significant proportion of these normal scan patients do not have PD. Later in the course of the illness, the diagnoses commonly confused with PD are progressive supranuclear palsy and multiple systems atrophy.[60,61] The difficulties posed by diagnosis early in the course of PD are largely overcome by more protracted periods of clinical observation of developing symptoms and response to dopaminergic therapy. The reported duration of observation for an accurate diagnosis in very early PD ranges from 3 to 12 months.

Delayed or misdiagnosed PD has several consequences. First, patients may be exposed to futile treatments with dopamine agents, often resulting in unnecessary side effects and cost. Many patients may undergo clinical testing with computed tomography (CT) or magnetic resonance imaging (MRI) to rule out other less likely disorders, resulting in inconvenience for the patient and higher costs. One overlooked aspect of inaccurate or delayed diagnosis is the fact that patients and families want to know their diagnosis as soon as possible to better understand the short- and long-term treatment options and prognosis.

In this setting, the introduction of DAT imaging agents for widespread clinical use in Europe provides the first *rule-in* imaging study for PS. The availability of ^{123}I FP-CIT (DAT scan) was preceded by a number of clinical investigations assessing the accuracy of dopamine transporter SPECT for distinguishing PD from conditions such as essential tremor. Some of these are summarized in Table 4.6 and despite the use of different imaging agents, such as ^{123}I FP CIT, ^{123}I β-CIT, ^{99m}Tc TRODAT, and ^{123}I IPT, these studies have consistently demonstrated outstanding sensitivity and specificity in the diagnosis of subjects with known PD.[62–66] Specifically, DAT imaging can distinguish patients with PD from those with drug-induced parkinsonism, gait disorders resembling PD, psychogenic parkinsonism, vascular parkinsonism, and dementia.

Table 4.6 Some diagnostic studies with dopamine transporter agents

Study	Tracer	Subjects	Findings	Comments
Parkinson Study Group[66]	^{123}I β-CIT	60 parkinsonism, 14 ET, 22 HS	Parkinsonism vs HS and ET: sensitivity = 0.98, specificity = 0.83	Multicenter, core lab visual read, quantitative read 0.96 sensitivity, 0.94 specificity
The ^{123}I FP-CIT Study Group[65]	^{123}I FP-CIT	128 parkinsonism, 27 ET, 35 HS	Parkinsonism sensitivity = 0.95, specificity = 0.93	Multicenter, core lab visual read
Huang, Lin, Lin, et al.[110]	^{99m}Tc TRODAT-1	34 PD, 17 HS	Good discrimination between PD and HS	Some group overlap of striatal uptake ratios
Mozley, Schneider, Acton, et al.[46]	^{99m}Tc TRODAT-1	42 PD, 61 HS	Good discrimination between PD and HS	Some group overlap of striatal uptake ratios
Schwarz, Linke, Kerner, et al.[111]	^{123}I IPT	28 PD, 9 HS	Excellent discrimination between PD and HS	Only one PD subject overlapped with control

The design of these trials has been criticized because the imaging evaluation is applied to a cohort of patients with defined disease compared with a control population. This is an unnatural scenario from the perspective of how a diagnostic imaging agent is used in the normal clinical sense in which patients in whom there is a suspicion but not a confirmed diagnosis of parkinsonism are referred for imaging evaluation to assist the clinical assessment.[67] A few studies have focused on this cohort, and additional studies are ongoing. In the largest published study to date, the Query study, community-based neurologists were asked to refer patients for imaging who had a relatively short duration of disease and an uncertain diagnosis. The patients were imaged with ^{123}I β-CIT SPECT imaging and followed for 6–12 months by a movement disorder specialist, who remained blinded to the imaging results. At the end of the evaluation period, the movement disorder specialist rendered a gold standard diagnosis, and this was compared with the diagnosis by the community neurologist, the initial diagnosis by the movement disorder specialist, and both qualitative and quantitative DAT imaging.[68] The results of this trial are summarized in Table 4.7. The study showed the highest concordance existed between the quantitative DAT imaging and the gold standard diagnosis, with a sensitivity of 93% and a specificity of 92%, followed by the qualitative interpretation of the scan, the initial movement disorder specialist's diagnosis, and finally the community neurologist's diagnosis.

Interestingly, the concordance between the imaging results and the movement disorder specialists' diagnosis improved with longer periods of clinical assess-

Table 4.7 Sensitivity and specificity of dopamine transporter imaging in patients with suspected parkinsonian syndrome referred by community-based neurologists

Final clinical diagnosis (*n* = 112)	PS	No PS	Sensitivity	Specificity
Baseline community neurologist				
PS	54	32	0.87	0.36
No PS	8	18	—	—
Baseline movement disorder expert				
PS	54	11	0.87	0.78
No PS	8	39	—	—
Three-month movement disorder expert				
PS	56	5	0.90	0.90
No PS	6	45	—	—
Baseline dopamine transporter imaging				
PS	58	4	0.93	0.92
No PS	4	46	—	—

PS, parkinsonian syndrome.

ment,[69] suggesting the blinded movement disorder specialist changed his or her diagnostic impression more in line with the imaging diagnosis as additional clinical information became available, such as response to medication, the development of more characteristic symptoms, and so forth. Overall, this study indicates that it is feasible to improve the accuracy and timeliness of diagnosis using imaging assessments. This type of study design has been incorporated into clinical trials evaluating the diagnostic performance of other DAT imaging agents in the context of trials supporting clinical approval.

Some investigators have questioned the clinical impact of making an earlier diagnosis in patients, as this could have limited influence on the actual clinical management. Many clinicians prefer to keep patients off medication as long as possible to minimize potential side effects, including dopaminergic side effects resulting from L-dopa. Others have argued that it may be of some benefit to rethink this strategy and start patients on medication earlier in that some studies suggest that patients initiated early with dopamine replacement therapies have a better clinical course than those for whom medications are withheld. Finally, the development of agents that might have actual disease-modifying effects places a heavy onus on early and accurate diagnosis. Assuming the intense drug development interest in this therapeutic approach will bear some fruit, there is a renewed emphasis placed on timely diagnosis, screening at-risk populations, and so forth as the goal in this case is to preserve as much function as possible by the rapid initiation of potential neuroprotective therapeutics.

Imaging studies with PET and SPECT presynaptic dopaminergic agents suggest that it is difficult to distinguish idiopathic PD from the Parkinson spectrum disorders, including multiple systems atrophy and progressive supranuclear palsy, as these disorders demonstrate deficits in striatal uptake. Some investigators have evaluated additional imaging measures, including the relative asymmetry of the left and right striatal uptake (tends to be greater in idiopathic PD) or the caudate-to-putamen ratio (tends to be higher in idiopathic PD), with mild success because of overlap on these adjunct measures between PD and the other Parkinson spectrum disorders. In addition, some studies have evaluated the concomitant presynaptic and postsynaptic assessment of the dopamine terminal in the striatum using D2/D3 receptor agents combined with presynaptic DAT or F-dopa.[70,71] Again, these studies have achieved some success in distinguishing between PD and parkinsonism, although the practical use and clinical need for these tests remain to be clarified.

More recently, interest has increased in identifying dopaminergic system deficits in patients with cognitive impairment in the context of movement abnormalities. A number of studies have shown the feasibility of distinguishing dementia with Lewy bodies from Alzheimer's dementia by identifying a dopaminergic deficit in the former. This indication has been approved in Europe for the commercially available DAT agent, ^{123}I FP-CIT.[72–74]

Monitoring Disease Progression and Drug Development Trials in Movement Disorders

A number of clinical studies have used PET and SPECT to monitor the progression of PD as well as assess drugs that have putative neuroprotective effects. These studies, using different imaging agents, have consistently demonstrated a loss of imaging signal on the order of 6%–13% per year.[14,50–54,75–78] The slowly insidious progression of PD makes it challenging to evaluate imaging signal loss, usually expressed as a percent reduction per year in individual subjects. Most studies of disease progression that have incorporated imaging measures have relied on large subject numbers. This is especially true for evaluating differences in disease progression in cohorts of subjects who are undergoing treatment with agents purported to engender reduction of an already small imaging signal loss. For such studies, a combination of adequate subject number and appropriate duration of evaluation are required based on the projected impact of the disease-modifying treatment.

The difficulties in applying neuroimaging as a biomarker of disease progression in individual PD patients is no less difficult than the challenge presented by using clinical measures for assessing changes over time. In addition to the fact that PD subjects progress slowly, with significant variability between patients, as well as within an individual's treatment course, standard clinical measures are strongly influenced by symptomatic medications. It is difficult to thoroughly wash out medications to obtain an objective assessment of native illness in patients with moderate PD symptoms.[6] Indeed, imaging markers of dopaminergic function have been proposed to provide an objective marker of disease status in this setting, assuming that the neuroimaging measure is unaffected by symptomatic treatment.

Consistent with some clinical studies suggesting more rapid progression of PD early in the illness course, one imaging study has demonstrated the loss of imaging signal is greater in the early course of illness.[50,75] Other factors that are important in the application of imaging biomarkers for assessing disease progression include: (1) effects of symptomatic drugs on imaging measures, (2) requirement for robust quantitative algorithms with a high degree of reproducibility, and (3) understanding factors unrelated to the density of target sites or dopamine nerve terminal integrity, which influence the quantitative signal described in Table 4.5.

Considering the issue of modulation of the imaging measures with symptomatic treatment, speculation exists that medications used for symptomatic management of PD patients may potentially influence the quantitative imaging measures, producing short-term regulatory changes of the target site. This is based on a large, but inconsistent animal literature in which short-term treatment in animal models in some studies provoked changes in density of binding. These data are problematic, however, in using suprathreshold dosing of dopaminergic medications such as L-dopa or dopamine agonists, short duration of treatment, different in vitro or ex vivo measures of binding, and lack of comparable models to PD. More recently, several studies have been undertaken to directly measure the potential of L-dopa or dopamine agonists used commonly in the symptomatic treatment to influence the dopamine transporter using SPECT imaging. In preliminary work published in abstract form, a group of de novo PD patients (total $n = 61$) were imaged at baseline with ^{123}I β-CIT; randomized to standardized treatment with L-dopa, pramipexole, or no treatment for 12 weeks; scanned; had medication washed out for 8 weeks; and scanned a third time. In this ongoing study (Table 4.8), using a within-subject measure of percent change in striatal binding ratio (a modified striatal target-to-occipital ratio), there were no effects seen following treatment or with washout compared with baseline. Although preliminary, these sorts of designs are most useful in directly testing the important question of potential factors influencing imaging measures of disease progression.

The imaging biomarker must demonstrate robust reproducibility for imaging serial changes in PD patients and the putative effects of neuroprotective or neurorestorative interventions. It is a prerequisite that quantitative approaches be used, and that those factors that influence variability in the measurement be minimized. Some of these factors are aging effects, already well understood for the DAT ligands in large studies of healthy aging controls,[79] genetic factors in which allelic variants of the dopamine transporter have been demonstrated to

Table 4.8 Effects of anti-Parkinson medication treatment on dopamine transporter imaging in Parkinson's disease patients

	Percent change	Standard deviation (%)	No.
Scan 1–2 (baseline to week 12 on medication)			
Untreated	+3.16	±7.3	19
Pramipexole	–3.92	±8.1	20
Carbidopa-levodopa	+3.28	±9.6	22
Scan 2–3 (weeks 12–20 after 8-week washout of medication)			
Untreated	+2.87	±7.0	14
Pramipexole	+1.55	±10.4	17
Carbidopa-levodopa	–2.00	±6.9	16

result in differences of radiotracer on the order of 8%–10%,[80] and other medication compounds that are known to directly influence or compete for the target site with the radiotracer. In addition, technical factors related to the PET or SPECT camera, intrinsic spatial and energy resolution, methods for reconstruction and filtering data, attenuation correction techniques, and so forth, all contribute to differences in the quantitative imaging measure. Some of these factors are less important in serial assessment of disease progression within a patient, whereas other factors are crucial given the small signal change. It is useful to note that all studies of PD progression using imaging measures have relied on large patient numbers. Only limited studies have focused on the clinical question: Can serial neuroimaging with dopaminergic biomarkers using PET or SPECT be used in an individual PD patient to provide a reliable measure of disease progression? If so, what is the minimal time between imaging required to provide reliable information given the properties of the imaging assay?

Returning to the question of neuroimaging to evaluate treatments designed to produce slowing of neuronal loss in PD, a number of recent studies using PET and SPECT have evaluated disease progression and long-term monitoring in PD patients. Two important studies were designed to evaluate the hypothesis that dopamine agonist drugs have neuroprotective effects in preclinical models.[12,14,81] One of these trials, the CALM-PD study was performed by the Parkinson's Study Group in the United States to evaluate clinical outcomes in approximately 300 patients initially treated with the dopamine agonist pramipexole compared with those started on L-dopa. A substudy used dopamine transporter imaging with ^{123}I β-CIT SPECT as one marker for disease progression in 82 patients who were scanned at baseline and approximately 2, 3, and 4 years later. Imaging showed that those patients originally randomized to pramipexole demonstrated less striatal binding ratio reduction at each of the post baseline time points at 2, 3, and 4 years compared with the group originally treated with L-dopa. There was approximately a 41% relative difference between the dopamine agonist and L-dopa groups. No correlation existed between the percent change in imaging and the change in clinical measures (UPDRS motor scores) at 2 years, but at 3 and 4 years a modest but significant correlation was shown.

A study of similar design to the CALM-PD trial was reported about the same time in a similar cohort of PD subjects, with similar findings. The REAL-PET study used ^{18}F-FDOPA PET in a multicenter trial to assess the effects of ropinirole, a dopamine agonist versus L-dopa on both clinical and imaging measures. Forty-five PD patients were imaged at baseline and followed for 2 years after randomization and imaged again at 2 years. Patients treated with ropinirole over 2 years had approximately a 13% loss of uptake on the ^{18}F-FDOPA scan, whereas the patients treated with L-dopa showed a 20% loss, for a relative difference of 35%. No correlation existed between the percent loss of signal on ^{18}F-dopa PET and UPDRS clinical ratings.

Even though the imaging findings from the CALM-PD and REAL-PET studies are consistent with the original hypothesis, that dopamine agonists are neuroprotective, they do not prove this to be the case. Because neither of these studies had a placebo control group, it is not possible to determine whether the imaging differences were caused by slowing of the rate of progression by the dopamine agonists, or hastening of the progression by L-dopa, some combination of these factors, or another explanation.[55] It is not possible to incorporate a placebo arm in a long-term trial of disease progression in PD owing to the requirement for symptomatic medication and ethical concerns about withholding therapy from patients. As a result, newer trial designs, including the staggered initiation of the neuroprotective drug, have been proposed and first studies reported.[19] In this design, PD cohorts are started on the neuroprotective drug at different times after enrollment in the trial. The symptomatic effects of the therapeutic agent may thus be distinguished from the neuroprotective effects because for agents with some component of neuroprotection, those started early will always have a better course than those started later. If the drug is purely symptomatic, it is argued, it does not matter when the drug is initiated as the two groups will converge on clinical measures with treatment.[82]

Another way to address this question of drug versus placebo is highlighted in the ELLDOPA trial. This study evaluated the dose-dependent effects of L-dopa treatment in 300 de novo PD patients studied over 9 months.[11] Because these PD patients were early in their diagnosis, it was possible to delay the initiation of treatment for a short period of time while remaining consistent with the clinical practice of many movement disorder specialists. In order to test the hypothesis that L-dopa, the most potent antiparkinsonian agent, may be neurotoxic, both clinical measures and imaging were performed in a substudy of 135 patients using ^{123}I β-CIT SPECT. Patients were randomized to either placebo, or one of three doses of L-dopa after an initial ^{123}I β-CIT SPECT scan, then followed for 9 months; they received a second SPECT scan at the end treatment and received medication washout for 2 weeks.

The clinical data show a dose-response effect of L-dopa treatment on change in the UPDRS total score for the four treatment groups. With the 2-week washout all groups demonstrated worsening of the UPDRS score at the end of the study, but the L-dopa–treated groups did not return to the same baseline as the placebo group. In the 135 patients who were scanned at baseline and 9 months, striatal binding ratios showed a nonsignificant trend for a larger percent reduction in the ratio in the high-dose L-dopa patients compared with the placebo group. Of note, 19 out of 135 patients had scans within the normal range. When the statistical analysis was redone with these 19 normal scans, the imaging became significant for a greater reduction of the imaging signal in the high-dose L-dopa group compared with placebo.

The ELLDOPA trial underscored two important controversies that are illustrative when considering the use of neuroimaging in disease progression trials. First, what does it mean when imaging measures and clinical measures of progression do not correlate, or worse, as in the ELLDOPA trial, produce potentially opposed conclusions? Second, how are patients with SWEDD, who still meet the operational definition of PD made by movement disorder experts, to be handled?

For the first point, the lack of correlation of imaging and clinical measures is not surprising, as most clinical assessment is performed when the patient is on medication or partially washed out from medication. However, in the ELLDOPA study, review of the clinical and imaging data would lead to entirely opposite conclusions regarding the primary study hypothesis; in the clinical instance, the fact that the UPDRS ratings did not return to the same level in the L-dopa–treated groups as the placebo group suggests that perhaps L-dopa is neuroprotective, in contradistinction to the initial hypothesis of the study and the results of the imaging component, which suggested that the greater loss of imaging signal is consistent with the idea that L-dopa is neurotoxic. This seeming conundrum can be explained by the short period of L-dopa washout, which does not permit full assessment of native disease. Alternatively, critics have speculated about the possibility of regulatory changes in DAT caused by L-dopa as an explanation for the discrepancy. From the perspective of drug development, an imaging signal may be useful, but neither necessary nor sufficient for establishing disease modification of putative neuroprotective drugs.

Considering the second controversy in these trials, how are we to understand a SWEDD or normal scan in subjects who meet diagnostic criteria for PD by movement disorder specialists? Some possibilities include: (1) the patient may not have PD, (2) the patient may have PD, but without a dopamine transporter or F-dopa deficit, or (3) imaging is not sensitive to alterations found in early disease.

Data from large ^{18}F-FDOPA PET and DAT PET and SPECT PD disease progression trials argue against imaging being insensitive in early disease. When SWEDD patients identified at baseline imaging are followed over 2 or more years, no change occurs between the baseline and repeat scans, i.e., the imaging results do not become abnormal in the patients. Specifically in the ELLDOPA (19 of 19) and REAL-PET (19 of 19) studies patient scans that were normal at baseline remained normal at follow-up. Other cross-sectional studies in early Parkinson's disease support the notion that imaging is exquisitely sensitive to changes in brain that may be manifest before the development of clinical symptoms. In every ^{18}F-FDOPA and DAT imaging study reported involving early PD patients the great majority of these patients are hemiparkinsonian, with symptoms detectable only on one side of the body. Both qualitative and quantitative imaging measures demonstrate bilateral changes.[83] The side contralateral to symptoms shows the greatest abnormality. Because these patients go on to develop bilateral disease with time and the progression of disease, this suggests imaging is sensitive to changes before the manifestation of symptoms.

Another indirect line of evidence cited to argue that SWEDD subjects do not have PD is the observation that the percentage of patients with normal scan or SWEDD results, among patients enrolled as meeting clinical criteria for PD, decreases as the duration of diagnosis of the patient at the time of enrollment increases from 6, 12, 18, and 23 months.[69] This could mean that the accuracy of clinical diagnosis improves with longer disease duration as more clinical information including treatment response is available to the movement disorder specialist.

Taken together, these studies suggest but do not prove that patients with SWEDD scan results most likely do not have PD, consistent with the clinical literature pointing to an approximately 10% misdiagnosis rate by movement disorder specialists in the evaluation of early PD. These studies have not supported a pathophysiologic entity of PD in the absence of imaging dopaminergic deficits or lack of sensitivity of the imaging measures. The final resolution of this controversy of normal scans among operationally diagnosed PD patients awaits the data from ongoing, long-term clinical follow-up of these patients. Nonetheless, the incorporation using PET or SPECT imaging of dopaminergic function as a screening criterion for enrollment into long-term disease-modification trials has been suggested. If the SWEDD scan ultimately proves to be a good means to separate PD from other diagnostic entities without detectable dopaminergic abnormality, the argument follows, then trial sizes could be smaller, and the population for whom the treatment is intended would be enrolled. This is especially important given the long duration and high costs of disease-modification therapeutic trials in PD.

New Targets, New Directions

The progress made in applying imaging in PD and its rapid incorporation into studies of the pathophysiology of disease progression and therapeutics stems from the long-understood phenomenon of dopaminergic degeneration of the nigral–striatal system. This knowledge fostered the development of current and powerful symptomatic medications. However, PD is not singularly and exclusively a disease of the degenerating dopamine neuron alone. An explosion has occurred in the development of new targets and potential mechanisms for new therapeutics in PD. The concomitant development of new radioligands to explore these targets in patients and evaluate the mechanisms of these drugs in vivo in a relevant patient population creates substantial opportunities for both expanding our knowledge of the alterations in PD, but also for speeding evaluation on the next generations of therapeutics. Other neurochemical systems are known to be involved, either directly or in response to dopaminergic functional loss. More recently, this concept has been expanded into a more fully articulated model by Braak and colleagues in reviewing pathologic brain specimens from PD, Alzheimer's disease, and other neurodegenerative disorders. The theory proposes a serial evolution of changes, occurring in multiple neuronal systems in susceptible nerve types, which begins in the more primitive brain structures including brain stem and progresses over time to involve anteromedial temporal mesocortex, then neocortex from prefrontal and high-order sensory association areas, to first-order sensory association and premotor areas, along with primary sensory and motor fields.[84,85]

These investigations and others suggest the utility of evaluating a range of newer brain targets, potentially accessible with in vivo imaging modalities such as PET, to directly explore newer pathophysiologic hypotheses in PD, as well as the mechanism for progression.[86,87]

Some specific areas of interest include: (1) characterizing alterations in other brain monoamine systems including norepinephrine, serotonin, as well as cholinergic systems; and (2) identifying markers of inflammation as a potential mechanism for promoting neurodegeneration. Both norepinephrine and serotonin are key neurochemical systems implicated in the Braak hypothesis of neurodegeneration. In addition, both norepinephrine and serotonin may play key roles in the depression and anxiety that commonly occur in PD. Depression occurs in approximately 45% of all patients with PD, reduces quality of life independent of motor symptoms, and seems to be underestimated in severity and undertreated. In fact, anxiety and depression may manifest as first symptoms of PD many years before motor symptoms. Norepinephrine may be involved in the autonomic dysfunction commonly occurring in PD and its variants.[88,89] Tricyclic and newer selective antidepressants including serotonin and norepinephrine reuptake inhibitors appear to be effective in treating depression in PD.[90,91] These agents have potency at the SERT and norepinephrine transporter. Limited studies have been performed with SERT agents in PD to date.

Cholinergic Markers and Cognitive Dysfunction

Cerebral cortical cholinergic deficits, including a decrease in choline acetyltransferase activity and severe losses of nicotinic binding sites as well as cell degeneration in the basal forebrain, have been demonstrated in PD as well as Alzheimer's disease and diffuse Lewy body disease.[92] A reduction in nicotinic receptor binding has been observed in putamen in PD and dementia with Lewy bodies (diffuse Lewy body disease).[93] These finding raise the potential role of nicotinic acetylcholine receptor subunits as neuroimaging targets for the assessment of cognitive deficits in PD. In particular, reports show a decrease in the $\alpha 4$ and $\alpha 7$ nicotinic acetylcholine receptor subunits in cortices of PD patients that turns out to be similar to recent findings in Alzheimer's disease patients. Furthermore, in vitro autoradiography investigating the distribution of 5-^{125}I-A-85380, a marker of $\alpha 4\beta 4$ nicotinic receptors, showed reductions of nicotinic receptors in postmortem brain tissue seen in the neurodegenerative disorders, Alzheimer's disease, diffuse Lewy body disease, and PD, but not in vascular dementia.[94]

Imaging Biomarkers for Inflammation

Numerous studies have demonstrated that the inflammatory process plays an important role in the pathology of chronic neurodegenerative disorders such as Alzheimer's disease, PD, and amyotrophic lateral sclerosis.[95–98] Markers of inflammation such as complement proteins, complement inhibitors, acute phase reactants, inflammatory cytokines, proteases, and protease inhibitors have been associated with the pathobiology of these disorders.[99] In the MPTP (1-methyl-4-phenyl-1,2,3,6-tetrahydropyridine) model of PD, reactive microglia are present, even 5–14 years after initiation of the toxic insult.[100,101] Moreover postmortem examination in PD reveals a loss of dopaminergic neurons in the substantia nigra associated with astrogliosis and the presence of activated microglial cells.[102] More recent evidence further suggests that PD may progress even when the initial cause of neuronal degeneration has disappeared, suggesting that toxic substances released by the glial cells may be involved in the propagation and perpetuation of neuronal degeneration.

Epidemiologic evidence supports a crucial role for neuroinflammation in the pathogenesis of neurodegenerative disorders. Several epidemiologic studies indicate that populations taking antiinflammatory drugs have a significantly reduced risk of Alzheimer's disease. In a prospective study of health professionals, use of aspirin significantly reduced risk of PD in this cohort.[103] The epidemiologic evidence of reduced risk of Alzheimer's disease and PD caused by antiinflammatory drugs has led to several clinical drug trials to further assess the potential benefit of nonsteroidal antiinflammatory drugs. In addition, other targets in the inflammatory cascade have been identified as potential therapeutic targets for neurodegenerative disorders.[104] Clinical trials investigating the potential benefit of antiinflammatory drugs in Alzheimer's disease have been inconclusive and those for PD have not yet been completed.

PET and SPECT have the potential to provide biomarkers with which to monitor the inflammatory process in PD and other neurodegenerative disorders. Several studies have used the peripheral benzodiazepine receptor located on microglia as a target to assess the onset and severity of neuroinflammation in neurodegenerative disorders. PET imaging using ^{11}C PK11195, a peripheral benzodiazepine receptor agent, has demonstrated increased uptake in patients with Alzheimer's disease, PD, multisystem atrophy, cortical basal ganglionic degeneration, and motor neuron disease.[105–109] Some studies suggest ^{11}C PK11195 may be useful at disease onset, but not to monitor progression.[106] Most recently, evidence suggests that ^{11}C PK11195 scan findings may correlate with disease severity as well as mark disease onset.[108]

Summary and Conclusions

The rapid elaboration of imaging biomarkers for PET and SPECT has resulted in significant changes in the potential approach to diagnosis and symptom management in the movement disorders, especially PD. The proliferation of readily available radiopharmaceuticals for assessing dopamine deficits raises the possibility of earlier and more accurate diagnosis with an algorithm that includes a rule-in diagnostic imaging examination. Significant unanswered questions remain with regard to the place of neuroimaging in such algorithms for at-risk screening and differential diagnosis. As novel therapeutics altering the course of disease progression come to the clinic, the need for better clinical assessment will become paramount. Finally, the elaboration of novel imaging targets provides the opportunity for more sophisticated understanding of the neurochemical basis of movement disorders beyond the dopamine system and may open novel areas of imaging research and, ultimately, therapeutics.

References

1. Yahr MD. Early recognition of Parkinson's disease. Hosp Pract (Off Ed) 1981;16:65–72, 77–80.
2. Fahn S. Description of Parkinson's disease as a clinical syndrome. Ann NY Acad Sci 2003;991:1–14.
3. Fahn S. Controversies in the therapy of Parkinson's disease. Adv Neurol 1996;69:477–486.
4. Uitti RJ, Baba Y, Wszolek ZK, et al. Defining the Parkinson's disease phenotype: initial symptoms and baseline characteristics in a clinical cohort. Parkinsonism Relat Disord 2005;11:139–145.
5. Lewis SJ, Foltynie T, Blackwell AD, et al. Heterogeneity of Parkinson's disease in the early clinical stages using a data driven approach. J Neurol Neurosurg Psychiatry 2005;76:343–348.
6. Jankovic J Progression of Parkinson disease: are we making progress in charting the course. Arch Neurol 2005;62:351–352.
7. Olanow CW. The scientific basis for the current treatment of Parkinson's disease. Annu Rev Med 2004;55:41–60.
8. Tetrud J. Treatment challenges in early stage Parkinson's disease. Neurol Clin 2004;22 (3 Suppl):S19–33.
9. Markham CH, Diamond SG. Long-term follow-up of early dopa treatment in Parkinson's disease. Ann Neurol 1986;19:365–372.
10. Wermuth L. Outpatient treatment of Parkinson's disease. Eur Neurol 1988;28:152–155.
11. Fahn S, Oakes D, Shoulson I, et al. Levodopa and the progression of Parkinson's disease. N Engl J Med 2004;351(24):2498–2508.
12 Dopamine transporter brain imaging to assess the effects of pramipexole vs levodopa on Parkinson disease progression. JAMA 2002;287:1653–1661.
13. Rakshi JS, Pavese N, Uema T, et al. A comparison of the progression of early Parkinson's disease in patients started on ropinirole or L-dopa: an 18F-dopa PET study. J Neural Transm 2002;109:1433–1443.
14. Whone AL, Watts RL, Stoessl AJ, et al. Slower progression of Parkinson's disease with ropinirole versus levodopa: the REAL-PET study. Ann Neurol 2003;54:93–101.
15. Swope DM. Rapid treatment of "wearing off" in Parkinson's disease. Neurology 2004;62 (6 Suppl 4):S27–31.
16. Obeso JA, Rodriguez-Oroz M, Marin C, et al. The origin of motor fluctuations in Parkinson's disease: importance of dopaminergic innervation and basal ganglia circuits. Neurology 2004;62(Suppl 1):S17–30.
17. Lyons KE, Pahwa R. Deep brain stimulation in Parkinson's disease. Curr Neurol Neurosci Rep 2004;4:290–295.
18. Breit S, Schulz JB, Benabid AL. Deep brain stimulation. Cell Tissue Res 2004;318:275–288.
19. Elm JJ, Goetz CG, Ravina B, et al. A responsive outcome for Parkinson's disease neuroprotection futility studies. Ann Neurol 2005;57:197–203.
20. Calne D, Schulzer M, Mak E, et al. Treatment for the progression of Parkinson's disease. Lancet Neurol 2005;4:206.
21. Schapira AH, Olanow CW. Neuroprotection in Parkinson disease: mysteries, myths, and misconceptions. JAMA 2004;291:358–364.
22. Schapira AH. Disease modification in Parkinson's disease. Lancet Neurol 2004;3:362–368.
23. Lang AE, Obeso JA. Challenges in Parkinson's disease: restoration of the nigrostriatal dopamine system is not enough. Lancet Neurol 2004;3:309–316.
24. Koller WC, Cersosimo MG. Neuroprotection in Parkinson's disease: an elusive goal. Curr Neurol Neurosci Rep 2004;4:277–283.
25. Johnston TH, Brotchie JM. Drugs in development for Parkinson's disease. Curr Opin Investig Drugs 2004;5:720–726.
26. Drucker-Colin R, Verdugo-Diaz L. Cell transplantation for Parkinson's disease: present status. Cell Mol Neurobiol 2004;24:301–316.

27. Dlamini Z, Mbita Z, Zungu M. Genealogy, expression, and molecular mechanisms in apoptosis. Pharmacol Ther 2004;101:1–15.
28. Clarke CE. Neuroprotection and pharmacotherapy for motor symptoms in Parkinson's disease. Lancet Neurol 2004;3:466–474.
29. Siderowf A, Newberg A, Chou KL, et al. [99mTc]TRODAT-1 SPECT imaging correlates with odor identification in early Parkinson disease. Neurology 2005;64:1716–1720.
30. Brooks DJ, Ibanez V, Sawle GV, et al. Differing patterns of striatal 18F-dopa uptake in Parkinson's disease, multiple system atrophy, and progressive supranuclear palsy. Ann Neurol 1990;28:547–555.
31. Boja JW, Patel A, Carroll FI, et al. [125I]RTI-55: a potent ligand for dopamine transporters. Eur J Pharmacol 1991;194:133–134.
32. Brooks DJ. Functional imaging in relation to parkinsonian syndromes. J Neurol Sci 1993;115:1–17.
33. Brucke T, Kornhuber J, Angelberger P, et-al. SPECT imaging of dopamine and serotonin transporters with [123I]beta-CIT. Binding kinetics in the human brain. J Neural Transm Gen Sect 1993;94:137–146.
34. Innis RB, Seibyl JP, Scanley BE, et al. Single photon emission computed tomographic imaging demonstrates loss of striatal dopamine transporters in Parkinson disease. Proc Natl Acad Sci USA 1993;90:11965–11969.
35. Wilson AA, DaSilva JN, Houle S. In vivo evaluation of [11C]- and [18F]-labelled cocaine analogues as potential dopamine transporter ligands for positron emission tomography. Nucl Med Biol 1996;23:141–146.
36. Scheffel U, Steinert C, Kim SE, et al. Effect of dopaminergic drugs on the in vivo binding of [3H]WIN 35,428 to central dopamine transporters. Synapse 1996;23:61–69.
37. Haaparanta M, Bergman J, Laakso A, et al. [18F]CFT ([18F]WIN 35,428), a radioligand to study the dopamine transporter with PET: biodistribution in rats. Synapse 1996;23:321–327.
38. Brownell AL, Elmaleh DR, Meltzer PC, et al. Cocaine congeners as PET imaging probes for dopamine terminals. J Nucl Med 1996;37:1186–1192.
39. Volkow ND, Ding YS, Fowler JS, et al. A new PET ligand for the dopamine transporter: studies in the human brain. J Nucl Med 1995;36:2162–2168.
40. Malison RT, Vessotskie JM, Kung MP, et al. Striatal dopamine transporter imaging in nonhuman primates with iodine-123-IPT SPECT. J Nucl Med 1995;36:2290–2297.
41. Lundkvist C, Halldin C, Swahn CG, et al. [O-methyl-11C]beta-CIT-FP, a potential radioligand for quantitation of the dopamine transporter: preparation, autoradiography, metabolite studies, and positron emission tomography examinations. Nucl Med Biol 1995;22:905–913.
42. Laruelle M, Wallace E, Seibyl JP, et al. Graphical, kinetic, and equilibrium analyses of in vivo [123I] beta-CIT binding to dopamine transporters in healthy human subjects. J Cereb Blood Flow Metab 1994;14:982–994.
43. Innis R, Baldwin R, Sybirska E, et al. Single photon emission computed tomography imaging of monoamine reuptake sites in primate brain with [123I]CIT. Eur J Pharmacol 1991;200:369–370.
44. Frey KA, Koeppe RA, Kilbourn MR. Imaging the vesicular monoamine transporter. Adv Neurol 2001;86:237–247.
45. Best SE, Sarrel PM, Malison RT, et al. Striatal dopamine transporter availability with [(123)I] beta-CIT SPECT is unrelated to gender or menstrual cycle. Psychopharmacology (Berl) 2005;183:181–189.
46. Mozley PD, Schneider JS, Acton PD, et al. Binding of [99mTc]TRODAT-1 to dopamine transporters in patients with Parkinson's disease and in healthy volunteers. J Nucl Med 2000;41:584–589.
47. Huang WS, Chiang YH, Lin JC, et al. Crossover study of (99m)Tc-TRODAT-1 SPECT and (18)F-FDOPA PET in Parkinson's disease patients. J Nucl Med 2003;44:999–1005.
48. Brooks DJ. Detection of preclinical Parkinson's disease with PET. Geriatrics 1991;46 (Suppl 1):25–30.
49. Seibyl JP, Marek KL, Quinlan D, et al. Decreased single-photon emission computed tomographic [123I]beta-CIT striatal uptake correlates with symptom severity in Parkinson's disease. Ann Neurol 1995;38:589–598.

50. Hilker R, Schweitzer K, Coburger S, et al. Nonlinear progression of Parkinson disease as determined by serial positron emission tomographic imaging of striatal fluorodopa F 18 activity. Arch Neurol 2005;62:378–382.
51. Au WL, Adams JR, Troiano AR, et al. Parkinson's disease: in vivo assessment of disease progression using positron emission tomography. Brain Res Mol Brain Res 2005;134:24–33.
52. Sossi V, de la Fuente-Fernandez R, Holden JE, et al. Changes of dopamine turnover in the progression of Parkinson's disease as measured by positron emission tomography: their relation to disease-compensatory mechanisms. J Cereb Blood Flow Metab 2004;24:869–876.
53. Seibyl JP. Single-photon emission computed tomography and positron emission tomography evaluations of patients with central motor disorders. Semin Nucl Med 2008;38:274–286.
54. Pirker W, Holler I, Gerschlager W, et al. Measuring the rate of progression of Parkinson's disease over a 5-year period with beta-CIT SPECT. Mov Disord 2003;18:1266–1272.
55. Morrish PK REAL and CALM: what have we learned. Mov Disord 2003;18:839–840.
56. Ito K, Morrish PK, Rakshi JS, et al. Statistical parametric mapping with 18F-dopa PET shows bilaterally reduced striatal and nigral dopaminergic function in early Parkinson's disease. J Neurol Neurosurg Psychiatry 1999;66:754–758.
57. Gelb DJ, Oliver E, Gilman S. Diagnostic criteria for Parkinson disease. Arch Neurol 1999;56:33–39.
58. Quinn N. Parkinsonism—recognition and differential diagnosis. BMJ 1995;310:447–452.
59. Meara J, Bhowmick BK, Hobson P. Accuracy of diagnosis in patients with presumed Parkinson's disease. Age Ageing 1999;28:99–102.
60. Hughes AJ, Daniel SE, Kilford L, et al. Accuracy of clinical diagnosis of idiopathic Parkinson's disease: a clinico-pathological study of 100 cases. J Neurol Neurosurg Psychiatry 1992;55:181–184.
61. Rajput DR. Accuracy of clinical diagnosis of idiopathic Parkinson's disease. J Neurol Neurosurg Psychiatry 1993;56:938–939.
62. Weng YH, Yen TC, Chen MC, et al. Sensitivity and specificity of 99mTc-TRODAT-1 SPECT imaging in differentiating patients with idiopathic Parkinson's disease from healthy subjects. J Nucl Med 2004;45:393–401.
63. Chou KL, Hurtig HI, Stern MB, et al. Diagnostic accuracy of [99mTc]TRODAT-1 SPECT imaging in early Parkinson's disease. Parkinsonism Relat Disord 2004;10:375–379.
64. Tzen KY, Lu CS, Yen TC, et al. Differential diagnosis of Parkinson's disease and vascular parkinsonism by (99m)Tc-TRODAT-1. J Nucl Med 2001;42:408–413.
65. Benamer TS, Patterson J, Grosset DG, et al. Accurate differentiation of parkinsonism and essential tremor using visual assessment of [123I]-FP-CIT SPECT imaging: the [123I]-FP-CIT study group. Mov Disord 2000;15:503–510.
66. Group PS. A multicenter assessment of dopamine transporter imaging with DOPASCAN/SPECT in parkinsonism. Parkinson Study Group. Neurology 2000;55:1540–1547.
67. Burn DJ, O'Brien JT. Use of functional imaging in Parkinsonism and dementia. Mov Disord 2003;18(Suppl 6):S88–95.
68. Jennings DL, Seibyl JP, Oakes D, et al. (123I) beta-CIT and single-photon emission computed tomographic imaging vs clinical evaluation in Parkinsonian syndrome: unmasking an early diagnosis. Arch Neurol 2004;61:1224–1229.
69. Seibyl J, Jennings D, Tabamo R, et al. The role of neuroimaging in the early diagnosis and evaluation of Parkinson's disease. Minerva Med 2005;96:353–364.
70. Varrone A, Marek KL, Jennings D, et al. [(123)I]beta-CIT SPECT imaging demonstrates reduced density of striatal dopamine transporters in Parkinson's disease and multiple system atrophy. Mov Disord 2001;16:1023–1032.
71. Kim YJ, Ichise M, Ballinger JM, et al. Combination of dopamine transporter and D2 receptor SPECT in the diagnostic evaluation of PD, MSA, and PSP. Mov Disord 2002;17:303–312.
72. Walker Z, Costa DC, Walker RW, et al. Striatal dopamine transporter in dementia with Lewy bodies and Parkinson disease: a comparison. Neurology 2004;62:1568–1572.
73. Small GW. Neuroimaging as a diagnostic tool in dementia with Lewy bodies. Dement Geriatr Cogn Disord 2004;17(Suppl 1):25–31.

74. O'Brien JT, Colloby S, Fenwick J, et al. Dopamine transporter loss visualized with FP-CIT SPECT in the differential diagnosis of dementia with Lewy bodies. Arch Neurol 2004;61:919–925.
75. Schwarz J, Storch A, Koch W, et al. Loss of dopamine transporter binding in Parkinson's disease follows a single exponential rather than linear decline. J Nucl Med 2004;45:1694–1697.
76. de la Fuente-Fernandez R, Sossi V, Huang Z, et al. Levodopa-induced changes in synaptic dopamine levels increase with progression of Parkinson's disease: implications for dyskinesias. Brain 2004;127(Pt 12):2747–2754.
77. Snow B. Objective measures for the progression of Parkinson's disease. J Neurol Neurosurg Psychiatry 2003;74:287.
78. Marshall V, Grosset D. Role of dopamine transporter imaging in routine clinical practice. Mov Disord 2003;18:1415–1423.
79. van Dyck CH, Seibyl JP, Malison RT, et al. Age-related decline in dopamine transporters: analysis of striatal subregions, nonlinear effects, and hemispheric asymmetries. Am J Geriatr Psychiatry 2002;10:36–43.
80. van Dyck CH, Malison RT, Jacobsen LK, et al. Increased dopamine transporter availability associated with the 9-repeat allele of the SLC6A3 gene. J Nucl Med 2005;46:745–751.
81. A randomized controlled trial comparing pramipexole with levodopa in early Parkinson's disease: design and methods of the CALM-PD Study. Parkinson Study Group. Clin Neuropharmacol 2000;23:34–44.
82. A controlled, randomized, delayed-start study of rasagiline in early Parkinson disease. Arch Neurol 2004;61:561-566.
83. Marek KL, Seibyl JP, Zoghbi SS, et al. [123I] beta-CIT/SPECT imaging demonstrates bilateral loss of dopamine transporters in hemi-Parkinson's disease. Neurology 1996;46:231–237.
84. Braak H, Del Tredici K, Rub U, et al. Staging of brain pathology related to sporadic Parkinson's disease. Neurobiol Aging 2003;24:197–211.
85. Braak H, Rub U, Gai WP, et al. Idiopathic Parkinson's disease: possible routes by which vulnerable neuronal types may be subject to neuroinvasion by an unknown pathogen. J Neural Transm 2003;110:517–536.
86. Kim SE, Choi JY, Choe YS, et al. Serotonin transporters in the midbrain of Parkinson's disease patients: a study with 123I-beta-CIT SPECT. J Nucl Med 2003;44:870–876.
87. Murai T, Muller U, Werheid K, et al. In vivo evidence for differential association of striatal dopamine and midbrain serotonin systems with neuropsychiatric symptoms in Parkinson's disease. J Neuropsychiatry Clin Neurosci 2001;13:222–228.
88. Dewey RBJr. Autonomic dysfunction in Parkinson's disease. Neurol Clin 2004;22(3 Suppl):S127–139.
89. Kaufmann H, Nahm K, Purohit D, et al. Autonomic failure as the initial presentation of Parkinson disease and dementia with Lewy bodies. Neurology 2004;63:1093–1095.
90. Schrag A. Psychiatric aspects of Parkinson's disease—an update. J Neurol 2004;251:795–804.
91. Lemke MR, Fuchs G, Gemende I, et-al. Depression and Parkinson's disease. J Neurol 2004;251(Suppl 6):VI/24–27.
92. Burghaus L, Schutz U, Krempel U, et al. Loss of nicotinic acetylcholine receptor subunits alpha4 and alpha7 in the cerebral cortex of Parkinson patients. Parkinsonism Relat Disord 2003;9:243–246.
93. Martin-Ruiz C, Lawrence S, Piggott M, et al. Nicotinic receptors in the putamen of patients with dementia with Lewy bodies and Parkinson's disease: relation to changes in alpha-synuclein expression. Neurosci Lett 2002;335:134–138.
94. Pimlott SL, Piggott M, Owens J, et al. Nicotinic acetylcholine receptor distribution in Alzheimer's disease, dementia with Lewy bodies, Parkinson's disease, and vascular dementia: in vitro binding study using 5-[(125)i]-a-85380. Neuropsychopharmacology 2004;29:108–116.
95. Frederickson RD, Brunden KK. New opportunities in AD research—roles of immunoinflammatory responses and glia. Alzheimer Dis Assoc Disord 1994;8:159–165.
96. Rogers J, Webster S, Lue LF, et al. Inflammation and Alzheimer's disease pathogenesis. Neurobiol Aging 1996;17:681–686.

97. McGeer EG, McGeer PL. The role of the immune system in neurodegenerative disorders. Mov Disord 1997;12:855–858.
98. Hirsch EC, Breidert T, Rousselet E, et al. The role of glial reaction and inflammation in Parkinson's disease. Ann NY Acad Sci 2003;991:214–228.
99. McGeer PL, McGeer EG. Inflammation and the degenerative diseases of aging. Ann NY Acad Sci 2004;1035:104–116.
100. McGeer PL, Schwab C, Parent A, et al. Presence of reactive microglia in monkey substantia nigra years after 1-methyl-4-phenyl-1,2,3,6-tetrahydropyridine administration. Ann Neurol 2003;54:599–604.
101. Langston JW, Forno LS, Tetrud J, et al. Evidence of active nerve cell degeneration in the substantia nigra of humans years after 1-methyl-4-phenyl-1,2,3,6-tetrahydropyridine exposure. Ann Neurol 1999;46:598–605.
102. Teismann P, Schulz JB. Cellular pathology of Parkinson's disease: astrocytes, microglia and inflammation. Cell Tissue Res 2004;318:149–161.
103. Chen H, Zhang SM, Hernan MA, et al. Nonsteroidal anti-inflammatory drugs and the risk of Parkinson disease. Arch Neurol 2003;60:1059–1064.
104. Asanuma M, Miyazaki I, Ogawa N. Neuroprotective effects of nonsteroidal anti-inflammatory drugs on neurodegenerative diseases. Curr Pharm Des 2004;10:695–700.
105. Cagnin A, Brooks DJ, Kennedy AM, et al. In-vivo measurement of activated microglia in dementia. Lancet 2001;358:461–467.
106. Gerhard A, Banati RB, Goerres GB, et al. [11C](R)-PK11195 PET imaging of microglial activation in multiple system atrophy. Neurology 2003;61:686–689.
107. Gerhard A, Watts J, Trender-Gerhard I, et-al. In vivo imaging of microglial activation with [11C](R)-PK11195 PET in corticobasal degeneration. Mov Disord 2004; 19(10):1221–1226.
108. Ouchi, Y, Yoshikawa E, Sekine Y, Futatsubashi M, Kanno T, Ogusu T, Torizuka T, Microglial activation and dopamine terminal loss in early Parkinson's disease. Ann Neurol 2005;57(2):168–175.
109. Turner MR, Cagnin A, Turkheimer FE, et al. Evidence of widespread cerebral microglial activation in amyotrophic lateral sclerosis: an [11C](R)-PK11195 positron emission tomography study. Neurobiol Dis 2004;15:601–609.
110. Huang WS, Lin SZ, Lin JC, et al. Evaluation of early-stage Parkinson's disease with 99mTc-TRODAT-1 imaging. J Nucl Med 2001;42:1303–1308.
111. Schwarz J, Linke R, Kerner M, et al. Striatal dopamine transporter binding assessed by [I-123] IPT and single photon emission computed tomography in patients with early Parkinson's disease: implications for a preclinical diagnosis. Arch Neurol 2000;57:205–208.
112. Reed J, Huang Z. Apoptosis pathways and drug targets. Nat Rev Drug Dis/Mol Cell Biol November 2004, www.nature.com/nrm/posters/apoptosis/index.html.
113. Marek K, SeibylJ.A molecular map for neurodegeneration. Science 2000;289:409–411.

Part II
Emerging Approaches Using PET

Chapter 5
Microstructural Imaging of Neurodegenerative Changes

Vladimir Kepe, Sung-Cheng Huang, Gary W. Small, Nagichettiar Satyamurthy, Jorge R. Barrio

Modern medical imaging techniques serve an important role in the diagnosis of neurodegenerative disorders. Assessment of structural changes, e.g., brain atrophy with magnetic resonance imaging (MRI) or computed tomography (CT), and functional changes, e.g., brain perfusion with single photon emission tomography (SPECT) or brain glucose utilization with positron emission tomography (PET), provide valuable information about the extent of cellular neurodegeneration processes in Alzheimer's disease (AD), frontotemporal dementia, Parkinson's disease, and other disorders. Neuronal loss, neuronal shrinkage, synaptic loss, and loss of neuronal projections contribute to the collapse of gray and white matter measurable as atrophy. At the same time, these neuronal changes compromise the integrity of the major neuronal circuits, which results in decreased function and decreased glucose utilization, which is measurable with ^{18}F-FDG PET.[1]

Cellular pathology in neurodegenerative disorders is paralleled or even preceded by deposition of pathologic intracellular and/or extracellular aggregates of disease-specific proteins, presenting another target for in vivo detection of brain's pathologic changes at early, presymptomatic stages. Because of the lack of suitable molecular probes that would specifically interact with inert structures of these aggregates in vivo, they had not been considered viable targets for in vivo imaging up until a decade ago. In the last decade, progress has been made in the field of AD imaging with development of several small molecule imaging probes with high binding affinity for β-amyloid plaques (and, in some cases, also neurofibrillary tangles [NFT]) in vivo, allowing detection of pathologic deposits in the brains of patients with AD with positron emission tomography (PET). This chapter focuses on development of imaging approaches for detection of molecular markers of neurodegeneration.

Alzheimer's Disease

Alzheimer's disease, the most common type of dementia in the elderly, is a progressive neurodegenerative disorder that gradually results in severe cognitive impairments that leave patients completely dependent on others.[2] AD manifests clinically as

D.H.S. Silverman (ed.), *PET in the Evaluation of Alzheimer's Disease and Related Disorders*,
DOI: 10.1007/978-0-387-76420-7_5,

impairment of a broad spectrum of cognitive processes, including verbal and nonverbal memory, language and semantic knowledge, attention and executive functions, and visuoperceptual and spatial abilities, all of which can be assessed with neuropsychological measures.[3] The prevalence of AD in different age groups in individuals older than 60 years doubles every 5 years, ranging from a little above 1% among 60–64 year olds to 40% among those over 85 years old, and will grow dramatically over the next three decades, barring discovery of a cure, with the maturing of the present middle-aged segment of the population.[4,5] The present financial burden exceeds $100 billion annually in the United States alone.[6]

Neuropathologic Hallmarks of Alzheimer's Disease

In his original report in 1907, Alois Alzheimer described the presence of two hallmark brain lesions, NFTs and senile plaques,[7] in the brain of a patient affected by the dementia syndrome that now carries his name.[8] Since then, it has become clear that the neuropathologic profile of AD is more complex and includes widespread neuronal loss, hippocampal granuvacuolar degeneration plus Hirano bodies, vascular changes, synaptic abnormalities, neurophil threads, and activation of glial cells[9]; however, β-amyloid–containing plaques and NFTs remain the most abundant neuropathologic lesions found in AD. Their average density in the cortex and hippocampus is significantly greater in AD than in normal aging or other neurodegenerative disorders. Neuropathologic deposits and neuronal losses are suitable targets for molecular imaging probes. Targeting initial neuronal loss in the most vulnerable areas, and early formation of β-amyloid plaques and NFTs leading to this neuronal loss may help to achieve early diagnosis and allow possible therapeutic intervention starting when damage to the brain is still limited and when the therapeutic interventions still have potential to protect the brain by arresting the progression of pathology.

β-Amyloid Plaques

β-Amyloid plaques appear as extracellular brain lesions composed mainly of water insoluble β-amyloid peptide aggregates.[10,11] β-Amyloid plaques are found throughout the AD neocortex as diffuse amorphous (noncongophilic) aggregates, and as dense focal (congophilic) fibrillar and dense core plaques.[12] A subset of β-amyloid plaques is also spatially co-localized with dystrophic neuritic processes and is thus referred to as *neuritic plaques*. These dystrophic neurites often include fibrillar aggregates of hyperphosphorylated microtubule-associated protein tau called *paired helical filaments*.[9,12] β-Amyloid peptides, 39–43 amino acid long peptides, are formed by β- and γ-secretase–mediated cleavage from a large transmembrane protein called *amyloid precursor protein*.[13] Detailed structural information about β-amyloid fibrils based on the high-resolution X-ray crystallography is not available because of the inability of insoluble β-amyloid fibrils to form single crystals.[14] Despite that fact, a considerable amount of information about the fibrillar nature of ex vivo β-amyloid fibrils is available from X-ray diffraction experiments, i.e., two distinctive diffraction bands at 4.7 and 10 Å were observed,[15,16] typical of fibrils with cross-β sheet secondary structure element.[10] Stacking of cross-β sheets leads to formation of protofilaments, which then bundled together twist around each other to form 7- to 10-nm–wide straight rigid fibrils, as demonstrated by electron microscopy.[17] Fibrils of synthetic β-amyloid (1–40), formed in vitro, resemble in vivo fibrils in terms of neurotoxic properties[18] and also ultrastructurally,[19,20] but this may not hold true for tau aggregates. β-Amyloid plaques are co-localized with a variety of proteinaceous and nonproteinaceous molecules, such as proteoglycans, inflammatory molecules, serum-related amyloid P component, ubiquitin, apolipoprotein E, low-density lipoprotein receptor–related protein, α2-macroglobulin, α1-antichymotripsin, and cholinesterases, among others.[21]

Neurofibrillary Tangles

The second pathologic hallmark of AD is NFTs found in vulnerable neuronal populations throughout the neocortex and subcortical structures. NFTs are cytoskeletal lesions largely composed of bundles of paired helical filaments and straight filaments, which are intraneuronal fibrillar aggregates of hyperphosphorylated microtubule-associated protein tau.[22] After the NFT-laden neurons die, extracellular *tombstone* tangles remain visible, keeping the shape of neurons in which they were formed (e.g., typical flame-like tangles originated in pyramidal neurons).[23] Hyperphosphorylated microtubule-associated protein tau aggregates into paired helical filaments, fibrillar structures 10–20 nm in width with 75- to 80-nm repeats, by forming a cross-β sheet with its repeat domain and with the rest of the peptide forming a largely unstructured *fuzzy* coat in which the cross-β sheet structure is embedded.[24] The presence of cross-β sheet in NFTs and in the in vitro assembled tau polymers has also been confirmed by the X-ray diffraction experiments.[15,25] NFTs undergo posttranslational modifications (e.g., proteolysis, glycation, cross-linking, amino acid racemization) and are spatially co-localized with a variety of proteins such as ubiquitin, proteoglycans, serum amyloid P component, kinases, other MAP proteins, and apolipoprotein E, among others.[26,27]

Early Neuronal Losses

AD is a neurodegenerative disease with progressive neuronal loss affecting vulnerable neuronal populations throughout the neocortex and subcortical structures in a complex pattern, which gets more extensive as the symptoms of AD worsen. In the advanced stages of the disease, when a diagnosis of probable AD can be made, the death toll in vulnerable populations of CNS neurons is already heavy and has spread to the cortical regions beyond the hippocampus, one of the critical sites of neuronal damage leading to dementia.[28,29] In the cortex, the pyramidal neurons furnishing long cortico-cortical projections are thought to be particularly vulnerable to neurodegeneration and synaptic loss, leading to disconnection of the association cortices.[30] In contrast, primary sensory and motor areas exhibit only limited degeneration.

The brain areas affected by substantial neuronal loss at the earliest stages of the disease are entorhinal cortex and hippocampus. The large pyramidal neurons in CA1 and subicular regions of hippocampus, and the neurons in layers II and IV of entorhinal cortex are particularly vulnerable.[30–32] These types of neurons predominantly use glutamate for neurotransmission and also receive glutamatergic inputs.

The extent of neuronal loss in these vulnerable populations is correlated with the degree of dementia in AD.[33,34] Gomez-Isla et al.[35] reported 57% neuronal loss in layer II of the entorhinal cortex of patients with very mild AD, and similar results have been reported by others.[36,37] Substantial loss (>50%) of neurons in hippocampal CA1 field of AD patients has also been observed,[36–39] and in severely affected AD patients the loss of CA1 neurons was reported to reach as high as 86%.[32] Rössler and colleagues[40] described a loss of 33% at Braak NFT stage IV and 51% at Braak NFT stage V. Neuronal losses are thus correlated with the presence of intraneuronal NFTs, but are not well correlated with amyloid deposition in the same areas.[28,40,41]

Patterns of Pathology Distribution and Progression in Alzheimer's Disease

The progressive nature of pathology in AD presents a unique challenge for any diagnostic method based on detection of β-amyloid plaques, NFTs, or both, as well as for any method that would monitor therapeutic treatments targeting those plaques and tangles. Such methods must be able to: (1) identify relatively low densities of proteinopathies in the affected areas present during the preclinical, nonsymptomatic AD stages, (2) accurately determine their amounts, and (3) detect the changes in the pattern of distribution and densities resulting from spreading of β-amyloid plaques and NFTs into new cortical areas.

The deposition of NFTs and β-amyloid plaques in AD has been studied extensively, and separate patterns have been proposed for evolution of NFT pathology and β-amyloid plaque pathology.[28,42] Braak and Braak[28] have proposed six stages of NFT pathology progression based on the spatial pattern of NFT distribution in the brain. In the initial stages (*transentorhinal* stages I and II), NFTs are observed only in entorhinal cortex; in the *limbic* stages III and IV, dense deposits of NFTs can be observed throughout the entire entorhinal cortex and hippocampal formation, with association areas of temporal lobe, cingulate gyrus, and orbito-frontal cortex having sparse deposits. In more advanced *cortical* stages V and VI, associated with fully developed dementia, NFTs finally spread throughout the neocortex, leaving only sensorimotor cortex relatively spared. Delacourte and colleagues[42] have proposed a ten-stage system (S1–S10) of NFT progression that more clearly defines the pattern of the expansion of NFT pathology through the neocortex after it progresses from the medial temporal lobe.

β-Amyloid plaque pathology develops in a pattern different from the NFT distribution and predominantly affects neocortical regions, with hippocampus and entorhinal cortex being affected to a lesser extent and at later stages of β-amyloid plaque progression. Braak and Braak[28] have proposed three stages of β-amyloid plaque progression. In stage A, the basal portions of temporal, frontal, and occipital lobes develop low densities of β-amyloid deposits. In stage B, almost all neocortical association areas develop medium densities of β-amyloid deposits. Finally, in stage C, densely packed β-amyloid deposits can be found throughout the whole neocortex and in numerous subcortical structures with relative sparing of primary sensory-motor areas. The patterns are shown in Fig. 5.1.

The model described by Braak and Braak is consistent with a detailed study of neuropathology distribution by Arnold et al.[43] in 39 brain areas of 11 patients with moderate to severe AD. Densities of NFTs and neuritic β-amyloid plaques were mapped out showing the degree of involvement of neocortex. The results corresponded to Braak NFT stages V/VI and Braak β-amyloid stage C. There was a gradient of NFT densities with limbic lobe (hippocampus and entorhinal cortex) > temporal lobe > frontal lobe > parietal lobe > occipital lobe. All primary sensory areas were relatively spared (Fig. 5.2). Neuritic β-amyloid plaques were distributed more uniformly in the neocortex with temporal, parietal, and occipital lobes more than frontal lobe. Similarly, Price et al.[44] determined in their moderately to heavily demented AD patients (Clinical Dementia Rating [CDR] scores 2 and 3) in a more limited number of analyzed areas that both NFTs and β-amyloid plaques were distributed densely throughout the cortex with caudate and putamen showing dense deposits of β-amyloid plaques. In very mildly demented patients (CDR score 0.5) the distribution of NFTs and β-amyloid plaques resembled that of more severely demented subjects, but lower densities of both pathologies were observed in all areas. The nondemented subjects had low levels of NFTs in CA1 region of hippocampus, entorhinal cortex and perirhinal cortex as well as in the anterior olfactory nucleus, and these densities increased with age. Low densities of β-amyloid plaques were found in isolated areas of lateral temporal cortex only in a small number of nondemented cases. The authors observed in an isolated nondemented case that the NFTs and β-amyloid plaque topography and densities were comparable to those observed in very mildly demented subjects.

A large-scale autopsy study of 1,258 brains from elderly patients for whom the clinical diagnosis was available (58 subjects had AD, 1,131 were not demented or were mildly impaired, and the remaining subjects had other types of dementias) demonstrated stark differences in densities of NFTs and β-amyloid plaques between the control group and the AD group in several brain regions (CA1 region of hippocampus, inferior temporal cortex, superior frontal cortex, and occipital cortex).[45]

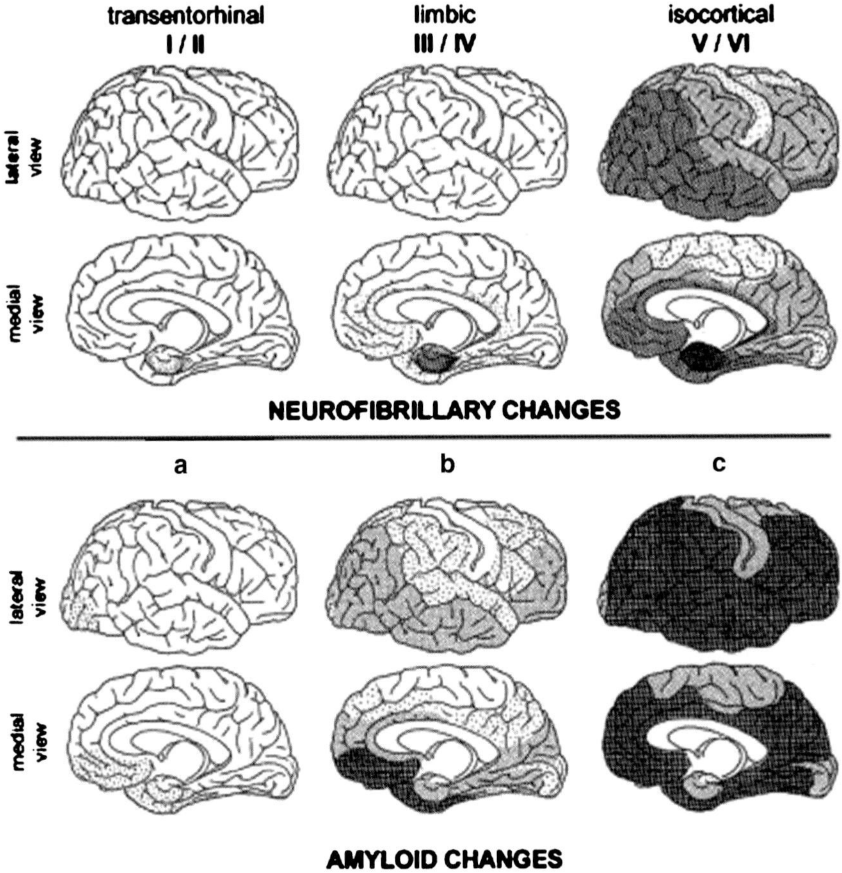

Fig. 5.1 Braak stages of pathology progression. Six stages of neurofibrillary tangle progression are shown in the upper rows. Transenthorinal NFT stages I and II (*left*) have tangles confined to transentorhinal and entorhinal areas. In limbic stages III and IV (*middle*) pathology engulfs the hippocampal formation and parts of the limbic lobe. In the final isocortical stages V and VI (*right*) neurofibrillary tangles are found throughout the neocortex. Three stages of β-amyloid pathology progression are show in the lower rows. The earliest β-amyloid plaques appear in the basal aspects of inferior aspects of temporal, occipital, and orbitofrontal cortices (Braak stage A, *left*); later pathology spreads to the rest of the cortex where it found at moderate level (Braak stage B, *middle*); and finally plaque densities reach high density throughout the neocortex (Braak stage C, *right*). Medial and lateral views are shown for each pattern of pathology distribution. (Adapted from Braak and Braak,[28] with permission.)

Reflecting the finding of Braak and Braak, these results showed presence of NFTs in CA1 region of hippocampus and in the inferior temporal cortex in a majority of the clinical AD cases (90% and 79%, respectively). NFTs were observed in 39% of AD cases in the superior frontal cortex and in 19% of AD cases in occipital lobe. These results also point to the gradual spreading of NFTs to the neocortex beyond the temporal lobe in AD patients with the disease progression. β-Amyloid plaques

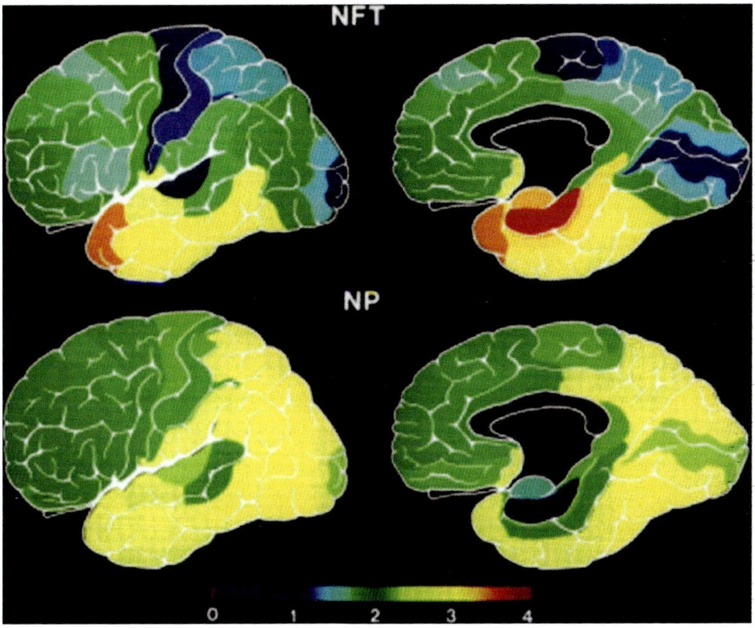

Fig. 5.2 Late stage Alzheimer's disease pathology distribution. Neurofibrillary tangles and neuritic β-amyloid plaques are widespread throughout the cortex at more advanced stages of Alzheimer's disease. NFTs (*upper row*) are most abundant in limbic and temporal lobes (red to yellow) followed by frontal and parietal lobes (green to light blue) and occipital lobe. Primary sensory areas are relatively spared (dark blue). Neuritic β-amyloid plaques (*lower row*) are distributed more uniformly with temporal, parietal, and occipital lobes (yellow) being higher than frontal lobe (green) and much higher than the limbic lobe (blue). Lateral view (*left column*) and medial view (*right column*) are shown for each type of pathology. (From Arnold et al.,[43] with permission.)

were observed extensively in certain neocortical regions (inferior temporal cortex, superior frontal cortex, occipital cortex) in 88–95% of AD cases, and β-amyloid plaques were present in the CA1 region of 85% of clinical AD subjects.

These studies demonstrate that both types of pathology are present to different degrees in the neocortex in symptomatic AD patients, with densities increasing with the severity of the disease. Interpretation of the in vivo imaging results requires good understanding of the spatial and temporal pattern of cortical neuropathology progression, i.e., topography of NFTs, β-amyloid plaques, and neuronal losses and their correlations with the cognitive performance and clinical symptoms of the disease.

Neuropathologic and clinical research support the idea that the pathologic processes leading to AD begin years before a clinical diagnosis of probable AD can be confirmed.[28,46,47] For example, Braak and Braak[47] have shown on a large sample of 2,661 autopsy brains from the general population (age range, 26–95 years) that NFTs are present in some individuals very early in adult life, e.g., among 141 subjects who died between ages 31 and 40 there were 34 (24%) who had at least a few NFTs in entorhinal cortex. The presence of diffuse amyloid deposits in neocortex in the same group has been demonstrated only in two cases.

Several studies that focused on cognitively normal control subjects have found that the majority of elderly subjects have some NFTs in the entorhinal cortex and in some cases also in perirhinal cortex (Brodmann area 35) and in the CA1/subicular region of hippocampus, consistent with Braak stages I–III.[29,48–50] The density of NFTs in these areas increases in an age-dependent manner, but it is significantly lower than observed in AD patients. β-Amyloid plaques were observed only in a smaller subgroup of these subjects in temporal cortex and occasionally also in other neocortical areas.

Knopman et al.[48] concluded that Braak NFT stage IV or above (i.e., spreading of NFTs to the neocortex) and presence of moderate levels of neuritic β-amyloid plaques in the neocortex (Braak amyloid stage B) should be considered as neuropathologic stages associated with dementia, either in preclinical stages or already manifested. In a similar fashion, Price and Morris[29] have reported that several cognitively normal subjects with CDR scores of 0 displayed the pattern and densities of NFTs and β-amyloid plaques typically found in subjects with very mild dementia (CDR score 0.5) and have therefore concluded that these were *preclinical* AD cases.

An important aspect of imaging in AD is to determine the neuropathology distribution in subjects who have developed the first symptoms of AD. Mild cognitive impairment (MCI) is a clinical category used to classify subjects who display isolated impairment in the area of memory or any other cognitive function, but who have otherwise preserved cognitive and functional abilities and do not meet criteria for the diagnosis of dementia.[51] This clinical category has been associated with a higher rate of conversion to AD, especially among the amnestic MCI subjects. In a study of pathology distribution in amnestic MCI subjects, Petersen et al.[52] reported that NFT pathology in hippocampus was more prevalent when compared with control subjects. The authors have frequently observed diffuse β-amyloid plaques, detected by Aβ immunohistochemistry, in the neocortex of both MCI and control subjects, but cored and neuritic plaques were observed less frequently. In contrast, AD patients had dense deposits of all types of β-amyloid plaques in the neocortex with NFTs distributed throughout the neocortex consistently with Braak stages IV, V, and VI. Jicha et al.[53] reported that among the amnestic MCI subjects who developed dementia, there was high prevalence of AD (71%) and these subjects displayed the NFT brain distribution consistent with Braak NFT stages > IV.

Although the protein aggregates in the majority of the cases are indicators of ongoing pathologic processes, they do not provide direct information on active cellular degeneration, which leads to symptomatology.[54] A low level of neurofibrillary deposition in the medial temporal lobe is part of normal aging without increased cellular pathology. In contrast, the medial temporal lobe is more heavily affected by NFT pathology (hippocampus, entorhinal cortex) and β-amyloid pathology (entorhinal cortex, perirhinal cortex, parahippocampal gyrus) in MCI and AD, with different degrees of both pathologies distributed in other cortical regions to a lesser degree in a limited number of areas in MCI and to a higher degree in all cortical areas in AD. Thus, imaging changes in pathologic deposit levels in medial temporal lobe can serve as an in vivo indicator of early stage of disease when cellular degeneration is still limited and opportunities for prevention and early treatment are still open. Cellular pathology in medial temporal lobe has been well correlated to NFT pathology and symptomatology of AD.[28,41]

PET Molecular Imaging of Neurodegenerative Changes

In vivo visualization of pathologic changes in AD is essential for early detection of disease and monitoring its progression or monitoring therapeutic intervention effects. Loss of connectivity and disconnection of neuronal circuits, loss of neurons in the vulnerable neuronal populations, and deposits of insoluble NFTs and β-amyloid plaques are three prominent types of pathologic changes in AD and important targets for detection. Synaptic and cellular degeneration, loss of projections, and demyelination are among the factors that contribute to disconnection on neuronal circuits, loss of function, and decrease in brain activity in the affected areas. Resulting decrease in brain glucose utilization can be assessed with 2-[^{18}F] fluoro-2-deoxy-*D*-glucose (^{18}F-FDG) PET, an important tool in the diagnosis of AD. The method has 93%–95% sensitivity and 89%–92% specificity for AD and progressive dementias in general.[55,56] The pattern of temporal, parietal, and posterior cingulate cortical glucose hypometabolism is a sign of early AD, showing the outcome of pathologic processes in the neuronal circuits projecting from and to the medial temporal lobe.[57]

PET imaging of different receptors, transporters, and enzymes presents opportunities for visualization of cellular pathology in vulnerable neuronal populations in different neurodegenerative disorders. For example, pathophysiologic changes in caudate/putamen in Parkinson's disease can be visualized by multiple tracers that target the production of dopamine via enzyme aromatic amino acid decarboxylase, the dopamine re-uptake from synapses via dopamine reuptake transporter, or dopamine receptors.[58] PET imaging of several brain neurotransmitter systems (e.g., cholinergic, dopaminergic, GABA-ergic, and serotoninergic) in AD has been described, yet the relationship between pathologic processes and density changes in these receptor populations are often very complex.[59] An example of such applications is visualization and quantification of 5-HT1A receptors in the medial temporal lobe in AD.[60] Glutamatergic large pyramidal neurons in hippocampus, carrying high levels of inhibitory 5-HT1A receptors on axonal hillocks, are one of the neuronal populations experiencing the earliest functional changes and neuronal loss in AD. Loss of these neurons causes decreases in 5-HT1A receptor densities, which can be measured in vivo with PET and appropriate 5-HT1A ligands.[61] Using 4-[^{18}F] fluoro-*N*-{2-[1-(2-methoxyphenyl)piperazinyl]ethyl}-*N*-(2-pyridinyl)benzamide (^{18}F-MPPF), a silent selective 5-HT1A receptor antagonist, with PET, the decline in densities was determined in eight AD patients, six subjects with MCIs and five control subjects.[60] Decreases in hippocampal ^{18}F-MPPF binding evident in MCI

(24%) and more dramatically in AD (49%) were associated with lower Mini Mental State Examination (MMSE) scores, lower cognitive performance, and higher levels of pathologic protein aggregate deposits as measured with ^{18}F-FDDNP PET. Since 5-HT1A receptors are also found on hippocampal interneurons and on other types of neurons in hippocampus, yet at much lower densities, these decreases may be caused by multiple factors. Because of the very high concentration of the receptors on pyramidal neurons, decreases in 5-HT1A receptor densities caused by neuronal loss of large pyramidal neurons are the major contributor to the total decline. Figure 5.3 illustrates typical ^{18}F-MPPF, ^{18}F-FDG and ^{18}F-FDDNP images for nondemented control subjects, MCI subjects, and severely affected AD patients.

Although the major pathologic hallmarks of AD are β-amyloid plaques and NFTs, compared with receptors, transporters, and enzymes, NFTs and β-amyloid plaques are inert structures without apparent functional activity, with the exception of β-sheet forming polymerization. (Cross-β sheet structure in the β-sheets results in a highly ordered arrangement of peptide monomers, with the hydrogen bond–linked peptide backbones and π–π stacking of the aromatic amino acid residues, as well as glutamic acid–lysine electrostatic interactions in the side chains probably constituting the target of these ligands.[62])

This lack of activity poses a serious challenge for development of molecular probes with specific binding to these structures.[63,64] Since the soluble monomeric peptides are in equilibrium with their oligomers and polymers forming fibrils, the monomeric peptides themselves (e.g., radiolabeled β-amyloid peptides[22,65]), or the monoclonal antibodies[66] raised against them would be top target choices in principle. Yet because of their protein nature and large size, these probes have very low

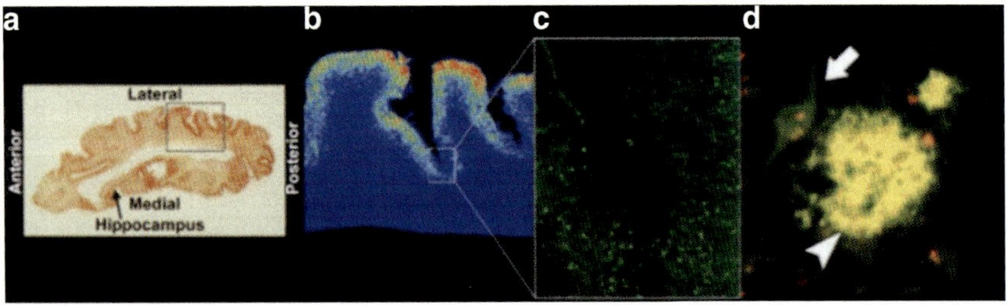

Fig. 5.3 PET imaging of pathologic changes in Alzheimer's disease (AD). Representative examples of ^{18}F-MPPF PET (*upper row*), ^{18}F-FDG PET (*middle row*), and ^{18}F-FDDNP PET (*lower row*) in a control (*left column*), and MCI (*middle column*), and an AD (*right column*). Warmer colors correspond to higher signal. ^{18}F-MPPF PET was used to measure the extent of AD-related neuronal loss in hippocampus; ^{18}F-FDDNP PET was used to detect and quantify the level of pathologic deposits; and ^{18}F-FDG PET was used to determine the regional brain glucose use. Note that a significant decrease in the 5-HT1A receptor density (cell loss) in an AD case (*right column*) is associated with strong metabolic decrease in parietal areas as measured with ^{18}F-FDG PET and with dense ^{18}F-FDDNP binding throughout the neocortex. (From Kepe et al.,[60] with permission.)

capacity to penetrate the blood–brain barrier and enter the brain, which significantly decreases their usefulness for in vivo imaging.

The blood–brain barrier is also an almost impenetrable barrier for charged histologic dyes such as Congo red and thioflavins, gold standards for visualization of β-amyloid plaques and NFTs in postmortem brain tissues in vitro. Nevertheless, these two histologic dyes have served as structural templates for development of a variety of β-amyloid–specific small molecule imaging agents with improved brain entry. Probes based on the Congo red core structure have been developed in radiolabeled form and used for in vitro and ex vivo tests, e.g., X-34,[67] methoxy-X04,[68] and BSB.[69]

Benzothiazole core structural element found in thioflavins served as a template for development of 2-[(4′-methylamino)phenyl]-6-hydroxybenzothiazole (PIB)[70] and 2-[(4′-methylamino)phenyl]benzothiazole.[71] Other core structural elements include imidazo[1,2-*a*]pyridine (IMPY[72–74]); benzofuran[75]; benzoxazole [IBOX,[76] BF-227 (2-(2-[2-dimethylaminothiazol-5-yl]ethenyl)-6-(2-[fluoro]ethoxy)-benzoxazole),[77] and styrylbenzoxazoles[78]]; acridine (BF-108)[79]; thiophenes[80]; flavones[81]; aurones[82]; and fluorenes.[83] Another family of β-amyloid–specific molecular probes are stilbenes 4-methylamino-4′-hydroxystylbene (SB-13),[84] BAY94–9172,[85] and other fluoroalkyl derivatives[86,87]; and diphenyltrienes.[88]

FDDNP (2-(1-{6-[(2-fluoroethyl)(methyl)amino]-2-naphthyl}ethylidene) malononitrile), a solvent viscosity and polarity sensitive probe, is a representative of a family of substituted naphthalenes with binding affinity for β-amyloid peptide aggregates and for NFTs.[89] A group of quinolines and benzimidazoles with preferential binding to hyperphosphorylated tau aggregates has also been described.[90] From this list, only ^{18}F-FDDNP,[89,91] ^{11}C-PIB,[92] ^{11}C-BTA-1,[71] ^{11}C-SB-13,[93] ^{18}F-BAY94–9172,[85] and ^{18}F-BF-227[7] have been used in PET imaging of human subjects with AD. In addition to these PET probes, the SPECT probe ^{123}I-IMPY has been used for determination of human dosimetry, opening the way for its clinical application.[94]

^{18}F-FDDNP (2-(1-{6-[(2–^{18}F-fluoroethyl)(methyl)amino]-2-naphthyl}-ethylidene)malononitrile)

^{18}F-FDDNP was the first radiolabeled PET molecular imaging probe to be successfully applied to in vivo visualization of NFTs and β-amyloid plaques in AD patients.[95–97] In vitro binding properties of ^{18}F-FDDNP to synthetic Aβ(1–40) fibrils were first determined by fluorescence titration of nonradioactive FDDNP.[96,98] These experiments, performed in 0.25% ethanol in phosphate-buffered saline, yielded apparent K_D values of 0.12 and 1.86 nM for two binding sites. ^{18}F-FDDNP binding values to brain homogenates from AD brains were determined to be $K_D = 0.75$ nM and $B_{max} = 144$ nM, performed in 1% ethanol in phosphate-buffered saline. Further experiments involved digital ^{18}F-FDDNP autoradiography of AD and control brain samples in 1% ethanol in saline, and correlation of the autoradiography results with

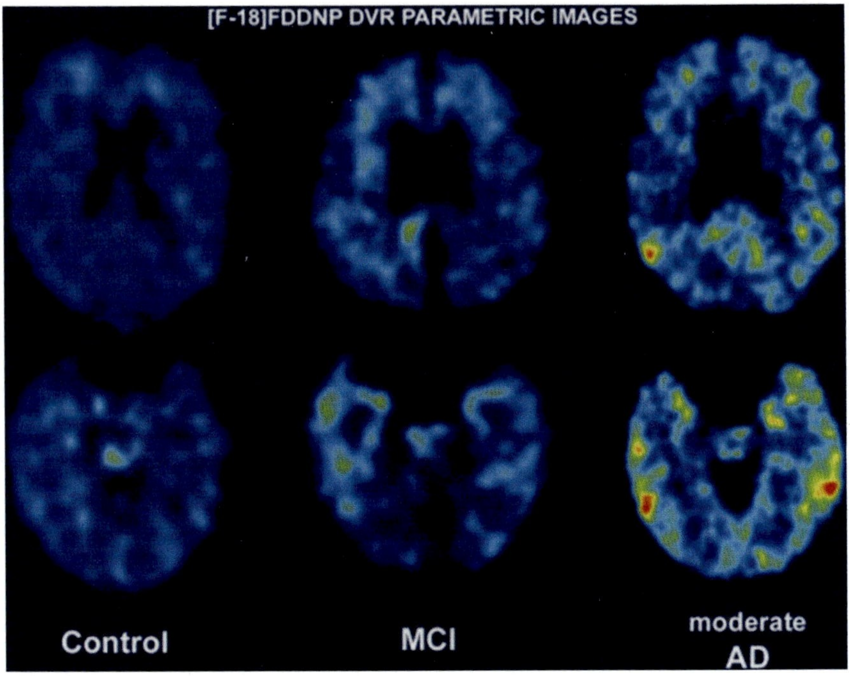

Fig. 5.4 In vitro detection of pathologic deposits with immunohistochemistry and FDDNP. **A.** Immunohistochemistry performed on a brain tissue slice from an Alzheimer's disease patient with Aβ and tau antibodies. **B.** ^{18}F-FDDNP autoradiography performed on the consecutive slice. **C.** Fluorescent properties of FDDNP allow detection of β-amyloid plaques and neurofibrillary tangles using fluorescence microscopy. Low magnification FDDNP fluorescence micrograph. **D.** High magnification fluorescent micrograph. (From Agdeppa et al.,[89] with permission.)

confocal fluorescence microscopy and immunohistochemistry in the AD brain specimens. ^{18}F-FDDNP binding was observed in different brain regions, most prominently in temporal and parietal cortices, matching the distribution of combined β-amyloid plaques and NFT immunostaining of adjacent slices (Fig. 5.4).

Several nonsteroidal anti-inflammatory drugs, such as naproxen and ibuprofen, share their binding site on in vitro formed β-amyloid fibrils with ^{18}F-FDDNP. This binding site is not occupied by diclofenac, Congo red, or thioflavin T as revealed in competitive binding assays.[99] Similarly, ^{18}F-FDDNP autoradiography blocking experiments on AD brain tissue samples showed that naproxen and ibuprofen completely blocked specific ^{18}F-FDDNP binding in the gray matter, but no such blocking was observed with diclofenac, Congo red or thioflavin T. These in vitro blocking experiments were paralleled by experiments demonstrating blockage of in vivo ^{18}F-FDDNP binding to β-amyloid deposits in the β-amyloid–rich brains of β-amyloid triple transgenic rats by pre-exposure to naproxen.[100]

FDDNP has also been applied as a histologic dye for visualization of different types of pathologic aggregates containing amyloid β-sheets such as prion amyloid plaques in Gerstmann-Sträussler-Scheinker disease, sporadic Creutzfeldt-Jakob disease, and variant Creutzfeldt-Jakob disease.[101,102] FDDNP has been shown to bind to the majority of fibrillar pathologic aggregates that display Congo red birefringence indicative of the presence of β-sheet type of aggregation.[101]

A necessary requirement for ^{18}F-FDDNP, or any other PET molecular imaging probe designed to visualize brain pathology at a very early stage of disease, is to be able to detect low levels of deposits localized to a small number of highly vulnerable areas (for early diagnosis) and to detect changes in densities and changes in spatial distribution of pathology over time (for monitoring of disease progression, therapeutic intervention, or both).

The medial temporal lobe is vulnerable to accumulation of both NFTs and β-amyloid plaques. High densities of NFTs are found in entorhinal cortex and throughout hippocampus in AD; β-amyloid plaques are especially prominent in entorhinal cortex, rhinal and perirhinal cortices, and parahippocampal gyrus. For this reason the first clinical ^{18}F-FDDNP PET study in nine AD subjects and seven control subjects specifically analyzed accumulation of ^{18}F-FDDNP in the medial temporal lobe areas. AD patients had significantly higher relative residence time values than controls, using pons as the internal reference region. Medial temporal lobe relative residence time values were also significantly correlated with MMSE scores.[95] A more recent clinical ^{18}F-FDDNP PET study, which also included a subset of subjects who were scanned longitudinally, included 83 age-matched subjects (25 AD patients, 28 MCI subjects, and 30 control subjects).[100] Quantification of ^{18}F-FDDNP binding data was performed with Logan graphical analysis using cerebellum as the reference region. Relative distribution volume (DVR) values were determined for the frontal lobe, parietal lobe, posterior cingulate gyrus, lateral temporal lobe, and medial temporal lobe. Detection of the pathology pattern in MCI subjects served to test the sensitivity of the method, and the follow-up study served to test the capacity of ^{18}F-FDDNP PET to detect the progression of pathology in subjects who experienced progression of disease between the baseline and follow-up scans. Comparison of the ^{18}F-FDDNP DVR values among the groups showed that the binding of the probe in all areas analyzed was significantly elevated in the AD patients when compared with controls. An average of all areas in the same subject was used as a global DVR measure. Representative examples of ^{18}F-FDDNP DVR parametric images are shown in Figure 5.2. The three subject groups were compared with respect to their global and regional ^{18}F-FDDNP binding values (DVR) using ANCOVAs. The Spearman rank correlation, a nonparametric measure of association between ranked pairs of observations, was used to test the strength of association between ^{18}F-FDDNP DVR values and neuropsychological performance.

The mean ^{18}F-FDDNP DVR values differed significantly among the three diagnostic groups: values were lower for the control group compared with the MCI group, which in turn had lower mean FDDNP binding compared with the AD group, for global DVR (control 1.07 ± 0.03; MCI 1.12 ± 0.01; AD 1.16 ± 0.02; ANOVA: $F(2,57) = 233.8$, $P < 0.001$), as well as for all regional values. Of particular interest were the results from the medial temporal lobe, where the MCI group significantly overlapped with the AD group. Global ^{18}F-FDDNP DVR values were inversely correlated with the results of cognitive tests (MMSE scores: $r_s = -0.75$; digit symbol test of the Wechsler adult intelligence test: $r_s = -0.65$). The pattern of pathology distribution in symptomatic AD subjects showed all areas affected, with medial and lateral temporal areas strongly affected in all cases and parietal and frontal lobes affected to varying degrees. This is consistent with the Braak NFT stages V/VI and β-amyloid plaque stage C, all of which are associated with AD. The pattern of ^{18}F-FDDNP binding observed in the MCI group was more variable, with fewer areas affected than in AD cases and with lower ^{18}F-FDDNP DVR values in the affected areas. Peterson and colleagues[52] determined that amnestic MCI patients with AD pathology have a higher prevalence of Braak stages III and IV than controls. In our study, the cognitively normal controls displayed uniformly low ^{18}F-FDDNP binding throughout most of the cortex, with some variability in the medial temporal lobe. ^{18}F-FDDNP PET analysis accurately identified three subject converters out of a total of 12 subjects in the longitudinal study. Two subjects converted from amnestic MCI to AD and one subject converted from control to amnestic MCI. This observed worsening of symptomatology was paralleled by observed increases in DVR values in affected areas and expansion of ^{18}F-FDDNP binding into previously unaffected areas. Global binding DVR value increased in nonconverters by up to 3%. The increases in global DVR values for converters ranged from 5.5% to 11.2% between baseline and the follow-up scan. Another control subject showed increased ^{18}F-FDDNP binding consistent with MCI, but his symptomatology did not reach criteria for AD, although this subject was considered to have *borderline* MCI. Figure 5.5 shows typical patterns of ^{18}F-FDDNP binding observed in this study.

^{18}F-FDDNP PET brain imaging was also expanded to examine prion diseases. In a recent report, PET imaging in two siblings from a family with known mutation of the PRNP gene (6 octapeptide repeat insertion mutation associated with Creutzfeldt-Jakob disease) was reported.[103] Both siblings were already demented at the time of the scans; one of them was scanned with ^{18}F-FDDNP and the other with ^{11}C-PIB. ^{18}F-FDDNP binding was observed in several cortical areas, but not the cerebellum. The level of ^{18}F-FDDNP signal was lower than in AD but higher compared with the control subjects. The ^{11}C-PIB scan was indistinguishable from controls.

^{11}C-6-OH-BTA-1 or ^{11}C-PIB. 2-[(4′-^{11}C-methylamino)phenyl]-6-hydroxy-benzothiazole

PET imaging using a hydroxylated benzothiazole derivative of thioflavin T ^{11}C-2-(4′-(^{11}C-methylaminophenyl)-6-hydroxybenzothiazole (^{11}C-6-OH-BTA, or ^{11}C-PIB), with in vitro affinity for Aβ aggregates in the low nanomolar range, was reported by Klunk et al.[92] In 16 AD subjects, ^{11}C-PIB retention was most prominently increased in frontal cortex and parietal areas and less in lateral temporal cortex. Medial temporal lobe ^{11}C-PIB accumulation was reported to

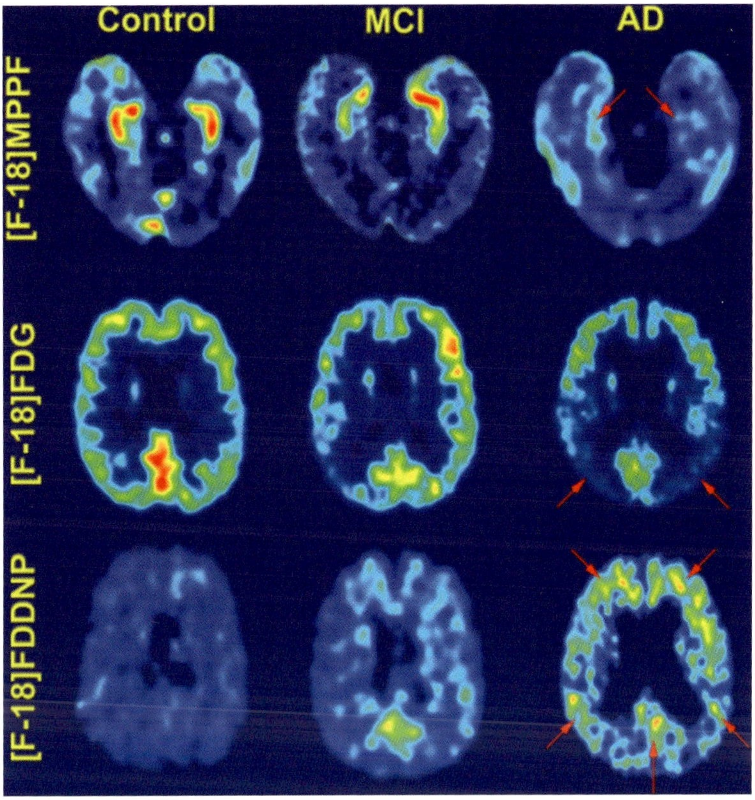

Fig. 5.5 Representative examples of ^{18}F-FDDNP relative distribution volume (DVR) parametric images. ^{18}F-FDDNP DVR parametric images were generated with Logan graphical analysis with cerebellum as reference region. ^{18}F-FDDNP PET detects changes in pathology caused by the disease progression: a control case (*left*) shows uniformly low ^{18}F-FDDNP binding; an MCI (*middle*) shows moderate levels of ^{18}F-FDDNP binding in medial and lateral temporal lobes, posterior cingulate gyrus, and low level of ^{18}F-FDDNP binding in the frontal lobe; an AD (*right*) shows high levels of ^{18}F-FDNP binding throughout the cortex with the most prominent binding in the lateral temporal lobe. Warmer colors represent higher values

be low. The control group consisted of three young subjects (all 21 years) and six older subjects (range, 59–77 years). Control subjects displayed low levels of gray matter binding, with white matter being higher than gray matter. An exception was one older control subject, who displayed elevated signal in a pattern indistinguishable from that seen in subjects with AD. Apart from this subject, no differences resulting from age were observed in the control group in cortex or the pons, which is known to lack Aβ aggregates. The observed increases in ^{11}C-PIB binding in AD patients were inversely correlated with decreases in regional brain glucose utilization observed in those patients.[92] A more recent study on the same 16 subjects from the AD group demonstrated no changes in ^{11}C-PIB accumulation with disease progression, although there was significant ^{18}F-FDG metabolic decline in three AD patients who also experienced cognitive decline.[104] Additional independent clinical ^{11}C-PIB PET studies[85,105–107] have confirmed the initial observations. A study by Mintun et al. in older control subjects (41 subjects) and AD subjects (10 subjects) showed that a global binding measure (mean cortical binding potential, an average of prefrontal cortex, gyrus rectus, lateral temporal, and precuneus regions) was clearly elevated in the AD group (0.633 ± 0.351) compared with older controls (0.098 ± 0.241).[105] Although the group means were well separated, there was one AD subject with very low binding potential value and two normal controls with values and binding patterns similar to those observed in the AD group.

MCI subjects were studied in a ^{11}C-PIB PET imaging study that compared 13 amnestic MCI subjects and 14 control subjects.[106] Region-of-interest-to-cerebellum ratios for frames 60–90 min were used to quantify ^{11}C-PIB binding. In group comparisons, the MCI subjects had 30%–40% higher ^{11}C-PIB signal in frontal, parietal, posterior cingulated, and lateral temporal areas. About half of MCI subjects had cortical signal in the AD range.

A ^{11}C-PIB PET imaging study by Jack et al.[107] of 20 cognitively normal controls, 17 amnestic MCI subjects, and 8 AD subjects also found that the AD group showed significantly higher global binding (ROI-to-cerebellum ratio of 40- to 60-min signal; an average of six cortical regions) compared with control and amnestic MCI groups. The values were 1.1 for normal controls, 1.6 for amnestic MCI subjects, and 2.2 for AD subjects. There was a large variability in the control and MCI groups, so that approximately 20% of control subjects and approximately 50% of MCI subjects had a global ^{11}C-PIB binding value higher than 1.5, which was set as a threshold for detecting AD.

Although ^{11}C-PIB clearly displays cortical binding in AD and separates clinical groups, on an individual level it also reveals some normal controls with AD levels of binding. Whether this represents early pathology has to be tested in longitudinal studies.

^{11}C-BTA-1. 2-[(4'-^{11}C-methylamino)phenyl]benzothiazole

^{11}C-BTA-1 is a derivative of ^{11}C-PIB lacking the 6-hydroxy group, making it less prone to metabolic degradation.[71] One report on PET imaging (one AD subject, and one normal control) was published, finding that ^{11}C-BTA-1 binding was relatively elevated in cortical areas of the AD subject. A larger clinical study, with AD, MCI, and control subjects, will be required to compare this tracer with ^{11}C-PIB.

^{11}C-SB-13. 4-(N-[C-11]methylamino)-4'-hydroxystilbene

^{11}C-SB-13 is a representative of the stilbene family of β-amyloid–specific molecular imaging probes.[93] The binding affinity of this compound to β-amyloid–containing brain homogenates was determined to be 2.4 ± 0.2 nM.[84] Five female AD patients and five female control subjects were scanned with ^{11}C-SB-13 and ^{11}C-PIB. The pattern of ^{11}C-SB-13 binding was very similar to binding observed with ^{11}C-PIB in the same subjects, in frontal, posterior temporal, and inferior parietal cortices. Both tracers separated ADs from controls as well.

^{18}F-BAY94–9172. trans-4-(N-methylamino)-4′-{2-[2-(2–^{18}F-fluoroethoxy)-ethoxy]ethoxystilbene

^{18}F-BAY94–9172 was developed as a radiofluorinated derivative of SB-13 and was reported to have binding $K_i = 6.7 \pm 0.3$ nM for tissue sample from an AD brain.[85,86] Fifteen mild AD subjects, 15 cognitively healthy controls, and 5 subjects with frontotemporal dementia were scanned with ^{18}F-BAY94–9172. Healthy controls and FTD patients generally showed only white matter binding, although three controls and one FTD patient had mild uptake in frontal cortex and precuneus. All AD patients showed widespread neocortical binding, which was greater in the precuneus/posterior cingulate and frontal cortex than in the lateral temporal and parietal cortex. There was relative sparing of sensorimotor, occipital, and medial temporal cortex. The ROI-to-cerebellum ratios were determined for 90–120 min and an average of values from six cortical regions was used as a measure of cortical binding. At 90–120 min after injection, higher neocortical SUVR values were observed in AD patients (2.0 ± 0.3) than healthy controls (1.3 ± 0.2; $P < 0.0001$) or FTD patients (1.2 ± 0.2; $P = 0.009$).

2-(2-[2–^{11}C-Dimethylaminothiazol-5-yl]ethenyl)-6-(2-[fluoro]-ethoxy)benzoxazole (^{11}C-BF-227)

BF-227 was developed as a molecular imaging probe with high affinity (4.3 ± 1.5 nM) for β-amyloid.[77] In its ^{11}C-methylated form it was used for amyloid PET imaging in 10 AD subjects and 11 healthy control subjects. All AD subjects had increased ^{11}C-BF-227 binding in cortical areas when compared with controls.

^{11}C-PIB, ^{18}F-BAY94–9172, and ^{11}C-SB-13 all demonstrated large differences in signal between amyloid-rich and unaffected areas, potentially allowing high sensitivity for detection of changes in pathologically affected areas of the brain. The earliest histologic changes in the AD brain are NFT deposits in the entorhinal cortex and hippocampus, most often without significant presence of β-amyloid deposits in the neocortex; therefore, detection of these changes requires a molecular imaging probe with the capacity to detect increased NFT densities. Finally, the NFT densities in several brain regions (entorhinal cortex, CA1 region of hippocampus, superior temporal cortex) have been repeatedly correlated with neuronal loss in the same regions, and with dementia severity and duration, whereas limited published data describe β-amyloid plaque density correlations with neuronal loss and memory decline.[108]

Imaging of Amyloid Deposits in Animal Models of Alzheimer's Disease

Another application of these tracers has been monitoring effects of emerging therapeutic interventions in animal models of disease.[109] Animal models of brain amyloidosis in AD are used for testing the interventions targeting β-amyloid aggregation. Availability of these models allows preliminary testing of new molecular imaging probes, and validation of their efficacy through comparison with actual levels and distribution of β-amyloid deposits in the brain. ^{18}F-FDDNP has been successfully used for in vivo micro-PET imaging of β-amyloid brain load in triple β-amyloid transgenic rats.[100] Parametric images based on Logan graphical analysis with the cerebellum as the reference region demonstrated that ^{18}F-FDDNP preferentially binds to the β-amyloid rich areas of the rat brain (frontal cortex and hippocampus) when compared with cerebellum, an area almost devoid of any plaques in these animals. In contrast, micro-PET imaging of β-amyloid deposits in Tg2576 β-amyloid transgenic mice[110] or PS1 and PS1/APP β-amyloid transgenic mice[111] with ^{11}C-PIB did not demonstrate ^{11}C-PIB binding in β-amyloid rich areas. One reason for this lack of ^{11}C-PIB binding in transgenic rodents may be the significantly lower number of binding sites for ^{11}C-PIB on β-amyloid fibrillar deposits in the rodent brains compared with β-amyloid fibrillar deposits found in AD patients.[111] More work is required in the future for proper validation of other molecular imaging probes in animal models of AD amyloidosis.

Conclusion

PET in conjunction with a set of molecular imaging probes targeting pathologic aggregates on the one hand and neuronal loss on the other can provide information about very early neurodegeneration that complements the information available from ^{18}F-FDG PET imaging in MCI and dementia. Different aspects of early distribution of pathology in the brain can be imaged with the agents discussed previously. Pyramidal neuronal loss in the medial temporal area can be quantified with ^{18}F-MPPF PET, giving information about an early site of atrophy. There is thus potential for early identification of disease processes using these agents and for monitoring of disease progression or efficacy of experimental therapeutic interventions.

Acknowledgments The authors would like to thank Dr. Linda Ercoli for directing neuropsychological testing and Dr. Prabha Siddarth for performing statistical analyses. Financial support from the Department of Energy (grant DE-FC03–02ER63420) is gratefully acknowledged.

References

1. Minoshima S. Imaging Alzheimer's disease: clinical applications. Neuroimaging Clin North Am 2003;13:769–780.
2. Evans DA. Estimated prevalence of Alzheimer's disease in the United States. Milbank Q 1990;68:267–289.

3. Salmon DP, Lange KL. Cognitive screening and neuropsychological assessment in early Alzheimer's disease. Clin Geriatr Med 2001;17:229–254.
4. Von Strauss EM, Viitane D, De Ronchi D, et al. Aging and the occurrence of dementia. Arch Neurol 1999;56:587–592.
5. Iqbal K. Alzheimer's Disease: Basic Mechanisms, Diagnosis, and Therapeutic Strategies. Chichester: Wiley, 1991.
6. Rice DP, Fillit HM, Max W, et al. Prevalence, costs, and treatment of Alzheimer's disease and related dementia: a managed care perspective. Am J Manag Care 2001;7:809–817.
7. Vickers JC, Dickson TC, Adlard PA, et al. The cause of neuronal degeneration in Alzheimer's disease. Prog Neurobiol 2000;60:139–165.
8. Alzheimer A. Über eine eigenartige Erkrankung der Hirnrinde. Allgem Zeitschr Psychiatrie 1907;64:146–148.
9. Lantos P, Cairns N. The neuropathology of Alzheimer's disease. In:O'Brien J, Ames D, Burns A (eds). Dementia, 2nd ed. London: Arnold, 2000:443–459.
10. Teplow DB. Structural and kinetic features of amyloid beta-protein fibrillogenesis. Amyloid 1998;5:121–142.
11. Selkoe DJ. Cell biology of the amyloid beta-protein precursor and the mechanism of Alzheimer's disease. Annu Rev Cell Biol 1994;10:373–403.
12. Dickson TC, Vickers JC. The morphological phenotype of β-amyloid plaques and associated neuritic changes in Alzheimer's disease. Neuroscience 2001;105:99–107.
13. Wisniewski T, Ghiso J, Frangione B. Biology of Aβ amyloid in Alzheimer's disease. Neurobiol Dis 1997;4:313–328.
14. Lansbury PT. A reductionist view of Alzheimer's disease. Accounts Chem Res 1996;29:317–321.
15. Kirschner DA, Abraham C, Selkoe DJ. X-ray diffraction from intraneuronal paired helical filaments and extraneuronal amyloid fibers in Alzheimer disease indicates cross-beta conformation. Proc Natl Acad Sci USA 1986;83:503–507.
16. Serpell LC. Alzheimer's amyloid fibrils: structure and assembly. Biochim Biophys Acta 2000;1502:16–30.
17. Malinchik SB, Inouye H, Szumowski KE, et al. Structural analysis of Alzheimer's β(1–40) amyloid: protofilament assembly of tubular fibrils. Biophys J 1998;74:537–545.
18. Seilheimer B, Bohrmann B, Nondolfi B, et al. The toxicity of the Alzheimer's beta-amyloid peptide correlates with a distinct fiber morphology. J Struct Biol 1997;119:59–71.
19. Miyakawa T, Katsuragi S, Watanabe K, et al. Ultrastructural studies of amyloid fibrils and senile plaques in human brain. Acta Neuropathol 1986;70:202–208.
20. Kirschner DA, Inouye H, Duffy LK, et al. Synthetic peptide homologous to beta protein from Alzheimer disease forms amyloid-like fibrils *in vitro*. Proc Natl Acad Sci USA 1987;84:6953–6957.
21. Atwood CS, Martins RN, Smith MA, et al. Senile plaque composition and posttranslational modification of amyloid-β peptide and associated proteins. Peptides 2002;23:1343–1350.
22. Lee VM, Goedert M, Trojanowski JQ. Neurodegenerative tauopathies. Annu Rev Neurosci 2001;24:1121–1159.
23. Braak E, Griffing K, Arai K, et al. Neuropathology of Alzheimer's disease: what is new since A. Alzheimer? Eur Arch Psychiatry Clin Neurosci 1999;249(Suppl 3):14–22.
24. Barghorn S, Davies P, Mandelkow E. Tau paired helical filaments from Alzheimer's disease brain and assembled *in vitro* are based on β-structure in the core domain. Biochemistry 2004;43:1694–1703.
25. von Bergen M, Barghorn S, Biernat J, et al. Tau aggregation is driven by a transition from random coil to beta sheet structure. Biochim Biophys Acta 2005;1739:158–166.
26. Mandelkow EM, Mandelkow E. Tau in Alzheimer's disease. Trends Cell Biol 1998;8:425–427.
27. Yen S-H, Liu W-K, Hall FL, et al. Alzheimer neurofibrillary lesions: molecular nature and potential roles of different components. Neurobiol Aging 1995;16:381–387.
28. Braak H, Braak E. Neuropathological staging of Alzheimer-related changes. Acta Neuropathol 1991;82:239–259.

29. Price JL, Morris JC. Tangles and plaques in nondemented aging and "preclinical" Alzheimer's disease. Ann Neurol 1999;45:358–368.
30. Morisson JH, Hof PR. Life and death of neurons in the aging brain. Science 1997;278:412–419.
31. Mann DMA. Pyramidal nerve cell loss in Alzheimer's disease. Neurodegeneration 1996;5:423–427.
32. Hof PR. Morphology and neurochemical characteristics of the vulnerable neurons in brain aging and Alzheimer's disease. Eur Neurol 1997;37:71–81.
33. Bobinski MJ, Wegiel M, Tarnawski M, et al. Relationships between regional neuronal loss and neurofibrillary changes in the hippocampal formation and duration and severity of Alzheimer disease. J Neuropathol Exp Neurol 1997;56:414–420.
34. Gomez-Isla T, Hollister R, West H, et al. Neuronal loss correlates with but exceeds neurofibrillary tangles in Alzheimer's disease. Ann Neurol 1997;41:17–24.
35. Gomez-Isla T, Price JL, McKeel DW, et al. Profound loss of layer II entorhinal cortex neurons distinguishes very mild Alzheimer's disease from nondemented aging. J Neurosci 1996;16:4491–4450.
36. Price JL, Ko AI, Wade MJ, et al. Neuron number in the entorhinal cortex and CA1 in preclinical Alzheimer's disease. Arch Neurol 2001;58:1395–1402.
37. Kordower JH, Chu Y, Stebbins GT, et al. Loss and atrophy of layer II entorhinal cortex neurons in elderly people with mild cognitive impairment. Ann Neurol 2001;49:202–213.
38. West MJ, Coleman PD, Flood DG, et al. Differences in the pattern of hippocampal neuronal loss in normal aging and Alzheimer's disease. Lancet 1994;344:769–772.
39. Fukutani Y, Kobayashi K, Nakamura I, et al. Neurons, intracellular and extracellular neurofibrillary tangles in subdivisions of the hippocampal cortex in normal aging and Alzheimer's disease. Neurosci Lett 1995;200:57–60.
40. Rössler M, Zarski R, Bohl J, et al. Stage-dependent and sector-specific neuronal loss in hippocampus during Alzheimer's disease. Acta Neuropathol 2002;103:363–369.
41. Giannakopoulos P, Herrmann FR, Bussiere T, et al. Tangle and neuron numbers, but not amyloid load, predict cognitive status in Alzheimer's disease. Neurology 2003;60:1495–1500.
42. Delacourte A, David JP, Sergeant N, et al. The biochemical pathway of neurofibrillary degeneration in aging and Alzheimer's disease. Neurology 1999;52:1158–1165.
43. Arnold SE, Hyman BT, Flory J, et al. The topographical and neuroanatomical distribution of neurofibrillary tangles and neuritic plaques in the cerebral cortex of patients with Alzheimer's disease. Cereb Cortex 1991;1:103–116.
44. Price JL, Davies PB, Morris JC, et al. The distribution of tangles, plaques and related immunohistochemical markers in healthy aging and Alzheimer's disease. Neurobiol Aging 1991;12:295–312.
45. Giannakopoulus P, Hof PR, Mottier S, et al. Neuropathological changes in the cerebral cortex of 1258 cases from a geriatric hospital: retrospective clinicopathological evaluation of a 10-year autopsy population. Acta Neuropathol 1994;87:456–468.
46. McKhann G, Drachman D, Folstein M, et al. Clinical diagnosis of Alzheimer's disease: report of the NINCDS-ADRDA Work Group under the auspices of the Department of Health and Human Services Task Force on Alzheimer's Disease. Neurology 1984;34:939–44.
47. Braak H, Braak E. Frequency of stages of Alzheimer-related lesions in different age categories. Neurobiol Aging 1997;18:351–357.
48. Knopman DS, Parisi JE, Salviati A, et al. Neuropathology of cognitively normal elderly. J Neuropathol Exp Neurol 2003;62:1087–1095.
49. Arriagada PV, Marzloff B, Hyman BT. Distribution of Alzheimer-type pathological changes in nondemented elderly individuals matches the pattern in Alzheimer's disease. Neurology 1992;42:1681–1688.
50. Guilloz et AL, Weintraub S, Mash DC, et al. Neurofibrillary tangles, amyloid, and memory in aging and mild cognitive impairment. Arch Neurol 2003;60:729–736.
51. Petersen R, Smith G, Waring S, et al. Mild cognitive impairment: clinical characterization and outcome. Arch Neurol 1999;56:303–308.

52. Petersen RC, Parisi JE, Dickson DW, et al. Neuropathologic features of amnestic mild cognitive impairment. Arch Neurol 2006;63:665–672.
53. Jicha GA, Parisi JE, Dickson DW, et al. Neuropathologic outcome of mild cognitive impairment following progression to clinical dementia. Arch Neurol 2006;63:674–681.
54. Price JL, Ko AI, Wade MJ, et al. Neuron number in the entorhinal cortex and CA1 in preclinical Alzheimer disease. Arch Neurol 2001;58:1395–1402.
55. Silverman DH, Small GW, Chang CY, et al. Positron emission tomography in evaluation of dementia: regional brain metabolism and long-term outcome. JAMA 2001;286:2120–2127.
56. Silverman DH, Truong CT, Kim SK, et al. Prognostic value of regional cerebral metabolism in patients undergoing dementia evaluation: comparison to a quantifying parameter of subsequent cognitive performance and to prognostic assessment without PET. Mol Genet Metab 2003;80:350–355.
57. Reiman EM, Caselli RJ, Yun LS, et al. Preclinical evidence of Alzheimer's disease in persons homozygous for the ε4 allele for apolipoprotein E. N Engl J Med 1996;334:752–758.
58. Minoshima S, Frey KA, Cross DJ, et al. Neurochemical imaging of dementias. Semin Nucl Med 2004;34:70–82.
59. Cohen RM. The application of positron-emitting molecular imaging tracers in Alzheimer's disease. Mol Imaging Biol 2007;9:204–216.
60. Kepe V, Barrio JR, Huang S-C, et al. Serotonin 1A receptors in the living brain of Alzheimer's disease. Proc Natl Acad Sci USA 2006;103:702–707.
61. Palmer AM, Middlemiss DN, Bowen DM. [3H]8-OH-DPAT binding in Alzheimer's disease: an index of pyramidal cell loss? In: Dourish CT, Ahlenius S, Hutson PHet-al., (eds) Brain 5-HT1A Receptors. New York: Ellis Horwood, 1997:286–299.
62. Makin OS, Atkins E, Sikorsky P, et al. Molecular basis for amyloid fibril formation and stability. Proc Natl Acad Sci USA 2005;102:315–320.
63. Shoghi-Jadid K, Barrio JR, Kepe V, et al. Imaging beta-amyloid fibrils in Alzheimer's disease: a critical analysis through simulation of amyloid fibril polymerization. Nucl Med Biol 2005;32:337–351.
64. Shoghi-Jadid K, Barrio JR, Kepe V, et al. Exploring a mathematical model for the kinetics of beta-amyloid molecular imaging probes through a critical analysis of plaque pathology. Mol Imaging Biol 2006;8:151–162.
65. Kurihara A, Pardridge WM. Abeta(1–40) peptide radiopharmaceuticals for brain amyloid imaging: (111)In chelation, conjugation to poly(ethylene glycol)-biotin linkers, and autoradiography with Alzheimer's disease brain sections. Bioconjug Chem 2000;11:380–386.
66. Friedland RP, Majocha RE, Reno JM, et al. Development of an anti-A beta monoclonal antibody for in vivo imaging of amyloid angiopathy in Alzheimer's disease. Mol Neurobiol 1994;9:107–113.
67. Styren SD, Hamilton RL, Styren GC, et al. X-34, a fluorescent derivative of Congo red: a novel histochemical stain for Alzheimer's disease pathology. J Histochem Cytochem 2000;48:1223–1232.
68. Klunk W, Bacskai BJ, Mathis CA, et al. Imaging Aβ plaques in living transgenic mice with multiphoton microscopy and methoxy-X04, a systemically administered Congo Red derivative. J Neuropathol Exp Neurol 2002;61:797–805.
69. Lee C-W, Zhuang Z-P, Kung M-P, et al. Isomerization of (Z,Z) to (E,E)1-bromo-2,5-bis-(3-hydroxycarbonyl-4-hydroxy)styrylbenzene in strong base: probes for amyloid plaques in the brain. J Med Chem 2001;44:2270–2275.
70. Mathis CA, Wang Y, Holt DP, et al. Synthesis and evaluation of 11C-labeled 6-substituted 2-arylbenzothiazoles as amyloid imaging agents. J Med Chem 2003;46:2740–2754.
71. Neumaier B, Deisenhofer S, Fürst D, et al. Radiosynthesis and evaluation of [11C]BTA-1 and [11C]3'-Me-BTA-1 as potential radiotracers for in vivo imaging of β-amyloid plaques. Nuklearmedizin 2007;46:271–280.
72. Kung M-P, Hou C, Zhuang, Z-P, et al. IMPY: an improved thioflavin-T derivative for *in vivo* labeling of β-amyloid plaques. Brain Res 2002;956:202–210.

73. Cai L, Chin FT, Pike VW, et al. Synthesis and evaluation of two 18F-labeled 6-iodo-2-(4′-*N*,*N*-dimethylamino)phenylimidazo[1,2-*a*]pyridine derivatives as prospective radioligands for β-amyloid in Alzheimer's disease. J Med Chem 2004;47:2208–2218.
74. Zeng F, Southerland JA, Voll RJ, et al. Synthesis and evaluation of two ^{18}F-labeled imidazo[1,--*a*]pyridine analogs as potential agents for imaging β-amyloid in Alzheimer's disease. Bioorg Med Chem Lett 2006;16:3015–3018.
75. Ono M, Kawashima H, Nonaka A, et al. Novel benzofuran derivatives for PET imaging of β-amyloid plaques in Alzheimer's disease brains. J Med Chem 2006;49:2725–2730.
76. Zhuang ZP, Kung M-P, Hou C, et al. IBOX(2-(4′-dimethylaminophenyl)-6-iodobenzoxazole): a ligand imaging amyloid plaques in the brain. Nucl Med Biol 2001;28:887–894.
77. Kudo Y, Okamura N, Furumoto S, et al. 2-(2-[2-Dimethylaminothiazol-5-yl]ethenyl)-6-(2-[fluoro]ethoxy)benzoxazole: a novel PET agent for in vivo detection of dense amyloid plaques in Alzheimer's disease patients. J Nucl Med 2007;48:553–561.
78. Okamura N, Suemoto T, Shimadzu H, et al. Styrylbenzoxazole derivatives for *in vivo* imaging of amyloid plaques in the brain. J Neurosci 2004;24:2535–2541.
79. Suemoto T, Okamura N, Shiomitsu T, et al. In vivo labeling of amyloid with BF-108. Neurosci Res 2004;48:65–74.
80. Chandra R, Kung M-P, Kung HK. Design, synthesis, and structure-activity relationship of novel thiophene derivatives for β-amyloid plaque imaging. Bioorg Med Chem Lett 2006;16:1350–1352.
81. Ono M, Yoshida N, Ishibashi K, et al. Radioiodinated flavones for in vivo imaging of β-amyloid plaques in the brain. J Med Chem 2005;48:7253–7260.
82. Ono M, Maya Y, Haratake M, et al. Aurones serve as probes of β-amyloid plaques in Alzheimer's disease. Biochem Biophys Res Comm 2007;361:116–121.
83. Lee C-W, Kung M-P, Hou C, et al. Dimethylamino-fluorenes: ligands for detecting β-amyloid plaques in the brain. Nucl Med Biol 2003;30:573–580.
84. Ono M, Wilson A, Nobrega J, et al. 11C-labeled stilbene derivatives as Aβ-aggregate-specific PET imaging agents for Alzheimer's disease. Nucl Med Biol 2003;30:565–571.
85. Rowe CC, Ackerman U, Browne W, et al. Imaging of amyloid β in Alzheimer's disease with 18F-BAY94–9172, a novel PET tracer: proof of mechanism. Lancet Neurol 2008;7:129–135.
86. Zhang W, Oya S, Kung M-P, et al. F-18 stilbenes as imaging agents for detecting β-amyloid plaques in the brain. J Med Chem 2005;48:5980–5988.
87. Zhang W, Oya S, Kung M-P, et al. F-18 Polyethylene glycol stilbenes as PET imaging agents targeting Aβ aggregates in the brain. Nucl Med Biol 2005;32:799–809.
88. Zhuang Z-P, Kung M-P, Kung HF. Synthesis of biphenyltrienes as probes for β-amyloid plaques. J Med Chem 2006;49:2841–2844.
89. Agdeppa ED, Kepe V, Liu J, et al. 2-Dialkylamino-6-acylmalononitrile substituted naphthalenes (DDNP Analogs): novel diagnostic and therapeutic tools in Alzheimer's disease. Mol Imaging Biol 2003;4:404–417.
90. Okamura N, Suemoto T, Furumoto S, et al. Quinoline and benzimidazole derivatives: candidate probes for in vivo imaging of tau pathology in Alzheimer's disease. J Neurosci 2005;25:10857–10862.
91. Small GW, Kepe V, Ercoli L, et al. FDDNP-PET scanning of cerebral amyloid and tau deposits in MCI. N Engl J Med 2006;355:2652–2663.
92. Klunk WE, Engler H, Nordberg A, et al. Imaging brain amyloid in Alzheimer's disease with Pittsburgh Compound-B. Ann Neurol 2004;55:306–319.
93. Verhoeff NP, Wilson AA, Takeshita S, et al. *In vivo* imaging of Alzheimer disease beta-amyloid with [11C]SB-13 PET. Am J Geriatr Psychiatry 2004;12:584–595.
94. Newberg AB, Wintering NA, Plössl K, et al. Safety, biodistribution and dosimetry of 123I-IMPY: a novel amyloid plaque-imaging agent for the diagnosis of Alzheimer's disease. J Nucl Med 2006;47; 748–754.
95. Shoghi-Jadid K, Small GW, Agdeppa ED, et al. Localization of neurofibrillary tangles and beta-amyloid plaques in the brains of living patients with Alzheimer disease. Am J Geriatr Psychiatry 2002;10:24–35.

96. Barrio JR, Huang S-C, Cole G, et al. PET imaging of tangles and plaques in Alzheimer disease with a highly hydrophobic probe. J Label Compd Radiopharm 1999;42(Suppl 1):S194–S195.
97. Agdeppa ED, Kepe V, Shoghi-Jadid K, et al. *In vivo* and *in vitro* labeling of plaques and tangles in the brain of an Alzheimer's disease patient: a case study. J Nucl Med 2001;42(Suppl):65P.
98. Agdeppa ED, Kepe V, Liu J, et-al. Binding characteristics of radiofluorinated 6-dialkylamino-2-naphthylethylidene derivatives as positron emission tomography imaging probes for β-amyloid plaques in Alzheimer's disease. J Neurosci 2001;21:RC189 (1–5).
99. Agdeppa ED, Kepe V, Petri A, et al. *In vitro* detection of (S)-naproxen and ibuprofen binding to plaques in the Alzheimer's brain using the positron emission tomography molecular imaging probe 2-(1-[6-[(2-[(18)F]fluoroethyl)(methyl)amino]-2-naphthyl]ethylidene) malononitrile. Neuroscience 2003;117:723–730.
100. Kepe V, Cole GM, Liu J, et al. [F-18]MicroPET imaging of β-amyloid deposits in the living brain of triple transgenic rat model of β-amyloid deposition. Mol Imaging Biol 2005;7:105.
101. Smid LM, Vovko TD, Popovic M, et al. The 2,6-disubstituted naphthalene derivative FDDNP labeling reliably predicts Congo red birefringence of protein deposits in brain sections of selected human neurodegenerative diseases. Brain Pathol 2006;16:124–130.
102. Bresjanac M, Smid LM, Vovko TD, et al. Molecular imaging probe 2-(1-{6-[(2-fluoroethyl) (methyl)amino]-2-naphthyl}-ethylidene)malononitrile labels prion plaques *in vitro*. J Neurosci 2003;23:8029–8033.
103. Boxer AL, Rabinovici GD, Kepe V, et al. Amyloid imaging in distinguishing atypical prion disease from Alzheimer disease. Neurology 2007;69:283–290.
104. Engler H, Forsberg A, Almkvist O, et al. Two-year follow-up of amyloid deposition in patients with Alzheimer's disease. Brain 2006;129:2856–2866.
105. Mintun MA, Larossa GN, Sheline YI, et al. [11C]PIB in a nondemented population: potential antecedent marker of Alzheimer disease. Neurology 2006;67:446–452.
106. Kemppainen NM, Aalto S, Wilson IA, et al. PET amyloid ligand [11C]PIB uptake is increased in mild cognitive impairment. Neurology 2007;68:1603–1606.
107. Jack CR Jr, Lowe VJ, Senjem ML, et al. ^{11}C PiB and structural MRI provide complementary information in imaging of Alzheimer's disease and amnestic mild cognitive impairment. Brain 2008;131:665–680.
108. Cummings BJ, Pike CJ, Shankle R, et al. Beta-amyloid deposition and other measures of neuropathology predict cognitive status in Alzheimer's disease. Neurobiol Aging 1996;17:921–933.
109. Sadowski M, Wisniewski T. Disease modifying approaches for Alzheimer's pathology. Curr Pharm Des 2007;13:1943–1954.
110. Toyama H, Ye D, Ichise M, et al. PET imaging of brain with β-amyloid probe, [11C]6-OH-BTA-1, in a transgenic mouse model of Alzheimer's disease. Eur J Nucl Med Mol Imaging 2005;32:593–600.
111. Klunk WE, Lopresti BJ, Ikonomovic MD, et al. Binding of the positron emission tracer Pittsburgh compound-B reflects the amount of amyloid-β in Alzheimer's disease brain but not in transgenic mouse brain. J Neurosci 2005;25:10598–10606.

Chapter 6
Amyloid Imaging with PET in Alzheimer's Disease, Mild Cognitive Impairment, and Clinically Unimpaired Subjects

William E. Klunk, Chester A. Mathis, Julie C. Price, Steven T. DeKosky, Brian J. Lopresti, Nicholas D. Tsopelas, Judith A. Saxton, and Robert D. Nebes

Public Health Impact

Since 1900, the percentage of Americans aged 65 or over has more than tripled (4.1% in 1900 to 12.4% in 2000), and the number has increased 11 times (from 3.1 to 35.0 million). The older population itself is getting older. In 2000, the 65–74 age group (18.4 million) was eight times larger than in 1900, but the 75–84 age group (12.4 million) was 16 times larger, and the 85 and older group (4.2 million) was 34 times larger. Although aging is the major risk factor for Alzheimer's disease (AD), most elderly do not meet clinical criteria for either dementia or mild cognitive impairment (MCI; see following discussion). In this chapter, we refer to these subjects as *clinically unimpaired*. Although they do not have AD or MCI, many clinically unimpaired elderly show decrements in cognitive performance in comparison with the young. Furthermore, a percentage of clinically unimpaired elderly (particularly those over 75 years) is found to have AD pathology after death; this has been termed *pathologic aging*.[1] These findings raise obvious questions: (1) Can we determine if the age-related cognitive decrements commonly found in clinically unimpaired elderly relate to the presence of varying amounts of amyloid pathology in these individuals? (2) Does the presence of amyloid pathology in clinically unimpaired elderly identify those who will develop a clinical diagnosis of AD? Determination of the nature, cause, and outcome of decreased cognitive performance in these elderly will be an essential component to improving the quality of life of our aging population.

Disclosure: GE Healthcare holds a license agreement with the University of Pittsburgh based on the technology described in this manuscript. Drs. Klunk and Mathis are co-inventors of PiB and, as such, have a financial interest in this license agreement.

D.H.S. Silverman (ed.), *PET in the Evaluation of Alzheimer's Disease and Related Disorders*, 119
DOI: 10.1007/978-0-387-76420-7_6, © Springer Science+Business Media, LLC 2009

Amyloid Imaging in Clinically Unimpaired Elderly

The finding of postmortem amyloid plaque deposition in the brains of individuals in whom the *absence* of clinical AD was well documented prior to their death[1] has been interpreted to both support[2] and refute[3] the hypothesis that deposition of beta-amyloid (β-amyloid) protein in the brain is the cause of AD.[4] This wide range of interpretations exists partly because of the lack of in vivo longitudinal data on the natural history of amyloid deposition. Such data could clarify whether cognitively normal individuals with brain amyloid deposition are destined to develop clinical dementia.

A current goal of several groups is to assess the in vivo prevalence of brain amyloid deposition in cognitively normal elderly subjects who do not meet clinical criteria for MCI or AD (i.e., clinically unimpaired). Although these elderly subjects do not meet clinical diagnostic criteria for cognitive impairment, previous studies have shown that a high percentage of these elderly have cognitive performance below that of young subjects with equal education (Fig. 6.1a).[5] We refer to these subjects as *low-normal performers* (Fig. 6.1a). It is important to assess whether in vivo evidence of amyloid deposition is associated with cognitive performance in the lower end of this normal range (i.e., being a low-normal performer; Fig. 6.1a). With increasing age, the cognitive performance of many individuals declines while still not meeting criteria for MCI or AD (i.e., cognitive decline below the threshold of clinical impairment). It also is important to assess whether evidence of amyloid deposition is associated with greater decrements in cognitive performance that could ultimately lead to conversion to MCI or AD over time (Fig. 6.1b).

Three fundamental questions can be addressed in amyloid imaging studies of clinically unimpaired elderly:

1. How common is amyloid deposition in clinically unimpaired elderly?
2. Is the greater variability of cognitive performance in the clinically unimpaired elderly (compared with the young) explained by the presence or absence of amyloid deposition?
3. Will clinically unimpaired elderly who have evidence of amyloid deposition invariably progress to a clinical diagnosis of MCI or AD within some reasonable amount of time?

Postmortem examinations of the brain have provided some insight to these questions. Autopsy studies suggest that the prevalence of amyloid deposition in nondemented elderly over the age of 75 is 40%–70%, with over 25% having amounts of amyloid typical of those seen in AD.[1,6,7] The correlation of amyloid deposition at autopsy with cognitive decline before death is controversial, and there are studies supporting both the presence[7] and absence[2] of this correlation. Despite the fact that some more recent postmortem studies have done well to minimize the sources of uncertainity,[2,7] the first two questions are difficult to fully answer with autopsy studies alone, because of the variable time lag between cognitive testing and death, and

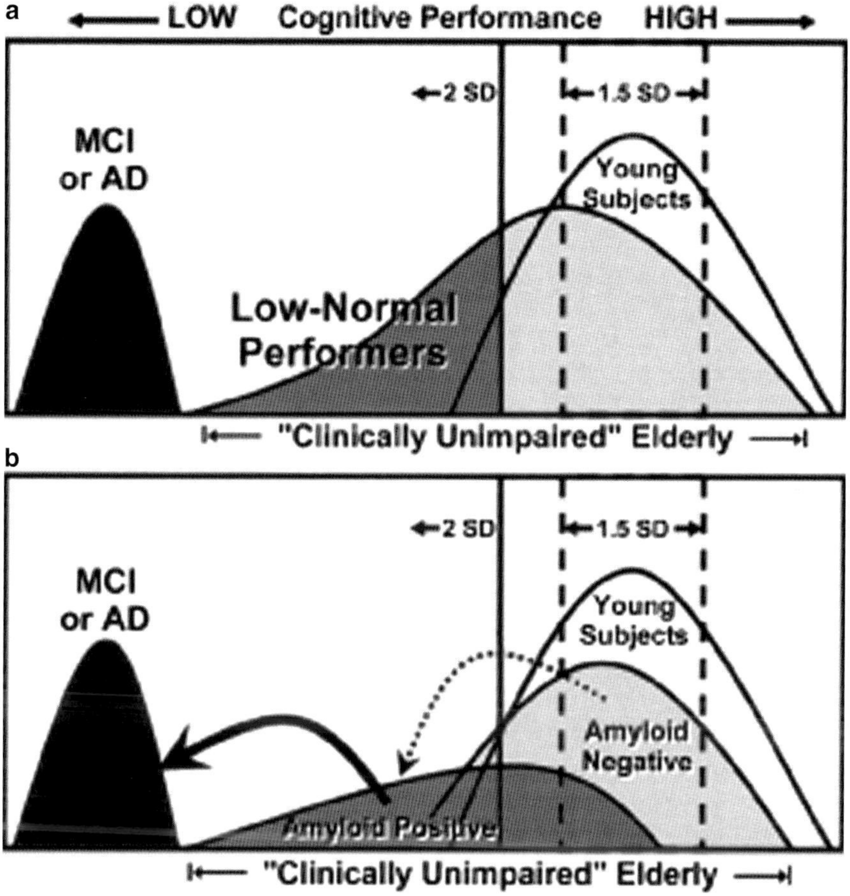

Fig. 6.1 Schematic of the distribution of cognitive performance measures in young subjects, *clinically unimpaired* elderly, and clinically affected individuals who meet criteria for mild cognitive impairment (MCI) or Alzheimer's disease (AD). **A.** Clinically unimpaired elderly show increased variability compared with young subjects, skewed toward poorer performance, but not reaching clinical criteria for MCI or AD. **B.** We hypothesize that much of the poorer performance of the elderly is explained by a subset who have amyloid deposition and that this amyloid-positive subset contains those individuals who may convert to MCI or AD over time (i.e., amyloid-negative subjects will become amyloid-positive before converting to MCI or AD)

the possible effect of the disease that ultimately led to death on cognition. By its nature, the third question cannot be addressed with an autopsy study, and a clear answer to this question will require a longitudinal study of individual subjects. This chapter explores amyloid imaging in MCI and dementia, with a special emphasis on the issues relating to amyloid imaging in clinically unimpaired elderly.

Role of Beta-Amyloid in the Pathophysiology and Treatment of Alzheimer's Disease

Amyloid-Beta and the Neuropathology of Alzheimer's Disease

Definitive diagnosis of AD relies on the demonstration of amyloid plaques and neurofibrillary tangles (NFTs) at autopsy.[8] Amyloid plaques are composed of 40–42 amino acid β-amyloid peptides.[9] NFTs are mainly composed of a hyperphosphorylated form of the microtubule-associated protein, tau.[10] Amyloid plaques occur earliest in the neocortex, where they are relatively evenly distributed.[11] Tangles appear first in limbic areas such as the transentorhinal cortex and progress in a predictable topographic pattern to the neocortex.[12,13] Arnold et al.[14] mapped the distribution of NFT and neuritic plaques (amyloid plaques surrounded by dystrophic neurites) in the brains of patients with AD. Compared with NFTs, neuritic plaques were generally more evenly distributed throughout the cortex, with the exceptions of notably fewer neuritic plaques in limbic periallocortex and allocortex (the areas with greatest NFT density). The cerebellum is notably free of neuritic plaques in AD, although diffuse amyloid deposits that do not label with fibrillar dyes such as Congo red are commonly observed in the cerebellum.[15,16]

Central Role of Amyloid-Beta in the Pathophysiology of Alzheimer's Disease

A growing consensus points to deposition of β-amyloid plaques as a central event in the pathogenesis of AD. This "amyloid cascade hypothesis" [4] states that the overproduction of β-amyloid, or the failure to clear β-amyloid, leads to AD primarily through β-amyloid deposition, which produces NFTs, inflammation, cell death, and ultimately the clinical symptoms such as memory impairment.[17] The single most important piece of evidence for the amyloid cascade hypothesis of AD is the demonstration that several different mutations in the β-amyloid precursor protein (APP) gene on chromosome 21, all lying in or near the β-amyloid peptide region, cause early onset AD.[17–19] Further genetic support for the amyloid cascade hypothesis comes from the finding that the most common form of early onset familial autosomal dominant disease (chromosome 14 mutations) is caused by mutations in the presenilin-1 (PS1) gene, which codes for a protein that is strongly implicated to be an essential component of the γ-secretase enzyme complex responsible for C-terminal cleavage of β-amyloid from APP.[20] Evidence is accumulating to suggest that small, soluble oligomers may be the most toxic species of β-amyloid in the human brain[21,22] and have been reported to cause memory deficits in experimental models.[23] However, for soluble β-amyloid oligomers to be removed from the extracellular space, it is likely that plaques also will have to be removed because they serve as a source of soluble β-amyloid. In AD brain, soluble forms of β-amyloid make up less than 1% of total brain β-amyloid.[4] Soluble and insoluble β-amyloid pools are in equilibrium, as supported by the fact that immunization of β-amyloid–depositing transgenic mice in a manner that produces antibodies specific for oligomeric β-amyloid leads to both marked reduction of oligomeric forms of β-amyloid and clearance of thioflavin-S positive plaque (i.e., fibrillar) forms of β-amyloid.[25,26] This suggests that any meaningful antiamyloid therapy will need to have a significant impact on insoluble brain β-amyloid deposits for there to be a long-lasting lowering of soluble β-amyloid. Such an effect should be detectable with agents that bind to fibrillar β-amyloid.

Amyloid-Beta Synthesis and Clearance as a Therapeutic Target

The metabolism of β-amyloid has become an important therapeutic target in AD research. A corollary of the amyloid cascade hypothesis is that prevention of β-amyloid accumulation in oligomers or plaques should prevent AD. Approaches to antiamyloid therapy have focused on both decreasing production and increasing clearance of β-amyloid. Attempts to decrease β-amyloid production involve inhibition of two distinct *secretase* enzymes responsible for cleavage of β-amyloid from its much larger precursor protein.[27] The β-secretase or β-amyloid cleaving enzyme (BACE) cleaves the N-terminus of β-amyloid and the γ-secretase enzyme complex cleaves the C-terminus.[28] Studies with transgenic mice that deposit β-amyloid plaques in their brain have shown that γ-secretase inhibitors can prevent amyloid deposition.[29]

Both β- and γ-secretase have proved to be difficult drug targets. γ-Secretase knockout mice are not viable. Inhibition of γ-secretase not only reduces the processing of APP to β-amyloid, but also reduces the processing of other γ-secretase substrates. The most important of the non-APP substrates appears to be Notch, a protein critical in cell proliferation and differentiation. Alteration of Notch metabolism produces marked gastrointestinal toxicity and reduced hematopoiesis in animals. Efforts are being made to develop γ-secretase inhibitors that have selectivity for APP processing over Notch, and some progress has been reported.[30] BACE-knockout mice are viable and appear to develop normally, making BACE look like the preferred secretase drug target.[31] However, BACE has proved difficult to inhibit potently with small molecules. This has been thought to be caused by the large catalytic site responsible for BACE cleavage of APP.[32,33] Despite the problems, progress toward human therapy has been made. Phase I human studies with γ-secretase inhibitors have been initiated.[34]

A second antiamyloid approach makes use of immunotherapy against β-amyloid. It is believed that this approach lowers β-amyloid levels by augmenting clearance of β-amyloid. The first iteration of the immunotherapeutic approach in clinical trials involved active immunization with β-amyloid 42 itself, along with an immunogenic adjuvant (QS-21). The combination of β-amyloid antigen and adjuvant was named AN-1792. Unfortunately, this AN-1792 trial was suspended because of a 6% incidence of a serious adverse event of meningoencephalitis[35,36] that may be related to the presence of cerebral amyloid angiopathy.[37] A report on a subset of patients suggested that successful immunization to β-amyloid slows cognitive decline,[38] but the results from the larger cohort showed a modest clinical effect.[36] The effects did seem related to the strength of the antibody response.[36] Surprisingly, high antibody titer also was linked to increased atrophy on magnetic resonance imaging, a finding that remains unexplained.[39] In addition to the clinical and imaging outcomes, key neuropathologic findings were reported in three autopsy cases from this AN-1792 trial. All three cases, one of which had no encephalitis, showed marked focal reduction of β-amyloid deposition,[40–42] providing proof-of-concept evidence that β-amyloid clearance can indeed occur in humans with AD. This has prompted more intense interest in further refinements of the immunotherapeutic antiamyloid approach such as passive immunization with anti-β-amyloid antibodies.[43,44] Such strategies may avoid many untoward effects of active immunization, including meningoencephalitis, although there has been a caution to the contrary.[45]

The Role of Amyloid Imaging

Rationale for Studying Amyloid Deposition in Mild Cognitive Impairment

MCI is a condition closely related to AD, being characterized by either isolated memory impairment or impairment in several cognitive domains, but not of sufficient severity to meet diagnostic criteria for AD.[46] Like AD, MCI is common, and the prevalence increases with age. In community samples, over 19% of subjects under age 75 and over 29% of subjects over age 85 were found to meet criteria for MCI.[47] MCI patients convert to AD at a rate of about 10%–15% per year,[48] and MCI may define a prodromal phase of AD.[49–51] Thus, in vivo identification of amyloid deposition in AD and MCI may have important implications for early diagnosis. The ability to follow an in vivo surrogate marker of amyloid deposition also may be critical to the timely development of the new antiamyloid therapies.

Rationale for Relating Amyloid Deposition and Cognition in Normal Aging

The rationale for studying amyloid deposition in normal aging, although perhaps less obvious, is equally important. At least three reasons exist to relate cognition and amyloid deposition in clinically unimpaired elderly: (1) definition of the prevalence of amyloid in clinically unimpaired elderly; (2) determination of how much of the greater variability of cognitive performance in the clinically unimpaired elderly (compared with the young) can be explained by the presence or absence of amyloid deposition; and (3) assessment of whether clinically unimpaired individuals with substantial amyloid deposition will invariably progress to clinical dementia.

Studies have attempted to address the first two questions with postmortem assessment of amyloid deposition, but there are obvious weaknesses to this approach. First, it is difficult to acquire cognitive testing close to the time of death, when the amyloid assessment is made. The time period between the last cognitive testing and death can vary by years in some studies. Even cognitive testing that occurs close to the time of death is problematic since any cognitive impairment present could be a result of the effects of the disease that led to the individual's death. Second, there is an additional selection bias added by the decision to agree to autopsy. This means that not all of the cognitively assessed group will be represented in the postmortem amyloid assessment. Finally, many of these studies involve cognitive testing that was not performed for the specific purposes of the study, but was gathered retrospectively as well. Frequently, the cognitive data available come from a simple cognitive screening tests such as the Mini Mental State Examination (MMSE)[52] and not measures that examine the specific components of cognition thought to be particularly affected by aging (e.g., information processing speed, working memory, inhibitory efficiency). Even when longitudinal data on cognitive performance are available,[53,54] it is not possible to link an age-related decrease in cognitive performance to a longitudinal increase in amyloid load (i.e., to establish causality) because amyloid load generally could only be determined at one time point—after death. All of these factors have hindered attempts to determine the role that amyloid deposition may play in the various cognitive decrements found. The ability to measure amyloid load at multiple time points in living individuals who are not close to death could be of great value.

Concept of Cognitive Reserve and Implications for Amyloid Imaging in Normal Aging

Increasing evidence suggests that individual characteristics such as premorbid intelligence and educational background have a major impact on the cognitive consequences of neuropathology. Individuals with greater premorbid intelligence and higher educational background are less sensitive to the initial effects of neuropathologic conditions such as AD.[55,56] This effect has been conceptualized as reflecting *cognitive reserve* or *brain reserve*, i.e., because of environmental enrichment, genetic endowment, or both, certain individuals have an elevated threshold for exhibiting the cognitive symptoms associated with neurologic disease.[57,58] For example, Bennett et al.[59] related the severity of senile plaques and NFTs present at autopsy to cognitive performance before death. They found that educational level moderated the cognitive effects of AD pathology such that more educated individuals showed less cognitive impairment per unit of AD pathology than did less educated persons. An in vivo study of AD subjects found a more advanced parieto-temporal blood flow deficit in highly educated subjects,[60] again suggesting that greater brain pathology is necessary to produce cognitive decrements (and perhaps onset of clinical symptoms) in highly educated individuals. Although the two previous studies looked at only AD patients, a third study focused on clinically unimpaired subjects and found increased cortical atrophy in clinically unimpaired subjects having higher education.[61] Once again, this suggests that highly educated individuals can maintain normal cognitive functioning despite a level of brain pathology that may produce symptoms in a less educated group. Results such as these require that one takes into account the premorbid intelligence and educational background (i.e., the brain reserve) of the subject when examining the relation of cognitive performance to brain pathology.

The concept of cognitive reserve has both positive and negative implications. It is certainly a positive feature that individuals with higher cognitive reserve might escape the symptoms of AD for a longer period of time. Given that AD normally occurs so late in life, this may allow these individuals to live out their normal lifespan without ever experiencing symptoms that an equivalent degree of brain pathology might cause in other individuals. On the negative side, these findings suggest that the pathology of AD would have an opportunity to become better established in individuals with greater cognitive reserve before the presence of this pathology can be detected. With the presently available treatment options, the implications of this are questionable. However, should an effective disease-modifying treatment such as an antiamyloid therapy become available, it is highly likely that such a treatment will be most effective early in the pathologic process before an extensive cascade of destruction has been established.

With respect to amyloid imaging, the notion of cognitive reserve is pertinent in at least two ways. First, as the studies of brain perfusion and atrophy described previously have reported, in a population of clinically unimpaired older individuals, we might expect to find the most amyloid pathology in those with the highest cognitive reserve (i.e., the most intelligent and highly educated). This is because a higher percentage of those individuals with the same level of detectable AD pathology but having lower premorbid cognitive reserve would already have become symptomatic and thus would not be found among the clinically unimpaired group. Second, the development of an effective disease-modifying therapy will make the detection of preclinical AD perhaps even more important to those with a higher cognitive reserve since they may not have a window of optimal treatment still available after the onset of their symptoms.

Postmortem Insights into Amyloid Pathology in Normal Aging

Prevalence and Degree of Amyloid Deposition in Normal Aging

The first reason to study in vivo amyloid deposition in normal aging is to define the prevalence of amyloid deposition in a normal elderly population. This is difficult to obtain with an autopsy study because of the reasons noted previously.

Preliminary findings from the *Nun Study* suggest that the prevalence of amyloid deposits in clinically unimpaired elderly may be on the order of 40% and that the presence of amyloid correlated with lower scores on several neuropsychological tests of memory function.[7] The ability to assess amyloid deposition in living subjects avoids these difficulties by: (1) allowing precise and detailed definition of cognitive function in healthy individuals within days of the assessment of amyloid deposition; and (2) not requiring a subsequent decision for autopsy, which may add a selection bias over and above that incurred in the selection of the group to be cognitively tested.

Price and Morris[6] have compiled one of the most extensively evaluated groups of clinically unimpaired and very mildly demented subjects clinically evaluated within a year before their death. Similar findings have been reported by Haroutunian et al.[62] These studies provide evidence that substantial amyloid deposition occurs in normal aging. Price and Morris reported the neuropathologic findings in 39 clinically unimpaired elderly subjects aged 51–93 and 15 very mildly demented subjects aged 75–95 and compared these with severely demented AD cases. Price and Morris found that all 13 clinically unimpaired cases under the age of 75 had no plaques whether examined with a sensitive modification of the Bielschowsky stain or with immunohistochemical stains for β-amyloid. The 26 clinically unimpaired cases over age 75 fell into three categories, unrelated to age. In eight subjects, aged 75–88, no plaques could be detected in any region. In 11 of 26 subjects aged 75–92, there were a very low number of plaques (approximately 2/mm^2), all of which were diffuse plaques. In 7 of 26 (27%) clinically unimpaired cases aged 75–93, there were more numerous plaques, and many were neuritic. Thus, 18 of 26 (69%) subjects over age 75 had some evidence of amyloid deposition and over 25% had amyloid deposition typical of AD. Very mildly demented patients showed numbers of plaques that were surprisingly similar to severely demented AD patients, although the type of plaques changed so that most plaques in severely demented patients were neuritic or cored. A corollary to the observation that patients at the threshold for clinical detection of AD (CDR = 0.5) already have extensive neuropathologic changes is the hypothesis that the pathologic process of AD must begin significantly before any cognitive change can be clinically detected; thus, Price and Morris hypothesized that the seven clinically unimpaired cases with numerous plaques may have been preclinical AD.[49,63] The availability of in vivo amyloid imaging probes such as those described in this chapter would make possible longitudinal imaging studies to test this hypothesis.

Further evidence for preclinical amyloid deposition comes from the study of Down syndrome patients. Having three copies of the β-amyloid precursor protein gene on chromosome 21, all Down syndrome patients develop amyloid pathology by their forties (many develop deposits earlier), and a large percentage show clinical dementia. Although the time course of amyloid deposition in AD is not known, evidence gained through postmortem study of Down syndrome subjects suggests that amyloid deposition begins over a decade prior to the clinical symptoms of dementia.[64,65]

Relationship of Amyloid Deposition to Age-Related Declines in Cognitive Performance

Identification of amyloid in normal elderly can address an important question regarding whether the greater variability of cognitive performance in the clinically unimpaired elderly (compared with the young) can be explained by the presence or absence of amyloid deposition, as is suggested by some postmortem studies.[7] With increasing age, cognitive performance tends to decline in persons who have no obvious neurologic or psychiatric illness—the *normal* old. However, the amount of age-related cognitive performance decline is not uniform across individuals; there is substantial intersubject variability,[5,66] especially at the lower end of the performance range. Thus, some older persons experience much greater age-related cognitive dysfunction than do others. This rise in intersubject variability could reflect the increased prevalence, in the older population, of individuals carrying significant cerebral amyloid loads. Even clinically unimpaired individuals have been shown to have a substantial number of amyloid plaques within their brain[2,67] and the prevalence of these plaques increases with age.[6,68]

The role that amyloid plays in producing age-related cognitive impairment in clinically unimpaired older persons is controversial. It is not clear that the amyloid found at autopsy in clinically unimpaired individuals has any relationship to the cognitive performance of these individuals. The few studies that have examined the relation of cognitive performance to the postmortem presence of amyloid in nondemented older individuals have produced conflicting conclusions. Several studies have used pathologic criteria to characterize small groups of clinically unimpaired individuals as having pathologically normal brains or brains with signs of preclinical AD (increased number of diffuse and neuritic plaques and NFTs). Hulette et al.[67] found that neuritic plaques were relatively common in clinically unimpaired individuals, and those who had them showed a tendency to perform more poorly on measures of memory and *executive* function than those without amyloid deposits in their brains. Green et al.[54] found that among 19 very old nondemented individuals who came to autopsy, those who had shown some cognitive performance decline (but not dementia) prior to death showed pathologic signs of AD, including plaques, whereas those whose cognitive status remained stable did not. By contrast, Goldman et al.[2] and Davis et al.[53] found no evidence that nondemented individuals with increased numbers of plaques showed poorer performance or a faster decline in performance than did individuals without plaques.

Information about the cognitive effects of amyloid deposition is important to our understanding of the cognitive changes that often occur during the normal aging process. It is possible that the research studies that have contributed to our present knowledge of the cognitive changes associated with normal aging have within their cohorts individuals with a substantial amyloid burden. Thus, our understanding of both the nature and severity of the cognitive decrements associated with normal aging may be distorted by the effects of a pathologic accumulation of amyloid in a subset of the population. If it turns out that part of the cognitive impairment currently thought to be intrinsic to normal aging actually relates to amyloid deposition, this raises the question as to the nature and amount of cognitive dysfunction present in older individuals without elevated amyloid levels. The availability of amyloid imaging allows this question to be examined directly. It also allows extensive longitudinal cognitive testing with much more assurance that serial measures of amyloid load will be available for correlation to the cognitive findings. This will be crucial for examining whether a longitudinal increase in amyloid eventually leads to MCI or AD. If antiamyloid therapies do become clinically available, we will need to know if clinically unimpaired individuals with evidence of a progressive amyloid deposition should be identified and treated.

Do Clinically Unimpaired Individuals with Amyloid Deposition Always Progress to Dementia?

The third reason for studying amyloid deposition in *normal* elderly is that we do not yet know whether all those who have substantial amyloid deposition without clinical symptoms of AD will eventually develop clinical AD if they survive for a reasonable period of time (e.g., 10 years). Some investigators have stated that amyloid deposition is responsible for the cognitive impairments seen in AD and that any older individuals with substantial amounts of brain amyloid, even if they presently score in the normal range on cognitive tasks, have preclinical AD.[49,50,63] Although there is evidence to support this notion, until now we have not had a tool that would allow the longitudinal studies necessary to test this hypothesis effectively.

Development of Amyloid Imaging Technologies

Preclinical Development

Establishing a post hoc reconstruction of the natural history of amyloid deposition had long been a goal of postmortem studies, but translation of this goal to in vivo human studies awaited the development of a suitable noninvasive technology suited to this purpose. For well over a decade, our laboratory has been interested in the development of a noninvasive method for direct and quantitative assessment of amyloid deposition in living subjects.[69–71] A number of other groups also have worked to develop radiolabeled amyloid-specific imaging agents, but early efforts were limited by poor brain entry, high levels of nonspecific binding, or low levels of specific binding in brain regions known to contain high concentrations of β-amyloid. Most groups used dyes known to bind amyloid deposits in postmortem tissue as the starting point. We reported that Crystamine G (CG), a lipophilic analog of the amyloid dye Congo red, possessed high affinity for β-amyloid fibrils and plaques,[72] but the penetration of an ^{125}I-labeled CG derivative into normal rat brain was low.[73] Similar results were reported using a ^{99m}Tc-labeled CG derivative.[74] More chemically distant analogs of CG composed of styrylbenzene salicylic acids, such as X-34, had high in vitro binding affinity to aggregated β-amyloid but low brain penetration in normal rodent brain.[75–77] Further modification of the structure by removing the carboxylic acid groups to provide Methoxy-X04 resulted in improved brain entry, but not to the degree typically necessary to provide a good noninvasive PET imaging agent.[76] To overcome the low brain penetration of the styrylbenzenes, we developed neutral carbon-11-labeled derivatives of another amyloid dye, thioflavin-T. Modification of the amyloid-binding histologic dye, thioflavin-T, led to the finding that neutral benzothiazole-anilines (BTAs) bound to amyloid with high affinity and crossed the blood–brain barrier very well.[78] The basic properties of the prototypical benzothiazole amyloid binding agent, termed BTA-1, and related derivatives have been described in detail.[79–81] These studies showed that these compounds could bind to amyloid with low nanomolar affinity, enter brain in amounts sufficient for imaging with PET, and clear rapidly from normal brain tissue. These data suggested benzothiazole derivatives could be good in vivo PET amyloid imaging agents. A structure activity study of a series of benzothiazoles suggested that a hydroxylated BTA-1 derivative had brain clearance properties typical of many useful PET radiotracers.[81] Therefore, this hydroxybenzothiazole was chosen as the lead compound for the first human trial of benzothiazole amyloid imaging agents performed in Uppsala, Sweden, in collaboration with Långström and colleagues.[82] For simplicity, the compound {*N*-methyl-^{11}C-}2-(4′-methylaminophenyl)-6-hydroxybenzothiazole was given the Uppsala University PET Centre code of Pittsburgh compound B (PiB). Preclinical studies showed that PiB bound to AD brain with a Kd of 1–2 nM, entered the brain rapidly (approximately 7% ID/g 2 min postintravenous injection in mice) and cleared rapidly from normal mouse brain (clearance t1/2 approximately 8 min) and baboon brain.[81] Using real-time in vivo multiphoton microscopy, benzothiazole amyloid imaging agents labeled individual amyloid plaques in transgenic mouse models of AD within 3 min after intravenous injection and cleared rapidly from normal brain parenchyma.[83]

The neuropathology of AD is characterized by abundant amyloid plaques and NFTs[8] and frequently includes α-synuclein deposits in the form of Lewy bodies or threads, making AD a *triple amyloidosis*.[84] Therefore, it is important to address the relative specificity of PiB for β-amyloid deposits given the co-deposition of NFT and the frequent occurrence of α-synuclein deposits. At the nanomolar concentrations attainable in human PET studies, PiB and related benzothiazole derivatives bind to homogenates of plaque- and cerebrovascular amyloid-containing AD brain frontal cortex at tenfold higher levels than the background binding observed in amyloid-free control brain frontal cortex.[85] Under these same conditions, benzothiazole compounds do not produce detectable binding to brain homogenates from the frontal cortex of *pure* brain with dementia with Lewy bodies (i.e., Lewy bodies and threads in the absence of β-amyloid plaques and NFT) or from the entorhinal cortex of a control brain with extensive entorhinal tangle pathology without plaque pathology (Braak II).[85] This suggests that any binding of benzothiazole compounds to tangles *cannot* be detected over background in vivo. The same appears true of α-synuclein pathology in the frontal lobe, although more complete studies with other brain areas with higher densities of Lewy bodies and threads will need to be completed to fully rule out a significant contribution of α-synuclein binding. Binding of PiB and related compounds to α-synuclein deposits is unlikely, however, since these compounds do not stain Lewy bodies in tissue sections (Klunk, unpublished observation). This indicates that the retention of PiB in vivo is primarily an indication of fibrillar β-amyloid deposition. Further studies suggest that PiB binds similarly to both β-amyloid 1–40 and β-amyloid 1–42 fibrils.[86]

Kung and coworkers developed similar radioiodinated thioflavin-T derivatives as potential β-amyloid imaging agents for single photon emission computed tomography (SPECT), and several of these compounds (e.g., IBOX and IMPY) show promise for this purpose with high binding affinities for aggregated β-amyloid and good penetration in mouse brain.[87–90]

Barrio and coworkers reported the synthesis of a lipophilic ^{18}F-radiolabeled tracer for PET imaging of plaques and NFTs in the brains of AD patients.[91,92] This tracer is a fluorinated derivative of a nonspecific cellular membrane dye, 1,1-dicyano-2-[6-(dimethylamino)naphthalen-2-yl]propene (DDNP). This agent is also capable of crossing the blood–brain barrier and entering brain tissue. The nature and degree of its specific binding to β-amyloid and NFTs has been partially characterized,[93] and ^{18}F-FDDNP has been used in one of the early human amyloid imaging studies (see Chapter 5 and the following discussion).

Several groups have taken a large biomolecule approach to amyloid imaging using either antibodies to β-amyloid[94–97] or labeled β-amyloid itself.[98–101] These approaches have not achieved sufficient transport of these large molecules across the blood–brain barrier.

Human Amyloid Imaging Studies

Anti-β-Amyloid Antibody Studies

The first in vivo attempt to image brain amyloid in humans used the anti-β-amyloid antibody approach.[97] The antibody was a monoclonal Fab fragment targeting β-amyloid protein residues 1–28 and was labeled with Tc-99m for SPECT detection. Six subjects with probable AD were studied at times from 0 to 24 h following injection. Disappointingly, SPECT images showed uptake around the head only in the scalp or bone mar row in all subjects. There was no evidence of cerebral uptake (i.e., no blood–brain barrier penetration) of the radiolabeled antibody.

^{18}F-FDDNP Studies

The second attempt to image amyloid in the brain of AD patients used the amyloid binding agent ^{18}F-FDDNP in an effort to specifically label amyloid deposits in nine AD patients and seven controls.[92,102] ^{18}F-FDDNP images from AD patients show similar patterns of retention in both cortical and white matter areas, such as the pons. Time–activity curves in an AD patient showed that, at steady-state (60–120 min postinjection), the absolute retention of ^{18}F-FDDNP in frontal, parietal, temporal, and occipital cortical areas exceeded the reference region, the pons, by 10%–15%. The area of highest retention at equilibrium was the hippocampus/amygdala/entorhinal cortex region, an area in which ^{18}F-FDDNP retention exceeded the reference region by approximately 30%. As noted, autopsy studies[14] showed that neuritic plaques are more densely concentrated in temporal and occipital lobes, whereas limbic areas, including the hippocampus/amygdala/entorhinal cortex region, contain the fewest neuritic plaques. Time–activity data from controls and cerebellar time–activity data from both controls and AD patients were not reported in the study by Shoghi-Jadid et al., but will be useful in determining the specificity of ^{18}F-FDDNP. Shoghi-Jadid et al. were able to demonstrate differences between AD patients and controls using a novel pharmacokinetic analysis procedure called the relative residence time (RRT). The RRT was significantly higher in AD patients and correlated significantly with memory scores when the data from AD patients representing a broad range of MMSE scores (8–28) were combined with control data.[102] RRT is sensitive to both peak and steady-state levels of tracer. Published time–activity data show that brain areas with nearly identical equilibrium levels of tracer such as temporal (RRT = 6.14) and occipital cortex (RRT = 0.37) can differ in RRT by over 1,600%. Inspection of the published time–activity curves[102] shows clearly that regional brain differences in the RRT values of AD patients were mainly dependent on differences in the early distribution of ^{18}F-FDDNP 5–10 min after injection of tracer, rather than by differences in steady-state brain levels at 60–120 min postinjection. Early distribution depends mainly on blood flow and brain permeability. Therefore, the blood-flow dependence of ^{18}F-FDDNP needs to be evaluated before imaging data can be clearly interpreted and specificity for either plaques or tangles can be judged.

Some of the uptake characteristics encountered with ^{18}F-FDDNP may stem from the very high lipophilicity of this tracer (logPoct = 3.92), which is a full log unit above the optimal value that has been previously proposed for effective brain imaging agents[103,104]; a very high blood–brain barrier permeability may cause brain uptake and clearance of a tracer to be more dependent on regional cerebral blood flow, causing it to behave more like a flow-imaging agent, while a low blood–brain barrier permeability may cause brain uptake of a tracer to be more dependent on blood–brain barrier integrity, causing it to behave like a contrast agent.

Reports by the UCLA group at several scientific meetings have indicated that the distribution volume ratio (DVR) for FDDNP covered a range of approximately 1–1.3 from control subjects through the most advanced AD subjects (group average differences were approximately 20%). This relatively narrow dynamic DVR range of 20%–30% for FDDNP can be compared with a dynamic DVR range of 1–3 (group average differences approximately 100%) over which PiB performs in control and AD subjects (see following discussion).

11c Sb-13

The properties of a stilbene derivative, 4-*N*-methylamino-4′-hydroxystilbene or SB-13, were recently reported.[105] In vitro, ^{3}H SB-13 bound specifically and with high affinity (Kd = 2.4 ± 0.2 nM) to cortical homogenates prepared from postmortem brain tissue samples of four patients with AD. In contrast, ^{3}H SB-13 did not specifically bind to homogenates of cerebellar and white matter tissues prepared from either AD or control brain tissue. In competition binding studies, BTA-1 displaced ^{3}H SB-13 binding to β-amyloid with an affinity (Ki = 6.9 nM) similar to that of SB-13 itself. FDDNP had 40-fold lower affinity (Ki = 294 nM) for ^{3}H SB-13 binding sites than BTA-1. This suggested that benzothiazoles, such as BTA-1 and PiB, share a binding site on the Aβ peptide with SB-13 for which FDDNP does not show high affinity.[106], ^{3}H SB-13 labeled Aβ plaques in sections of human AD cortex, but showed little binding to control brain. These favorable in vitro properties supported continued investigation of SB-13 as a potential molecular imaging probe for the noninvasive assessment of brain amyloid deposition in human subjects.

SB-13 was labeled with carbon-11 for in vivo investigations in five female AD subjects and six healthy controls using PET.[105] These same subjects were imaged with PiB to provide a basis of comparison for ^{11}C SB-13. Venous blood samples were drawn throughout the first 70 min of PET data acquisition to characterize the metabolism of ^{11}C SB-13 and to provide an approximation of the arterial input function for quantitative data analysis. To estimate nonspecific binding of ^{11}C SB-13, cerebellum was used as a reference region since it contains little fibrillar amyloid deposits in AD and can be assumed to be nearly devoid of ^{11}C SB-13 specific binding. Cerebellar time–activity data showed similar retention of ^{11}C SB-13 in AD patients and controls, supporting the use of cerebellum as a reference region. Clearance of cerebellar radioactivity after injection of ^{11}C SB-13 was slower than that observed for PiB in the same subjects, with ^{11}C SB-13 exhibiting an approximately 3:1 ratio in the peak to 90-min radioactivity concentrations, compared with approximately 8:1 for PiB. Increased retention of ^{11}C SB-13 was observed in AD subjects compared with controls in cortical areas known to contain significant amyloid deposits in AD, such as the frontal cortex. Across the four cortical areas assessed in this investigation (frontal, temporal, parietal, and occipital), standardized uptake values (SUVs) were determined from 40 to 120 min postinjection emission data and AD cortical averages exceeded control averages by a ratio of 1.44:1.75, with the greatest difference observed in left frontal cortex. In the same subjects, the ratio of AD to control SUV values for PiB ranged from 1.96 to 2.52, which was also maximal in the left frontal cortex. It is likely that the improved distinction between AD and control subjects using PiB is the result of more rapid clearance of nonspecific binding. Although the pattern of retention of ^{11}C SB-13 appeared to mirror that of PiB, the latter provides a greater dynamic range and improved differentiation of AD subjects from controls. This distinction becomes critical when the goal is to evaluate subjects in the very early stages of amyloid deposition, including clinically unimpaired elderly.

Pittsburgh Compound B (Initial Uppsala Studies)

The first human studies with PiB were presented in preliminary form in 2002[83] and were followed by the first full report in 2004.[107] The initial study included 16 probable AD patients (65.9 ± 11 years; 12.3 ± 4 years education), six elderly age-matched controls (69.0 ± 7 years; 12.7 ± 4 years education), and three 21-year-old controls (young controls). The young controls were included because of the near certainty that these young subjects would be truly plaque-negative. Dementia severity in the probable AD group, as evaluated by the MMSE, varied from moderate (MMSE = 18) to very mild/questionable (MMSE = 29), with a mean MMSE of 24.9 ± 3.4. Subjects were administered approximately 300 MBq (8 mCi) of PiB and dynamic PET data were acquired for 60 min. In that study, neither magnetic resonance imaging (MRI) nor arterial blood samples were obtained for anatomic co-registration and input function determination; analyses of these studies were limited to semiquantitative SUV measures of PiB uptake. Nevertheless, striking differences in PiB retention were observed between control and AD subjects in brain areas known to contain significant amyloid deposits in AD (e.g., frontal cortex and parietal cortex).[107] The six elderly control subjects had a brain entry and clearance pattern indistinguishable from that of the three young controls. This permitted young and elderly control groups to be combined to form a unified healthy control group for comparison with the AD patients. As a group, the control subjects showed rapid entry and clearance of PiB from all cortical and subcortical gray matter areas, including the cerebellar cortex (Fig. 6.2). Cerebellum, noted previously as lacking fibrillar amyloid plaques in AD, showed nearly identical uptake and clearance of PiB in healthy control and AD groups (Fig. 6.2a). Subcortical white matter showed lower entry and slower clearance in both healthy control subjects and AD

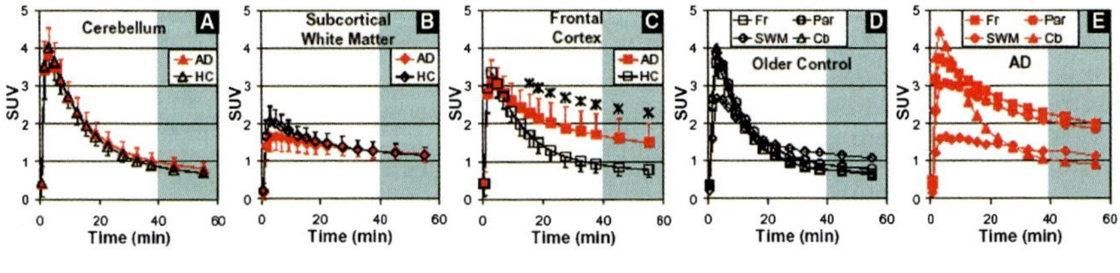

Fig. 6.2 Pittsburgh compound B (PiB) is differentially retained only in amyloid-laden cortical areas of Alzheimer's disease (AD) brain. Standardized uptake values (SUV) demonstrating brain entry and clearance of PiB. **A–C.** Averaged SUV values for all healthy control (HC) subjects (*open, black symbols*; $n = 9$) and all AD patients (*filled, red symbols*; $n = 15$) in cerebellum, subcortical white matter and frontal cortex. **D–E.** brain entry and clearance in cerebellum (*triangles*), subcortical white matter (*diamonds*), frontal cortex (*squares*), and parietal cortex (*circles*) for an older control subject (*D*) and an AD patient (*E*). Error bars represent one standard deviation (SD) and are too small to be seen in some of the healthy control subject data in (*A–C*). Asterisks indicate a significant difference between AD and healthy control values ($P < 0.006$). Shaded areas highlight the 40–60 time period used for the summed SUV data displayed in 6.5. (From Klunk et al.,[107] with permission.)

patients compared with cortical and subcortical gray matter areas (Fig. 6.2b). In contrast, the AD patients had marked retention of PiB compared with healthy control subjects in areas of the brain known to contain high levels of amyloid deposits in AD (Figs 6.2c–e), such as parietal and frontal cortices.[11,14]

The regional distribution of PiB retention was clearly different in AD patients compared with the healthy control subjects (Fig. 6.3). PiB accumulation in AD patients as a group was most prominent in cortical association areas and lower in

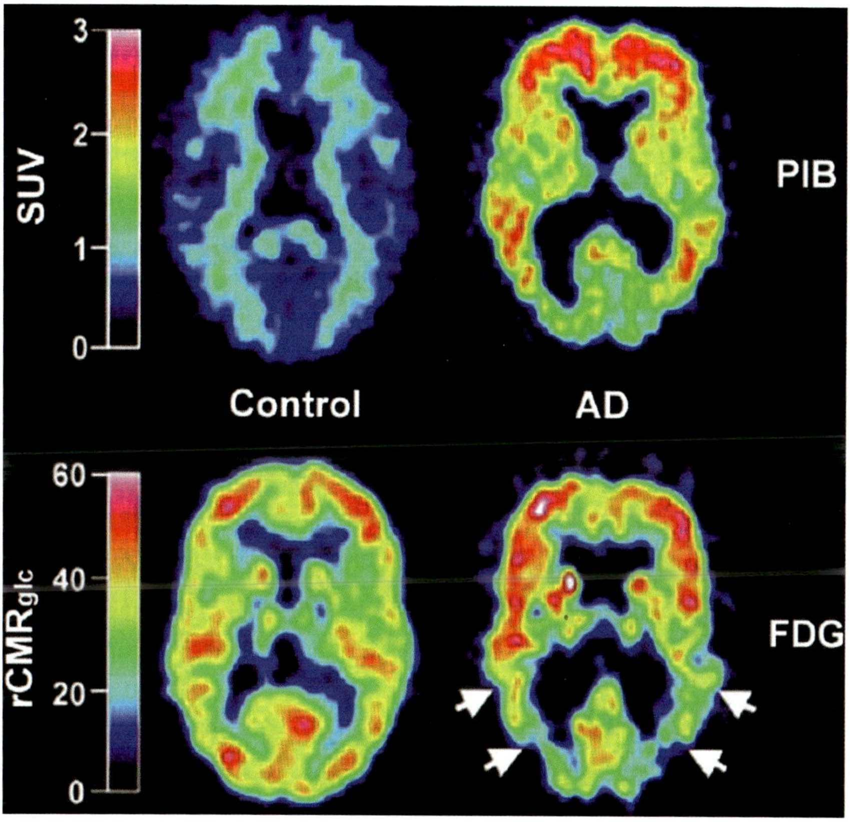

Fig. 6.3 Pittsburgh compound B (PIB) standardized uptake values (SUV) images demonstrate a marked difference between PIB retention in Alzheimer's disease (AD) patients and healthy control subjects. PET images of a 67-year-old healthy control subject (*left*) and a 79-year-old AD patient (AD6; MMSE = 21; *right*). *Top*: SUV PIB images summed over 40–60 min; *bottom*: FDG rCMRglc images (μmol/min/100 mL). The left column shows lack of PIB retention in the entire gray matter of the HC subject (*top left*) and normal FDG uptake (*bottom left*). Nonspecific PIB retention is seen in the white matter (*top left*). The right column shows high PIB retention in the frontal and temporoparietal cortices of the AD patient (*top right*) and a typical pattern of FDG hypometabolism present in the temporoparietal cortex (*arrows; bottom right*) along with preserved metabolic rate in the frontal cortex. PIB and FDG scans were obtained within 3 days of each other. (From Klunk et al.,[107] with permission.)

white matter areas, a pattern consistent with that described in postmortem studies of amyloid deposition in AD brain.[11] PiB images from healthy control subjects showed little or no PiB retention in cortical areas, leaving the subcortical white matter regions highest in relative terms. In absolute terms, the accumulation of PiB in white matter was essentially the same in AD patients and healthy control subjects (Fig. 6.2b).

A series of axial and sagittal SUV images provides a three-dimensional sense of the regional distribution of PiB retention (Fig. 6.4). The marked difference between PiB retention in the AD patient and the healthy control subject is apparent throughout most of the forebrain. High PiB retention was widely distributed in the frontal cortex of the AD patient, but intense PiB retention also was observed in temporal

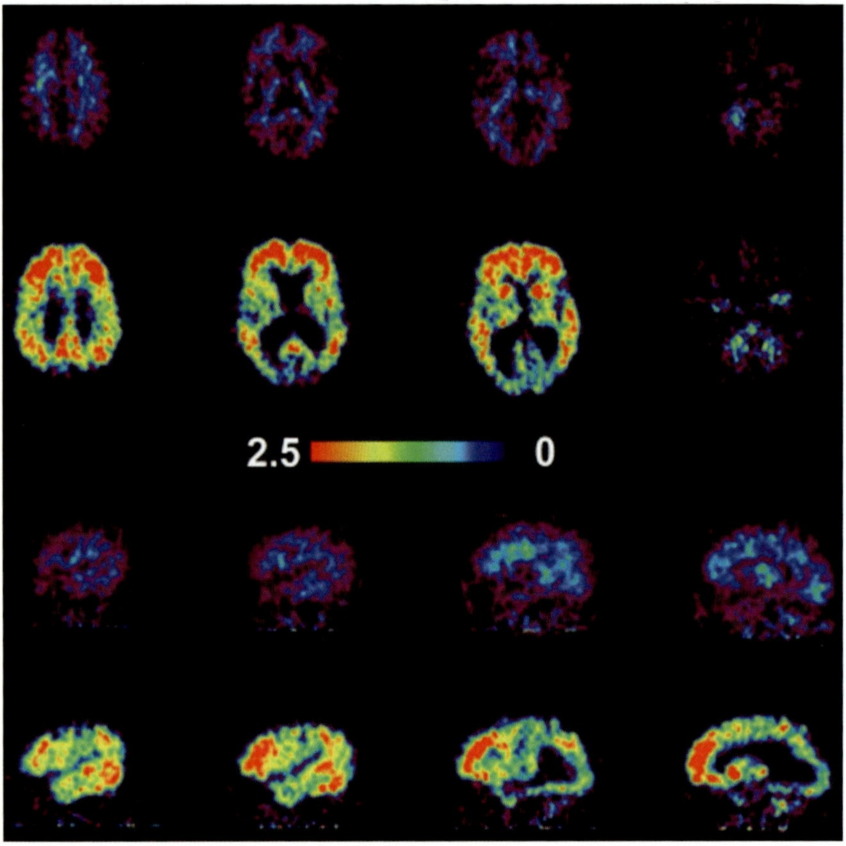

Fig. 6.4 Serial planes demonstrate the topography of Pittsburgh compound B (PiB) retention. Axial (*top two rows*) and sagittal (*bottom two rows*) standardized uptake values PiB images of the subjects shown in Figure 6.3. The healthy control subject data are shown in rows 1 and 3. The AD patient data are shown in rows 2 and 4. The reference region, the cerebellum, can best be appreciated in the images at the far right. The cerebellar peduncles (white matter) show some nonspecific retention, but the cerebellar cortex shows negligible retention. Scale bar indicates relative levels of PiB standardized uptake values. (From Klunk et al.,[107] with permission.)

and parietal cortices, part of the occipital cortex, and in the striatum. Lateral temporal cortex appeared to have greater PiB accumulation than mesial temporal areas. Consistent with previous reports of extensive amyloid deposition in the striatum of virtually all AD patients,[7,108–110] the striatum of AD patients had significantly higher PiB retention than healthy control subjects. Cerebellar cortex (Fig. 6.4) showed little PiB retention and was similar in AD patients and healthy control subjects. In general, the observed pattern of PiB retention in AD subjects was consistent with the pattern of amyloid plaque deposition described in postmortem studies of AD brain,[11,14] except that PiB retention typically predominated in frontal cortex. It should be noted, however, that frontal cortex did not always show the highest PiB retention in a given subject, and mean levels of frontal PiB retention exceeded parietal levels by less than 10%.

Three patients diagnosed as probable AD had high MMSE scores (28–29) and showed no significant deterioration over the 2- to 4-year follow-up period (i.e., MMSE remained 28–29). These atypical subjects had levels of PiB retention in cortical regions typical of controls (open triangles shown in Fig. 6.5), although they were retained in the AD group for all analyses. Other mild AD patients with similar clinical profiles showed typical AD-like changes in PiB retention and rCMRglc. It was unclear whether PiB was simply insensitive to the amount of amyloid deposits in the brains of these three atypical AD patients with MMSE scores of 28–29, or whether PiB imaging had correctly identified subjects without amyloid deposits in whom the clinical diagnosis of AD was incorrect and could or would not be confirmed by postmortem evaluation. In the elderly control group, the oldest subject (76 years) consistently showed the highest cortical PiB retention and the lowest cortical rCMRglc (boxed circles shown in Fig. 6.5). This subject had not expressed any subjective memory complaints and performed within the normal range on the neuropsychological test battery except for difficulty copying a complex cube. This type of case, which could be described as an asymptomatic amyloid-positive case, highlights the issue of specificity versus early detection. One possibility could be that a high PiB signal was obtained in the absence of amyloid deposits (i.e., a false-positive result). If this finding does represent the true presence of amyloid in an asymptomatic individual, the question becomes whether substantial amyloid deposition can be found as part of the normal aging process in subjects who will never develop AD[63] or is increased amyloid deposition always a sign of preclinical AD.[2,49,111] The ability to follow PiB retention longitudinally as an in vivo measure of amyloid deposition provides a new tool through which we may be able to answer this question in a manner that postmortem studies cannot.

Human Pittsburgh Compound B PET Studies in Alzheimer's Disease and Mild Cognitive Impairment

PiB PET studies have been performed at the University of Pittsburgh PET Facility (and other institutions) across a wide variety of research protocols. Subjects studied

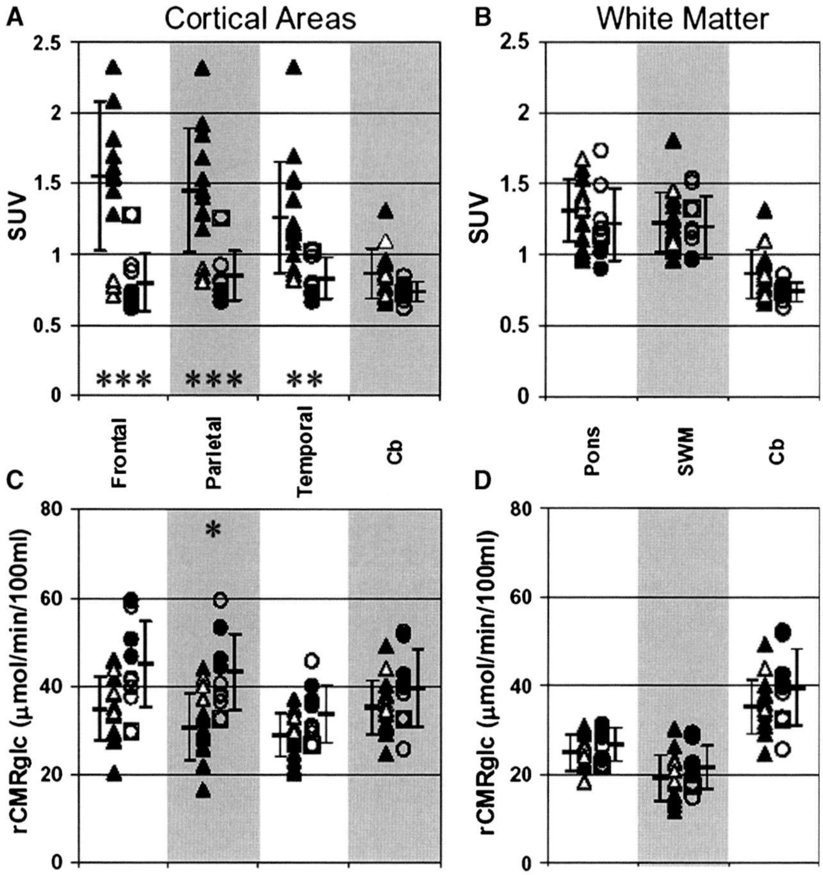

Fig. 6.5 Differences in Pittsburgh compound B (PiB) retention between Alzheimer's disease patients and healthy control (HC) subjects can be quantified and are statistically significant. Accumulation of PiB and rCMRglc in selected regions is shown. Average PiB standardized uptake values (SUV) were summed over 40–60 min in cortical areas (*A*) or white matter areas (*B*) and compared with cerebellum. Values for FDG uptake were calculated with the Gjedde-Patlak method in cortical areas (*C*) or white matter areas (*D*) and compared with cerebellum. The mean and 1 SD are indicated with the error bars beside the individual points. HC subjects: circles; $n = 9$; filled circles represent the three young HC subjects; boxed circle represents the outlier in the HC group (oldest subject). AD patients: triangles; $n = 15$ (SUV) or $n = 16$ (FDG); open triangles represent the three outliers in the AD group. AD mean and SD values include all 15 (SUV) or 16 (FDG) AD subjects; $P < 0.01$ (*); $P < 0.002$ (**); $P < 0.0002$ (***). (From Klunk et al.,[107] with permission.)

in Pittsburgh have been recruited and evaluated at the Alzheimer's Disease Research Center and received their diagnosis in a consensus conference of experienced neurologists, psychiatrists, neuropsychologists, and clinicians according to published criteria.[112] PiB PET imaging (ECAT HR + PET scanner, 13 ± 3 mCi, 90 min) was performed and arterial blood was collected throughout the PiB study for the determination of the plasma input function and radiolabeled metabolites.

Region-of-interest sampling and atrophy correction of the PET data were performed using coregistered MRIs. (MR scans were not performed in the Uppsala PiB studies, and only 60 min of PiB imaging data were acquired.) Region-of-interest sampling included posterior cingulate/precuneus, frontal, parietal, and lateral temporal cortices, subcortical white matter, and cerebellum (CER, nonspecific reference). Analyses provided PiB distribution volume and DVR values as measures of PiB retention, where DVR is the regional distribution volume normalized to the CER distribution volume. Comparative analyses were performed using either arterial (ART), image-based carotid, or CER data as input. Given the small sample sizes in the initial Pittsburgh study ($n = 15$), nonparametric statistical methods were used to assess group differences.[113]

Fully Quantitative Results

Fully quantitative PiB PET studies[113] were conducted in five AD, five MCI, and five control subjects (five subjects were retested within 20 days). Good agreement was observed between fully quantitative compartmental and Logan DVR values (e.g., posterior cingulate/precuneus: $r = 0.89$, slope = 0.91); the Logan results were less variable than the compartmental. Nonspecific PiB retention was similar across subjects ($n = 15$, Logan CER DV: 3.63 ± 0.48). As much as a twofold greater retention of PiB was observed in AD cortical areas relative to controls ($P < 0.05$). PiB retention in MCI subjects appeared heterogeneous and either "AD-like" or "control-like." The mean test/retest variation was approximately 6% in primary areas. The Logan analysis with 90 min of emission data and metabolite-corrected arterial input functions (ART90) proved stable, valid, and robust for parametric image generation (DVR images) and voxel-based statistical analyses.

Simplified Analyses

Because of the technical demands associated with arterial input function determination and metabolite correction, it is advantageous to identify simplified methods of analysis that provide outcome measure estimates that both compare well to ART90 and allow simpler methods of data acquisition (e.g., omission of arterial blood collection and metabolite corrections). We conducted a comparative study in 24 subjects, aiming to examine the potential usefulness of simplified PiB PET methods that involved shorter PET scan acquisitions and the use of image data to approximate the arterial input function.[114] Several simplified methods provided valid and reasonable alternatives to arterial input function data. A particular advantage of the SUV-based reference region ratio methods (SUVR) is that all of the data necessary for the analysis can be obtained by having the subject in the scanner during a 50-min (e.g., 40–90 min after injection) time window. The comparable performance of the

SUVR60 method using a 20-min (40–60 min) window suggests that it may be possible to optimize or shorten the 40- to 90-min window even further, without significant loss of performance. This may be especially important for the study of severe AD patients, who may not be able to tolerate a full 90 min of emission data acquisition. In addition to shorter scan time, other advantages of the SUVR method include simplicity of application (making it more applicable to multisite studies), very good test-retest reproducibility (±5.0%), and a large dynamic range (evidenced by a positive bias vs. ART90).[114]

PiB studies at Pittsburgh also have included FDG scans on the same day and ^{15}O water regional blood flow measures in a subset of subjects. ^{15}O Water studies showed regional PiB retention was not strongly influenced by blood flow, in fact PiB retention is inversely related to blood flow.[115] PiB retention correlated inversely to metabolism (FDG) in precuneus and frontal cortex, but FDG had a lower dynamic range. In separating mild AD and MCI cases from control subjects, voxel-based methods produced more robust group differences with PiB than with FDG.[116] Interestingly, PiB retention in MCI subjects did not cluster between the ranges of PiB retention observed in controls and AD patients, but was distributed across the entire range. Approximately 25% of MCI subjects showed no evidence of PiB retention and appeared control-like, approximately 60% had AD-like PiB retention, and only the remaining 15% had PiB retention intermediate between the control and AD range.[114] Additional cross-sectional and longitudinal studies using PiB to evaluate β-amyloid deposition in the normal aging process, MCI progression (or nonprogression) to AD, and early onset familial AD are underway at Pittsburgh, and other PiB studies in cerebral amyloid angiopathy, vascular dementia, frontotemporal dementia, and to monitor antiamyloid therapeutic strategies are underway at several PET centers throughout the world. A study comparing PiB retention to β-amyloid (1–42) in cerebrospinal fluid in AD demented, non-AD demented, and control subjects has recently been reported[117] and offers important insights into the combined use of PiB and peripheral biomarkers of AD.

Pittsburgh Compound B Studies in Clinically Unimpaired Elderly

At least five groups have reported preliminary findings from PiB-PET amyloid imaging studies of clinically unimpaired elderly.[107,118–121] Each group has reported that approximately 20% of clinically unimpaired subjects over the age of 70 show in vivo evidence of amyloid deposition. Although this number is lower than the number of similarly aged individuals who have any amyloid deposition at autopsy, it is consistent with the report of approximately 25% with AD-like amyloid pathology.[6] In most cases, the amyloid deposits appeared first in the precuneus or frontal cortex. An example of a cognitively normal control with very mild PiB retention in the left frontal lobe at baseline and more extensive deposition at 2 years is in shown in Figure 6.6. Further follow-up is warranted because at present there is no proof

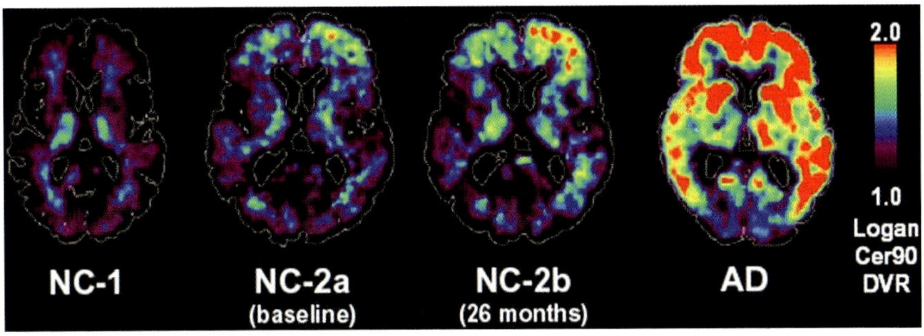

Fig. 6.6 Pittsburgh compound B (PiB) retention is detectable in some clinically unimpaired elderly. PiB-PET distribution volume ratio images of a cognitively normal control without PiB retention (NC-1), a cognitively normal control with a small amount of PiB retention mainly in frontal cortex at baseline (NC-2a) and increased deposition 26 months later (NC-2b) compared with a typical Alzheimer's disease (AD) patient. DVR, distribution volume ratio

that this type of amyloid deposition will progress to that seen in AD or that this amyloid deposition will ever result in cognitive deterioration.

Fagan et al. compared cerebrospinal fluid β-amyloid 42 levels of clinically diagnosed control and dementia subjects to PiB-PET imaging.[117] Of interest to the application of amyloid imaging to normal elderly, they found that all three cognitively normal subjects with low cerebrospinal fluid β-amyloid also had high PiB retention. Although the range of β-amyloid 42 values formed a continuum that made it difficult to define a cutoff, PiB retention showed a clear separation between normal and increased levels.

Rentz et al. reported preliminary findings from a PiB-PET study of nine highly intelligent older adults (American version of the Nelson Adult Reading Test IQ = 127; mean age = 74; CDR = 0).[120] When their neuropsychological test scores were adjusted for IQ, five subjects were reclassified as having memory impairment for their ability, whereas four remained in the normal range. Two of the five high-IQ–memory impaired subjects had PiB binding in the range of AD subjects. The remaining three had PiB binding in the range of normal controls. Rentz et al. offer the hypothesis that, similar to a subset of MCI subjects, a subset of highly intelligent adults with subtle memory impairment has evidence of amyloid deposition and may represent cases of prodromal AD. Most recently, Alzenstein et al. studied 43 subjects from a community-based sample who were between 65 and 88 years old, and considered to be cognitively normal.[121] Substantial PiB retention was identified in 21% of the subjects. Those subjects did not perform neurocognitively worse than the subjects who showed normal levels of PiB retention. It was suggested that the data indicated the ability of the elderly to remain cognitively normal despite significant amyloid burden. Longitudinal follow-up in such studies will be necessary to determine whether the presence of PiB retention in cognitively normal people above age 65 has predictive value with respect to their subsequent clinical course.

Summary

The PET tracer PiB has been shown to selectively label amyloid in vivo and distinguishes AD patients from amyloid-negative control subjects. It can also be used to differentiate MCI subjects according to the amount of labeling seen. Amyloid deposition, as indexed by PiB retention, also can be detected in clinically unimpaired elderly. Studies in clinically unimpaired elderly seek to address three overarching questions concerning the (1) prevalence, (2) cognitive impact, and (3) diagnostic outcome of amyloid deposits in these apparently normal individuals. Answers to these questions may lend important new insights into the validity of the amyloid cascade hypothesis,[4] and aid our understanding of the significance of amyloid deposition in nondemented individuals. This understanding will become important as effective antiamyloid therapies emerge. If it becomes clear that preclinical amyloid deposition progresses to clinical AD with high frequency, then it will become important to identify and treat nondemented, amyloid-positive individuals. It is at this early stage that antiamyloid therapies are most likely to be effective. It also is at this stage that treatment could actually prevent clinical symptoms before they occur. If we are to make significant changes in the currently projected, ominous course of AD in developed countries, it is likely that we will need to adopt a preclinical approach to this dementia.

Acknowledgments The authors thank E. Halligan, the staff at the University of Pittsburgh Alzheimer's Disease Research Center (C. McConaha, E. Eror, L. Macedonia, and M. Oakley) and PET facility (S. Hulland, J. Ruszkiewicz, P. McGeown, D. Ratica, K. Malone, S. Kendro, N. Flatt, and J. Gallo) for their efforts in conducting and analyzing these studies. We are indebted to our subjects and their families for their selfless contributions that made this work possible. Financial support for this work was provided by grants from The National Institutes of Health (R01 AG018402, P50 AG005133, K02 AG001039, R01 AG020226, R01 MH070729, K01 MH001976, R37 AG025516, and P01 AG025204), The Alzheimer's Association (TLL-01-3381), The US Department of Energy (DE-FD02-03 ER63590), and GE Healthcare, Inc.

References

1. Dickson DW, Crystal HA, Mattiace LA, et al. Identification of normal and pathological aging in prospectively studied nondemented elderly humans. Neurobiol Aging 1992;13:179–189.
2. Goldman WP, Price JL, Storandt M, et al. Absence of cognitive impairment or decline in preclinical Alzheimer's disease. Neurology 2001;56:361–367.
3. Terry RD, Masliah E, Salmon DP, et al. Physical basis of cognitive alterations in Alzheimer's disease: synapse loss is the major correlate of cognitive impairment. Ann Neurol 1991;30:572–580.
4. Hardy JA, Higgins GA. Alzheimer's disease: the amyloid cascade hypothesis. Science 1992;256:184–185.
5. Rabbitt P. Does it all go together when it goes? The Nineteenth Bartlett Memorial Lecture. Q J Exp Psychol A 1993;46:385–434.
6. Price JL, Morris JC. Tangles and plaques in nondemented aging and "preclinical" Alzheimer's disease. Ann Neurol 1999;45:358–368.
7. Wolf DS, Gearing M, Snowdon DA, et al. Progression of regional neuropathology in Alzheimer disease and normal elderly: findings from the Nun study. Alzheim Dis Assoc Dis 1999;13:226–231.

8. Mirra SS, Heyman A, McKeel D, et-al. The Consortium to Establish a Registry for Alzheimer's Disease (CERAD). Part II. Standardization of the neuropathologic assessment of Alzheimer's disease. Neurology 1991;41:479–486.
9. Iwatsubo T, Odaka A, Suzuki N, et al. Visualization of A beta 42(43) and A beta 40 in senile plaques with end-specific A beta monoclonals: evidence that an initially deposited species is A beta 42(43). Neuron 1994;13:45–53.
10. Goedert M. Tau protein and the neurofibrillary pathology of Alzheimer's disease. Trends Neurosci 1993;16:460–465.
11. Thal DR, Rub U, Orantes M, et al. Phases of A β-deposition in the human brain and its relevance for the development of AD. Neurology 2002;58:1791–1800.
12. Braak H, Braak E. Neuropathological staging of Alzheimer-related changes. Acta Neuropathol 1991;82:239–259.
13. Delacourte A, David JP, Sergeant N, et al. The biochemical pathway of neurofibrillary degeneration in aging and Alzheimer's disease. Neurology 1999;52:1158–1165.
14. Arnold SE, Hyman BT, Flory J, et al. The topographical and neuroanatomical distribution of neurofibrillary tangles and neuritic plaques in the cerebral cortex of patients with Alzheimer's disease. Cereb Cortex 1991;1:103–116.
15. Joachim CL, Morris JH, Selkoe DJ. Diffuse senile plaques occur commonly in the cerebellum in Alzheimer's disease. Am J Pathol 1989;135:309–319.
16. Yamaguchi H, Hirai S, Morimatsu M, et al. Diffuse type of senile plaques in the cerebellum of Alzheimer-type dementia demonstrated by beta protein immunostain. Acta Neuropathol 1989;77:314–319.
17. Hardy J, Duff K, Hardy KG, et al. Genetic dissection of Alzheimer's disease and related dementias: amyloid and its relationship to tau. Nat Neurosci 1998;1:355–358.
18. Tanzi RE, Kovacs DM, Kim TW, et al. The gene defects responsible for familial Alzheimer's disease. Neurobiol Dis 1996;3:159–168.
19. Price DL, Sisodia SS. Mutant genes in familial Alzheimer's disease and transgenic models. Ann Rev Neurosci 1998;21:479–505.
20. Xia W, Ostaszewski BL, Kimberly WT, et al. FAD mutations in presenilin-1 or amyloid precursor protein decrease the efficacy of a gamma-secretase inhibitor: evidence for direct involvement of PS1 in the gamma-secretase cleavage complex. Neurobiol Dis 2000;7:673–681.
21. Walsh DM, Klyubin I, Fadeeva JV, et al. Naturally secreted oligomers of amyloid beta protein potently inhibit hippocampal long-term potentiation in vivo. Nature 2002;416:535–539.
22. Caughey B, Lansbury PT. Protofibrils, pores, fibrils, and neurodegeneration: separating the responsible protein aggregates from the innocent bystanders. Annu Rev Neurosci 2003;26:267–298.
23. Lesne S, Koh MT, Kotilinek L, et al. A specific amyloid-beta protein assembly in the brain impairs memory. Nature 2006;440:352–357.
24. Lue LF, Kuo YM, Roher AE, et al. Soluble amyloid beta peptide concentration as a predictor of synaptic change in Alzheimer's disease. Am J Pathol 1999;155:853–862.
25. Glabe CG. Conformation-dependent antibodies target diseases of protein misfolding. Trends Biochem Sci 2004;29:542–547.
26. Zhou J, Fonseca MI, Glabe CG, et al. Age-related decline in the clearance of plaques by A β-immunotherapy in murine model of Alzheimer's disease using either fibrillar or a novel oligomeric A β as an immunogen. Society for Neuroscience Abstracts 2004, 716.9.
27. Olson RE, Copeland RA, Seiffert D. Progress towards testing the amyloid hypothesis: inhibitors of APP processing. Curr Opin Drug Dis Dev 2001;4:390–401.
28. Nunan J, Small DH. Regulation of APP cleavage by alpha-, beta- and gamma-secretases. FEBS Lett 2000;483:6–10.
29. Dovey HF, John V, Anderson JP, et al. Functional gamma-secretase inhibitors reduce beta-amyloid peptide levels in brain. J Neurochem 2001;76:173–181.
30. Petit A, Pasini A, Alves Da Costa C, et al. JLK isocoumarin inhibitors: selective gamma-secretase inhibitors that do not interfere with notch pathway in vitro or in vivo. J Neurosci Res 2003;74:370–377.

31. Roberds SL, Anderson J, Basi G, et al. BACE knockout mice are healthy despite lacking the primary beta-secretase activity in brain: implications for Alzheimer's disease therapeutics. Hum Mol Genet 2001;10:1317–1324.
32. Dewachter I, Van Leuven F. Secretases as targets for the treatment of Alzheimer's disease: the prospects. Lancet Neurol 2002;1:409–416.
33. Wang W, Reichert P, Beyer BM, et al. Crystallization of glycosylated human BACE protease domain expressed in *Trichoplusia ni*. Biochim Biophys Acta 2004;1698:255–259.
34. Siemers E, Skinner M, Dean RA, et al. Safety, tolerability, and changes in amyloid beta concentrations after administration of a gamma-secretase inhibitor in volunteers. Clin Neuropharmacol 2005;28:126–132.
35. Orgogozo JM, Gilman S, Dartigues JF, et al. Subacute meningoencephalitis in a subset of patients with AD after Abeta42 immunization. Neurology 2003;61:46–54.
36. Gilman S, Koller M, Black RS, et al. Clinical effects of A β immunization (AN1792) in patients with AD in an interrupted trial. Neurology 2005;64:1553–1562.
37. Gandy S, Walker L. Toward modeling hemorrhagic and encephalitic complications of Alzheimer amyloid-beta vaccination in nonhuman primates. Curr Opin Immunol 2004;16:607–615.
38. Hock C, Konietzko U, Streffer JR, et al. Antibodies against β-amyloid slow cognitive decline in Alzheimer's disease. Neuron 2003;38:547–554.
39. Fox NC, Black RS, Gilman S, et al. Effects of A β immunization (AN1792) on MRI measures of cerebral volume in Alzheimer disease. Neurology 2005;64:1563–1572.
40. Nicoll JA, Wilkinson D, Holmes C, et al. Neuropathology of human Alzheimer disease after immunization with amyloid- β peptide: a case report. Nat Med 2003;9:448–452.
41. Ferrer I, Boada R, Sanchez G, et al. Neuropathology and pathogenesis of encephalitis following amyloid-beta immunization in Alzheimer's disease. Brain Pathol 2004;14:11–20.
42. Masliah E, Hansen L, Adame A, et al. A β vaccination effects on plaque pathology in the absence of encephalitis in Alzheimer disease. Neurology 2005;64:129–131.
43. DeMattos RB, Bales KR, Cummins DJ, et al. Peripheral anti-A β antibody alters CNS and plasma A β clearance and decreases brain A β burden in a mouse model of Alzheimer's disease. Proc Natl Acad Sci USA 2001;98:8850–8855.
44. Bard F, Barbour R, Cannon C, et al. Epitope and isotype specificities of antibodies to beta-amyloid peptide for protection against Alzheimer's disease-like neuropathology. Proc Natl Acad Sci USA 2003;100:2023–2028.
45. Lee EB, Leng LZ, Lee VM, et al. Meningoencephalitis associated with passive immunization of a transgenic murine model of Alzheimer's amyloidosis. FEBS Lett 2005;579:2564–2568.
46. Petersen RC. Mild cognitive impairment as a diagnostic entity. J Intern Med 2004;256: 183–194.
47. Lopez OL, Jagust WJ, DeKosky ST, et al. Prevalence and classification of mild cognitive impairment in the Cardiovascular Health Study Cognition Study. Arch Neurol 2003;60:1385–1389.
48. Larrieu S, Letenneur L, Orgogozo JM, et al. Incidence and outcome of mild cognitive impairment in a population-based prospective cohort. Neurology 2002;59:1594–1599.
49. Morris JC, Price AL. Pathologic correlates of nondemented aging, mild cognitive impairment, and early-stage Alzheimer's disease. J Mol Neurosci 2001;17:101–118.
50. Morris JC, Storandt M, Miller JP, et al. Mild cognitive impairment represents early-stage Alzheimer disease. Arch Neurol 2001;58:397–405.
51. Petersen RC, Stevens JC, Ganguli M, et al. Practice parameter: early detection of dementia: mild cognitive impairment (an evidence-based review). Report of the Quality Standards Subcommittee of the American Academy of Neurology. Neurology 2001;56:1133–1142.
52. Folstein M, Folstein S, McHugh PR. Mini-mental state: a practical method for grading the cognitive state of patients for the clinician. J Psychiatry Res 1975;12:189–198.
53. Davis DG, Schmitt FA, Wekstein DR, et al. Alzheimer neuropathologic alterations in aged cognitively normal subjects. J Neuropathol Exp Neurol 1999;58:376–388.
54. Green MS, Kaye JA, Ball MJ. The Oregon brain aging study: neuropathology accompanying healthy aging in the oldest old. Neurology 2000;54:105–113.
55. Schmand B, Smit JH, Geerlings MI, et al. The effects of intelligence and education on the development of dementia. A test of the brain reserve hypothesis. Psychol Med 1997;27:1337–1344.

56. Stern Y, Albert S, Tang MX, et al. Rate of memory decline in AD is related to education and occupation: cognitive reserve. Neurology 1999;53:1942–1947.
57. Satz P. Brain reserve capacity on symptom onset after brain injury: a formulation and review of evidence for threshold theory. Neuropsychology 1993;7:273–295.
58. Stern Y. What is cognitive reserve? Theory and research application of the reserve concept. J Int Neuropsychol Soc 2002;8:448–460.
59. Bennett DA, Wilson RS, Schneider JA, et al. Education modifies the relation of AD pathology to level of cognitive function in older persons. Neurology 2003;60:1909–1915.
60. Stern Y, Alexander GE, Prohovnik I, et al. Inverse relationship between education and parieto-temporal perfusion deficit in Alzheimer's disease. Ann Neurol 1992;32:371–375.
61. Coffey CE, Saxton JA, Ratcliff G, et al. Relation of education to brain size in normal aging: implications for the reserve hypothesis. Neurology 1999;53:189–196.
62. Haroutunian V, Perl D, Purohit D, et al. Regional distribution of neuritic plaques in the non-demented elderly and subjects with very mild Alzheimer's disease. Arch Neurol 1998;55:1185–1191.
63. Morris JC, Storandt M, McKeel DWJr, et al. Cerebral amyloid deposition and diffuse plaques in "normal" aging: evidence for presymptomatic and very mild Alzheimer's disease. Neurology 1996;46:707–719.
64. Hyman BT. Down syndrome and Alzheimer disease. Prog Clin Biol Res 1992;379:123–142.
65. Hyman BT, West HL, Rebeck GW, et al. Neuropathological changes in Down's syndrome hippocampal formation. Effect of age and apolipoprotein E genotype. Arc Neurol 1995;52:373–378.
66. Morse CK. Does variability increase with age? An archival study of cognitive measures. Psychol Aging 1993;8:156–164.
67. Hulette CM, Welsh-Bohmer KA, Murray MG, et al. Neuropathological and neuropsychological changes in "normal" aging. J Neuropathol Exp Neurol 1998;57:1168–1174.
68. Price JL. Diagnostic criteria for Alzheimer's disease. Neurobiol Aging 1997;18:S67–S70.
69. Klunk WE, Debnath ML, Pettegrew JW. Development of small molecule probes for the beta-amyloid protein of Alzheimer's disease. Neurobiol Aging 1994;15:691–698.
70. Klunk WE. Biological markers of Alzheimer's disease. Neurobiol Aging 1998;19:145–147.
71. Mathis CA, Wang Y, Klunk WE. Imaging beta-amyloid plaques and neurofibrillary tangles in the aging human brain. Curr Pharm Des 2004;10:1469–1492.
72. Klunk WE, Debnath ML, Pettegrew JW. Chrysamine-G binding to Alzheimer and control brain: autopsy study of a new amyloid probe. Neurobiol Aging 1995;16:541–548.
73. Mathis CA, Mahmood K, Debnath ML, et al. Synthesis of a lipophilic radioiodinated ligand with high affinity to amyloid protein in Alzheimer's disease brain tissue. J Label Comp Radiopharm 1997;40:94–95.
74. Dezutter NA, Dom RJ, de Groot TJ, et al. 99mTc-MAMA-chrysamine G, a probe for beta-amyloid protein of Alzheimer's disease. Eur J Nucl Med 1999;26:1392–1399.
75. Styren SD, Hamilton RL, Styren GC, et al. X-34, a fluorescent derivative of Congo red: a novel histochemical stain for Alzheimer's disease pathology. J Histochem Cytochem 2000;48:1223–1232.
76. Klunk WE, Bacskai BJ, Mathis CA, et al. Imaging Abeta plaques in living transgenic mice with multiphoton microscopy and methoxy-X04, a systemically administered Congo red derivative. J Neuropathol Exp Neurol 2002;61:797–805.
77. Wang Y, Mathis CA, Huang G-F, et al. Synthesis and ^{11}C-labelling of (E,E)-1-(3′,4′-dihydroxystyryl)-4-(3′-methoxy-4′-hydroxystyryl) benzene for PET imaging of amyloid deposits. J Label Comp Radiopharm 2002;45:647–664.
78. Klunk WE, Wang Y, Huang GF, et al. Uncharged thioflavin-T derivatives bind to amyloid-beta protein with high affinity and readily enter the brain. Life Sci 2001;69:1471–1484.
79. Mathis CA, Bacskai BJ, Kajdasz ST, et al. A lipophilic thioflavin-T derivative for positron emission tomography (PET) imaging of amyloid in brain. Bioorg Med Chem Lett 2002;12:295–298.
80. Wang Y, Mathis CA, Huang G-F, et al. Synthesis and evaluation of 2-(3′-iodo-4′-amino)-6-hydroxy-benzothiazole for in vivo quantitation of amyloid deposits in Alzheimer's disease. J Mol Neurosci 2002;19:11–16.

81. Mathis CA, Wang Y, Holt DP, et al. Synthesis and evaluation of 11C-labeled 6-substituted 2-arylbenzothiazoles as amyloid imaging agents. J Med Chem 2003;46:2740–2754.
82. Engler H, Nordberg A, Blomqvist G, et al. First human study with a benzothiazole amyloid-imaging agent in Alzheimer's disease and control subjects. Neurobiol Aging 2002;23(1S):S429.
83. Bacskai BJ, Hickey GA, Skoch J, et al. Four-dimensional multiphoton imaging of brain entry, amyloid binding, and clearance of an amyloid-beta ligand in transgenic mice. Proc Natl Acad Sci USA 2003;100:12462–12467.
84. Trojanowski JQ, Mattson MP. Overview of protein aggregation in single, double, and triple neurodegenerative brain amyloidoses. Neuromusc Disord 2003;4:1–6.
85. Klunk WE, Wang Y, Huang GF, et al. The binding of 2-(4′-methylaminophenyl)benzothiazole to postmortem brain homogenates is dominated by the amyloid component. J Neurosci 2003;23:2086–2092.
86. Klunk WE, Lopresti BJ, Ikonomovic MD, et al. Binding of the positron emission tomography tracer Pittsburgh compound-B reflects the amount of amyloid-beta in Alzheimer's disease brain but not in transgenic mouse brain. J Neurosci 2005;25:10598–10606.
87. Zhuang ZP, Kung MP, Hou C, et al. IBOX(2-(4′-dimethylaminophenyl)-6-iodobenzoxazole): a ligand for imaging amyloid plaques in the brain. Nucl Med Biol 2001;28:887–894.
88. Zhuang ZP, Kung MP, Hou C, et al. Radioiodinated styrylbenzenes and thioflavins as probes for amyloid aggregates. J Med Chem 2001;44:1905–1914.
89. Ono M, Wilson A, Nobrega J, et al. 11C-labeled stilbene derivatives as Abeta-aggregate-specific PET imaging agents for Alzheimer's disease. Nucl Med Biol 2003;30:565–571.
90. Zhuang ZP, Kung MP, Wilson A, et al. Structure-activity relationship of imidazo[1,2-a] pyridines as ligands for detecting beta-amyloid plaques in the brain. J Med Chem 2003;46:237–243.
91. Barrio JR, Huang SC, Cole GM, et al. PET imaging of tangles and plaques in Alzheimer's disease with a highly hydrophilic probe. J Label Comp Radiopharm 1999;42:S194–S195.
92. Barrio JR, Huang SC, Cole GM, et al. PET imaging of tangles and plaques in Alzheimer's disease. J Nucl Med 1999;40(S):70P.
93. Agdeppa ED, Kepe V, Liu J, et al. Binding characteristics of radiofluorinated 6-dialkylamino-2-naphthylethylidene derivatives as positron emission tomography imaging probes for beta-amyloid plaques in Alzheimer's disease. J Neurosci 2001;21:RC18995.
94. Majocha RE, Reno JM, Friedland RP, et al. Development of a monoclonal antibody specific for beta/A4 amyloid in Alzheimer's disease brain for application to in vivo imaging of amyloid angiopathy. J Nucl Med 1992;33:2184–2189.
95. Bickel U, Lee VM, Trojanowski JQ, et al. Development and in vitro characterization of a cationized monoclonal antibody against beta A4 protein: a potential probe for Alzheimer's disease. Bioconjugate Chem 1994;5:119–125.
96. Friedland RP, Majocha RE, Reno JM, et al. Development of an anti-A beta monoclonal antibody for in vivo imaging of amyloid angiopathy in Alzheimer's disease. Mol Neurobiol 1994;9:107–113.
97. Friedland RP, Kalaria R, Berridge M, et al. Neuroimaging of vessel amyloid in Alzheimer's disease. Ann NY Acad Sci 1997;826:242–247.
98. Maggio JE, Stimson ER, Ghilardi JR, et al. Reversible in vitro growth of Alzheimer disease beta-amyloid plaques by deposition of labeled amyloid peptide. Proc Natl Acad Sci USA 1992;89:5462–5466.
99. Saito Y, Buciak J, Yang J, et al. Vector-mediated delivery of 125I-labeled beta-amyloid peptide A beta 1–40 through the blood-brain barrier and binding to Alzheimer disease amyloid of the A beta 1–40/vector complex. Proc Natl Acad Sci USA 1995;95:10227–10231.
100. Ghilardi JR, Catton M, Stimson ER, et al. Intra-arterial infusion of [125I]A beta 1–40 labels amyloid deposits in the aged primate brain in vivo. Neuroreport 1996;7:2607–2611.
101. Wengenack TM, Curran GL, Poduslo JF. Targeting Alzheimer amyloid plaques in vivo. Nat Biotechnol 2000;18:868–872.

102. Shoghi-Jadid K, Small GW, Agdeppa ED, et al. Localization of neurofibrillary tangles and beta-amyloid plaques in the brains of living patients with Alzheimer disease. Am J Geriatr Psychiatry 2002;10:24–35.
103. Dishino DD, Welch MJ, Kilbourn MR, et al. Relationship between lipophilicity and brain extraction of C-11-labeled radiopharmaceuticals. J Nucl Med 1983;24:1030–1038.
104. Gupta SP. QSAR studies on drugs acting at the central nervous system. Chem Rev 1989;89:1765–1800.
105. Verhoeff NP, Wilson AA, Takeshita S, et al. In-vivo imaging of Alzheimer disease beta-amyloid with [11C]SB-13 PET. Am J Geriatr Psychiatry 2004;12:584–595.
106. Kung MP, Hou C, Zhuang ZP, et al. Binding of two potential imaging agents targeting amyloid plaques in postmortem brain tissues of patients with Alzheimer's disease. Brain Res 2004;1025:98–105.
107. Klunk WE, Engler H, Nordberg A, et al. Imaging brain amyloid in Alzheimer's disease with Pittsburgh Compound-B. Ann Neurol 2004;55:306–319.
108. Braak H, Braak E. Alzheimer's disease: striatal amyloid deposits and neurofibrillary changes. J Neuropathol Exp Neurol 1990;49:215–224.
109. Suenaga T, Hirano A, Llena JF, et al. Modified Bielschowsky stain and immunohistochemical studies on striatal plaques in Alzheimer's disease. Acta Neuropathol 1990;80:280–286.
110. Brilliant MJ, Elble RJ, Ghobrial M, et al. The distribution of amyloid beta protein deposition in the corpus striatum of patients with Alzheimer's disease. Neuropathol Appl Neurobiol 1997;23:322–325.
111. Schmitt FA, Davis DG, Wekstein DR, et al. "Preclinical" AD revisited: neuropathology of cognitively normal older adults. Neurology 2000;55:370–376.
112. Lopez OL, Becker JT, Klunk W, et al. Research evaluation and diagnosis of probable Alzheimer's disease over the last two decades: I. Neurology 2000;55:1854–1862.
113. Price JC, Klunk WE, Lopresti BJ, et al. Kinetic modeling of amyloid binding in humans using PET imaging and Pittsburgh Compound-B. J Cereb Blood Flow Metab 2005;25:1528–1547.
114. Lopresti BJ, Klunk WE, Mathis CA, et al. Simplified quantification of Pittsburgh compound B amyloid imaging PET studies: a comparative analysis. J Nucl Med 2005;46:1959–1972.
115. Price JC, Ziolko SK, Weissfeld LA, et al. [O-15]Water and PIB PET imaging in Alzheimer's disease and mild cognitive impairment. 53rd Annual Meeting of the Society of Nuclear Medicine, 2006.
116. Ziolko SK, Weissfeld LA, Klunk WE, et al. Evaluation of voxel-based methods for the statistical analysis of PIB PET amyloid imaging studies in Alzheimer's disease. Neuroimage 2006;15;33:94–102.
117. Fagan AM, Mintun MA, Mach RH, et al. Inverse relation between in vivo amyloid imaging load and cerebrospinal fluid Abeta(42) in humans. Ann Neurol 2006;59:512–519.
118. Villemagne VL, Rowe CC, Macfarlane S, et al. *Imaginem oblivionis:* the prospects of neuroimaging for early detection of Alzheimer's disease. J Clin Neurosci 2005;12:221–230.
119. Mintun MA, LaRossa GA, Sheline YI, et al. [^{11}C]PIB in a nondemented population: potential antecedent marker of Alzheimer disease. Neurology 2006;67:446–452
120. Rentz DM, Becker JA, Moran EK, et al. Amyloid imaging with Pittsburgh compound-B (PIB) in AD, MCI, and highly intelligent older adults. AAN Abstracts 58th Annual Meeting, 2006:S21.002.147.
121. Aizenstein HJ, Nebes RD, Saxton JA, et al. Frequent amyloid deposition without significant cognitive impairment among the elderly. Arch Neurol. 2008;65:1509–1517.

Part III
Atlas

Chapter 7
Interpretive Practice Atlas

Daniel H.S. Silverman, Victoria Lau, Cheri Geist, and Erin Siu

The interpretive practice atlas that follows has not been designed to serve as a typical atlas, in the sense of presenting a set of prototypical examples of a wide variety of clinical entities. Rather, it has been designed to provide actual clinical cases involving a series of brain positron emission tomography (PET) imaging sets that pose interpretive challenges that readers can realistically and repeatedly expect to face in most current clinical environments—where often the patient's symptoms are mild or even questionable at the time of initial evaluation and the associated metabolic findings may be subtle.

Because of the value and, frequently, the complexity of integrating clinical and imaging data, we have concentrated on cases in which substantial neuropsychological and other clinical context for the imaging studies is presented, with respect to both the situation of the patients leading up to acquisition of brain PET, as well as close subsequent follow-up, usually for years after the time of initial PET scanning, and in some cases extending all the way to autopsy-confirmed diagnoses. Moreover, these cases often involve acquisition of a second PET scan, allowing the reader to see clinical changes or stability, as well as cerebral metabolic changes or stability, over a period of years, and how they relate to each other. We have also concentrated on cases involving the most common diagnoses, although a few cases involving rarer pathologic entities are included, and we have provided several examples of scans that turned out to be normal or near normal, so that the reader can develop a stronger sense of the ranges of physiologic variation to be seen.

Most importantly, the cases are designed to provide the opportunity for practice of clinical brain PET imaging interpretive skills. To this end, the images are presented primarily in full plane sets, allowing the reader to examine an entire scan to assess what, if any, metabolic abnormalities are to be noted in each patient's brain, and not as a handful of preselected planes, or laden with *give-away* arrows that

D.H.S. Silverman (ed.), *PET in the Evaluation of Alzheimer's Disease and Related Disorders*,
DOI: 10.1007/978-0-387-76420-7_7,

point out in advance the pertinent features of the scan. As it is becoming increasingly common in clinical settings for physicians to include in their interpretive process the use of analysis software packages designed to visually represent comparisons of patients' brain PET scans to normal databases, the majority of the cases presented here are also complemented by such images, thus providing the opportunity to gain practice in integrating visual assessments with quantifying data, along with salient clinical information, in carrying out the interpretations. PET scans have been processed by the package that has been in longest use under approval by the United States Food and Drug Administration as a software product dedicated to analysis of brain PET data, NeuroQ, which is described briefly here for those unfamiliar with the software and its display format.

Analytic Software

The NeuroQ package is a commercially available product distributed by Syntermed, Inc. (Atlanta, GA), under a software license from the University of California, where it was developed by the author and colleagues. The software automatically and rapidly calculates the amount of activity region by region throughout the patient's brain and compares the amount of activity in each region with the expected amount of activity based on comparison to a database derived from PET scans of normal subjects. It then redisplays the PET data using a two-dimensional color scale, which simultaneously represents the magnitude and statistical significance of those quantitative comparisons. A brain region that is very normal in activity will appear bright blue, a brain region that is very abnormal will appear bright red, and a region with an abnormality that may be statistically significant but of lesser magnitude will be represented as some intermediate shade in the blue–purple–red spectrum, with a unique one-to-one color mapping that represents both the magnitude and the statistical significance for each regional comparison.

Case Study 1

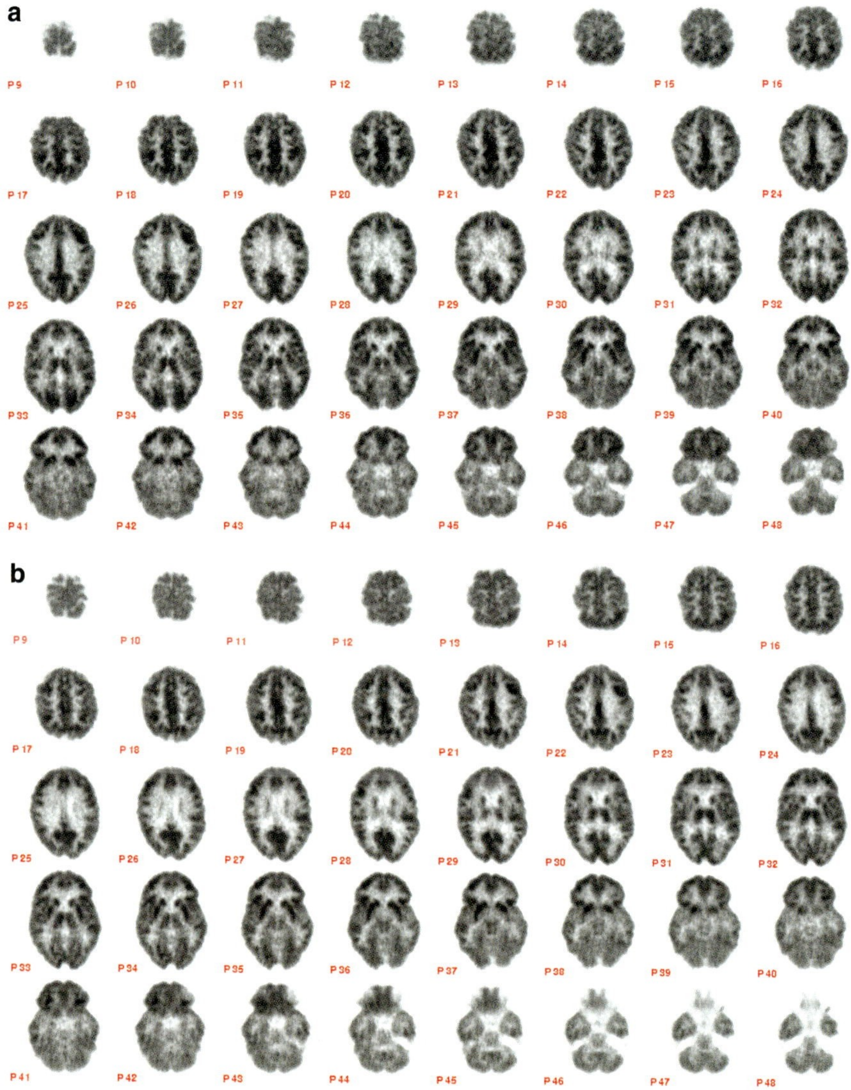

Fig. 7.1 **A.** Brain FDG PET of 60-year-old woman with symptoms of memory decline. **B.** A PET scan performed 20 months later shows improved neuropsychological performance

Indication

Ms. F, a right-handed woman, was 60 years old at the time of initial evaluation. She is an executive in the motion picture industry, with 13 years of education. She has a maternal family history of dementia, most likely of the Lewy Body type. She does not drink alcohol and denies illicit drug use. On presentation, Ms. F noted some gradual memory decline, particularly with respect to name and telephone number retrieval. At that time, a neuropsychological evaluation suggested signs of cognitive decline, as indicated by poor performances on tasks involving delayed verbal memory and encoding of rote verbal information, scoring as low as the first percentile on the latter.

Scan 1 Interpretation

The patient's initial PET scan showed a normal distribution of FDG, with no evidence of neurodegenerative disease (Fig. 7.1a).

Follow-up Visit

Ms. F's follow-up neuropsychological evaluation 20 months later showed that with respect to her earlier memory deficits, she demonstrated relative improvement on all tasks, including immediate and delayed verbal and visual memory recall. In addition, she was scoring at a consistent or improved performance level with respect to tasks of orientation, attention and concentration, language, executive functioning, psychomotor speed, visual spatial functioning, and abstract reasoning.

Scan 2 Interpretation

The patient's follow-up FDG PET scan, nearly unchanged from that of her initial one, indicated slightly less metabolism in the left temporal cortex than the right, and very mild occipital hypometabolism, although these findings are not clearly beyond the range of normal variation (Fig. 7.1b). The gross structure of the brain is normal. FDG distribution throughout the cortex is symmetric and unremarkable, with the expected pattern of relatively higher uptake in the posterior cingulate cortex intact. The pattern of FDG uptake in the basal ganglia, thalamus, and cerebellum is also within normal limits.

Teaching Point

Ms. F's initial clinical evaluation, including formal neuropsychological testing, was concerning, as demonstrated by her impaired performances on delayed verbal memory tasks. However, on clinical follow-up 2 years later, she had relative improvement on most tests, including all memory tasks. This finding was consistent with the patient's initial FDG PET scan, which showed a normal pattern of brain metabolism, with no evidence of neurodegenerative disease. In this case, Ms. F's initial clinical evaluation was ambiguous, leaving it unclear whether her performance on some neuropsychological tests was attributable to factors related to a progressive disease process. FDG PET administered on initial evaluation accurately suggested that her symptoms were unrelated to a progressive dementing disorder (with a sensitivity for detecting both early neurodegenerative disease[1,2] and also any clinical progression that would occur over the next 3 years of 93–95%[1,3,4]). This was confirmed by the patient's clinical follow-up evaluation 2 years later, as well as by a repeat PET scan.

Case Study 2

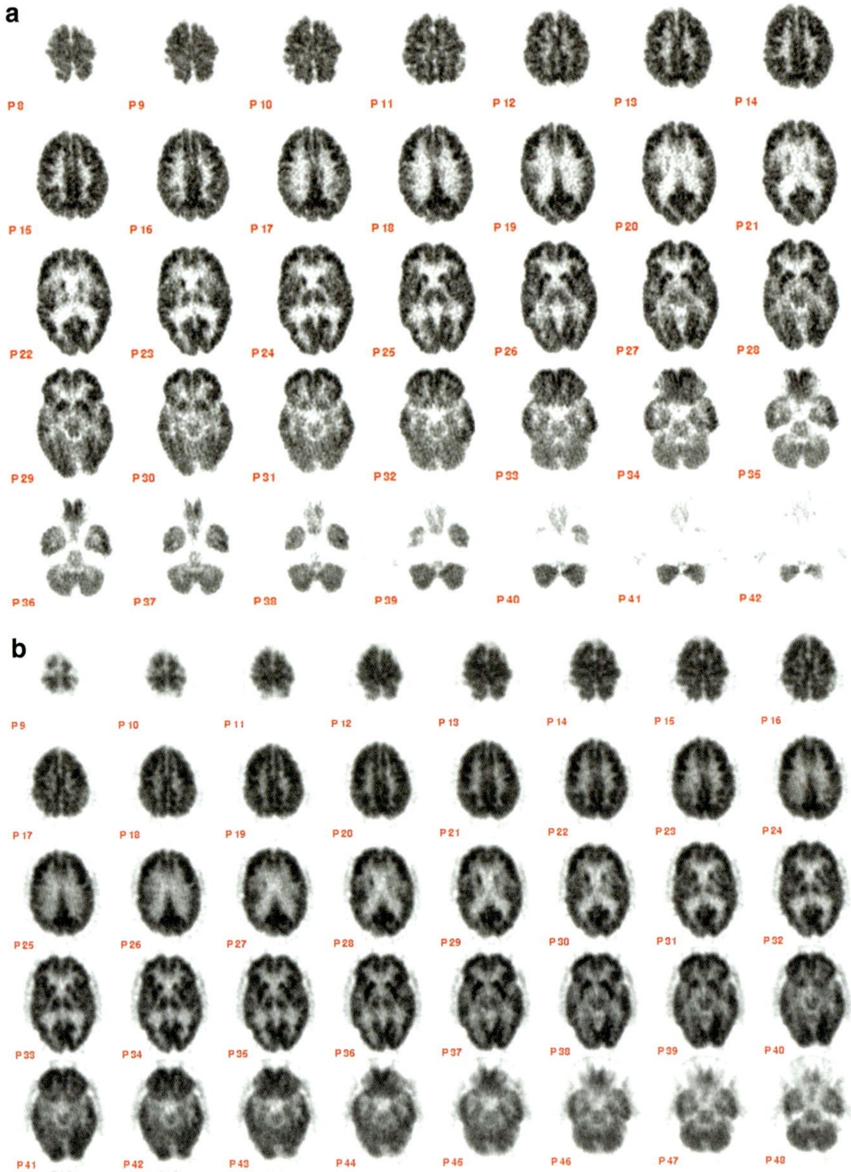

Fig. 7.2 **A.** Brain FDG PET of a cognitively normal 77-year-old man. **B.** A PET scan performed 5 years later shows decline in neuropsychological performance

Indication

Dr. S, a right-handed man, was a 77-year-old retired physician at the time of initial evaluation. With a history of depression dating back approximately 50 years, he had been medicated to treat mild depression and to achieve "deceleration of memory loss. In addition, he had a history of minimal carcinoma of the prostate, along with 'difficulties hearing.'" He denied alcohol abuse, illicit drug use, and any family history of dementia.

At the time of his initial examination, Dr. S was found to be cognitively normal on comprehensive clinical and neuropsychological evaluations and had a normal FDG PET scan (Fig. 7.2a). Five years later, he returned for complaints of difficulty with short-term memory, with symptoms starting approximately 2–3 years previously. He scored a 27/30 on the MMSE and performed well in tasks involving attention and concentration, psychomotor speed, and executive functioning. However, although his scores of semantic and phonemic fluency fell within normal ranges, they fell below expectations when taking into account his superior premorbid functioning. In addition, Dr. S struggled with most memory tasks, performing as low as the 16th percentile on delayed recall of word pairs. The patient was subsequently diagnosed with age consistent memory impairment.

Scan Interpretation

Follow-up FDG PET indicated right parietal, temporal, and occipital hypometabolism, as well as slight left inferior parietal and posterior cingulate hypometabolism (Fig. 7.2b). Preserved FDG uptake occurred in the remainder of the cortex and in noncortical structures.

Teaching Point

Dr. S's performance on memory tasks, including visual and verbal memory, are lower than expected, given his superior premorbid functioning and normal findings on his initial clinical evaluation several years ago. His neuropsychological evaluation 5 years later was also inconclusive for cognitive decline, and results of the follow-up FDG PET scan showed a significant change in brain metabolism compared with his initial FDG PET scan. Results from the clinical evaluation, even during his follow-up examination, suggested that he was performing within normal limits for age. However, taking into account his superior premorbid functioning and previous academic attainment, together with the results of FDG PET, the findings are consistent with the cognitive deficits representing early neurodegenerative disease. The pattern of posterior-predominant hypometabolism is consistent with Alzheimer's changes,[5,6] and the mild occipital hypometabolism raises the possibility of early involvement of Lewy bodies as well.[5]

Case Study 3

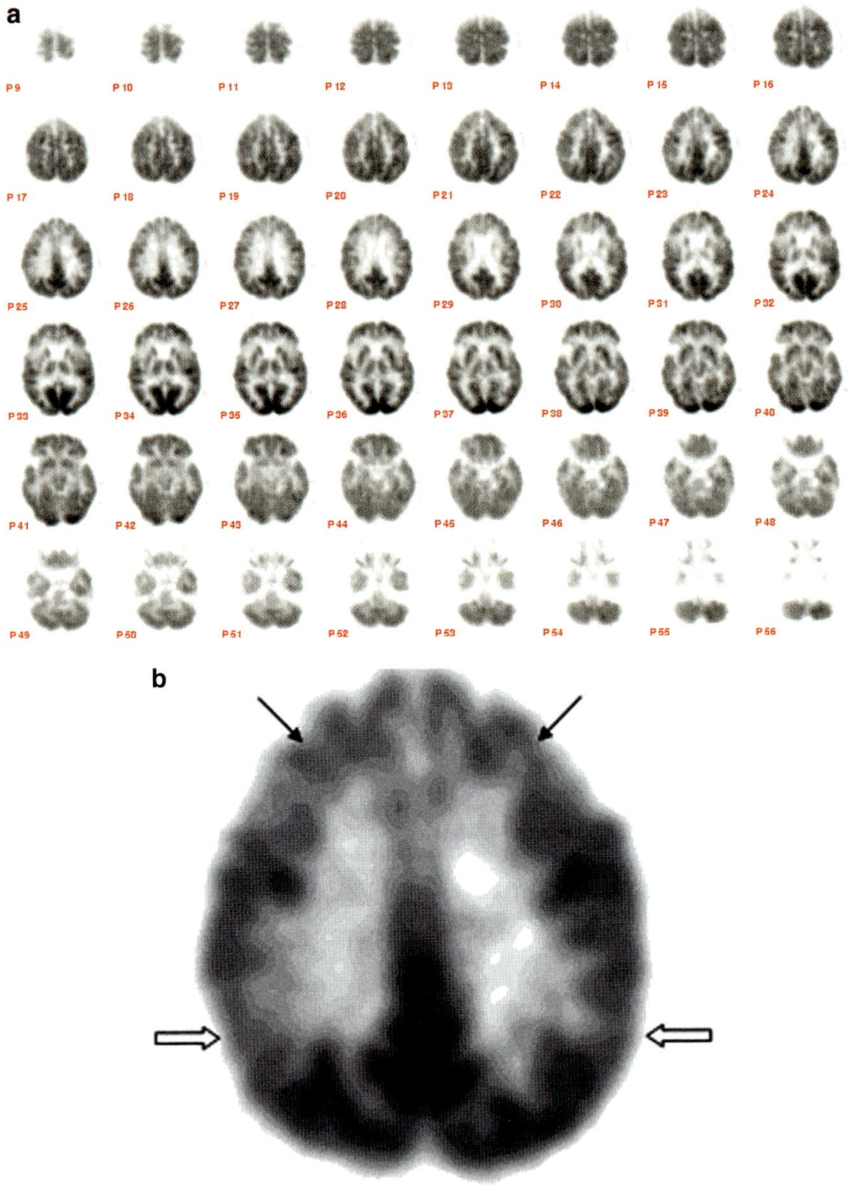

Fig. 7.3 **A.** Brain FDG PET of 60-year-old man with onset of behavioral, personality, and cognitive changes. **B.** Mild parietal hypometabolism (*open arrows*, right worse than left), and more extensive bilateral hypometabolism of the prefrontal cortex (*closed arrows*). **C.** Mild right anterior temporal hypometabolism. **D.** Quantitative (NeuroQ) assessment showing significant hypometabolism in the frontal cortex (>6 standard deviations below normal controls)

c

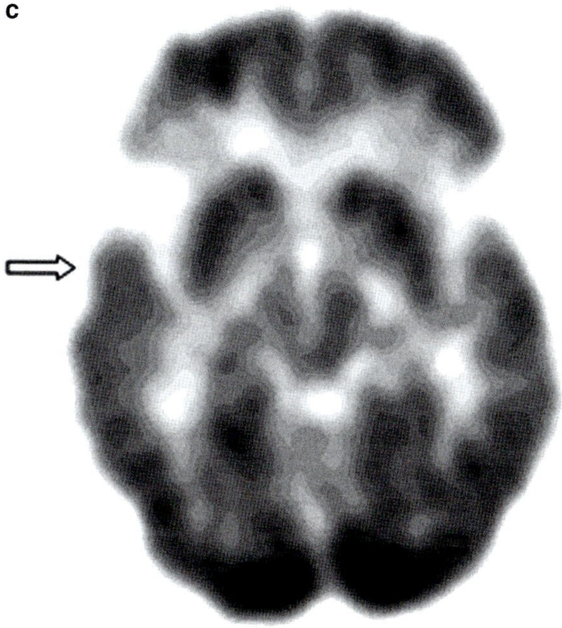

b

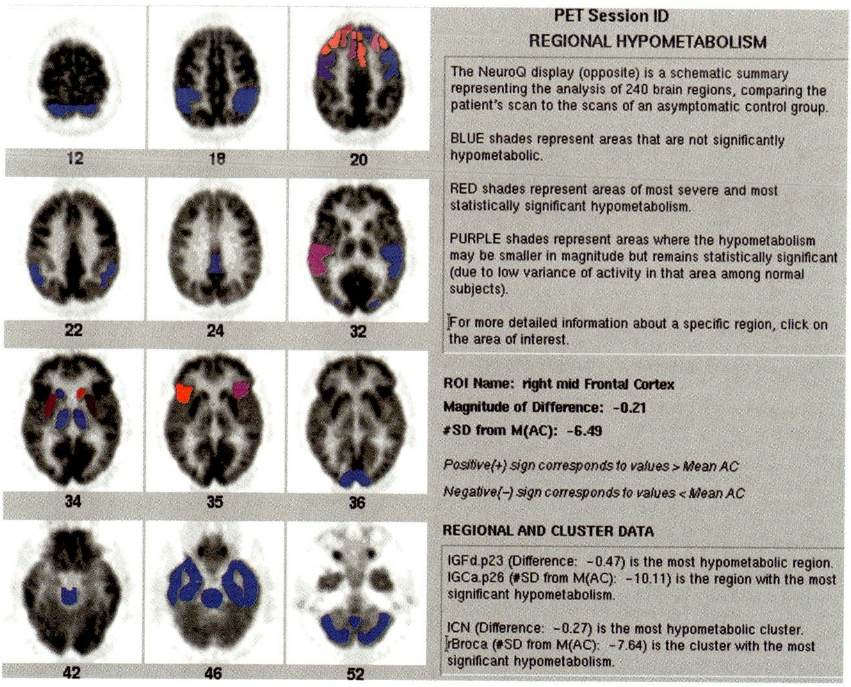

Fig. 7.3 (continued)

Indication

Mr. S was 60 years old when first evaluated for the acute onset of behavioral and personality changes. The patient had completed a grade school diploma in Jordan and had lived in the United States for the past two decades. Three years before his initial visit, he had begun experiencing several episodes of lightheadedness and nonvertiginous dizziness that had required a visit to the emergency room. During that time, Mr. S had elevated blood pressures and had experienced at least one episode of syncope. Since then, he experienced a lack of motivation and decreased initiation of motor behavior and speech. Subsequently, his business had suffered because of his decreased executive functioning and lack of judgment. At the time of his evaluation, he was noted to occasionally erupt in spontaneous laughter and sit with a vacant look for long periods of time, interacting only minimally. In addition, the clinician noted that his memory seemed to be impaired. On the other hand, Mr. S's ability for mathematical processing remained intact, and he was able to learn new information and keep up with current events fairly well. In terms of medical history, Mr. S was positive for malignant hypertension and irritable bowel syndrome. He reported no surgeries, medical ailments, illnesses, or conditions. In addition, his laboratory screen results, obtained 1 year before his examination, were normal with the exception of a slightly low hematocrit level (40). Mr. S reported occasional use of alcohol and a history of smoking before quitting over a decade ago.

On comprehensive neuropsychological testing, Mr. S was reluctant to comply or stay on track and answered with single word answers when questioned directly. He was unable to concentrate, completed only some language tasks, and refused to follow through on current events and abstract testing because of his failure to initiate behavior. He achieved a MMSE score of 21/30. Mr. S was assessed with frontal lobe syndrome, with ischemic insult to the frontal region, and frontotemporal dementia as considerations. Brain magnetic resonance imaging (MRI) at the time of his initial evaluation revealed "no structural abnormalities."

Scan Interpretation

FDG PET (Fig. 7.3a) revealed diffuse hypometabolism in the parietal and right anterior temporal regions (see open arrows in Figs. 7.3 b and c). PET also demonstrated bilateral frontal hypometabolism (see closed arrows in Fig. 7.3b). In addition, the posterior cingulate cortex was only mildly hypometabolic, the sensorimotor cortex was relatively spared, and the visual cortex appeared to be well preserved. These findings were supported through quantitative (NeuroQ analysis; Fig. 7.3d).

Follow-up Visit

Mr. S returned 3 months after his initial evaluation, whereupon he achieved a MMSE score of 23/30. On testing, the clinician noted that he sat quietly and stared vacantly. He again responded with short phrases and single words when asked direct questions, and he was unable to complete any language-related tasks. Mr. S's performance on most aspects of the neuropsychological battery remained relatively unchanged from his initial evaluation. The clinician thought that Mr. S's diagnosis was most consistent with frontotemporal dementia, such as Pick's disease.

Teaching Point

Mr. S experienced an acute onset of behavioral and personality change that was unexplained by his general history, physical examination, or laboratory screen. Although the patient's MRI revealed no structural abnormalities, FDG PET was able to detect clear patterns of cerebral metabolism most consistent with frontotemporal dementia.[7,8]

Case Study 4

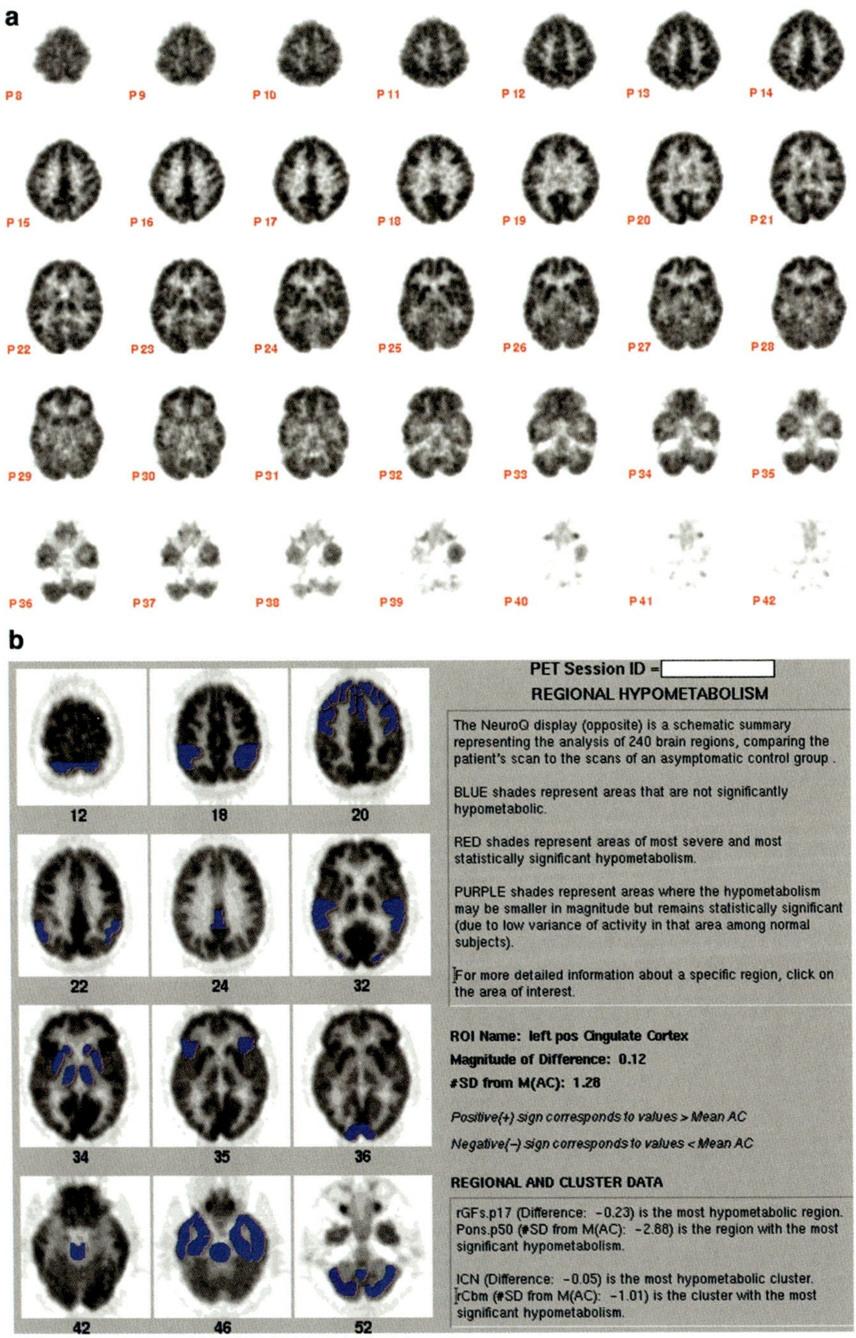

Fig. 7.4 **A.** Brain FDG of 54-year-old woman with mild memory complaints. **B.** Quantitative (NeuroQ) assessment showing no areas of significant hypometabolism.

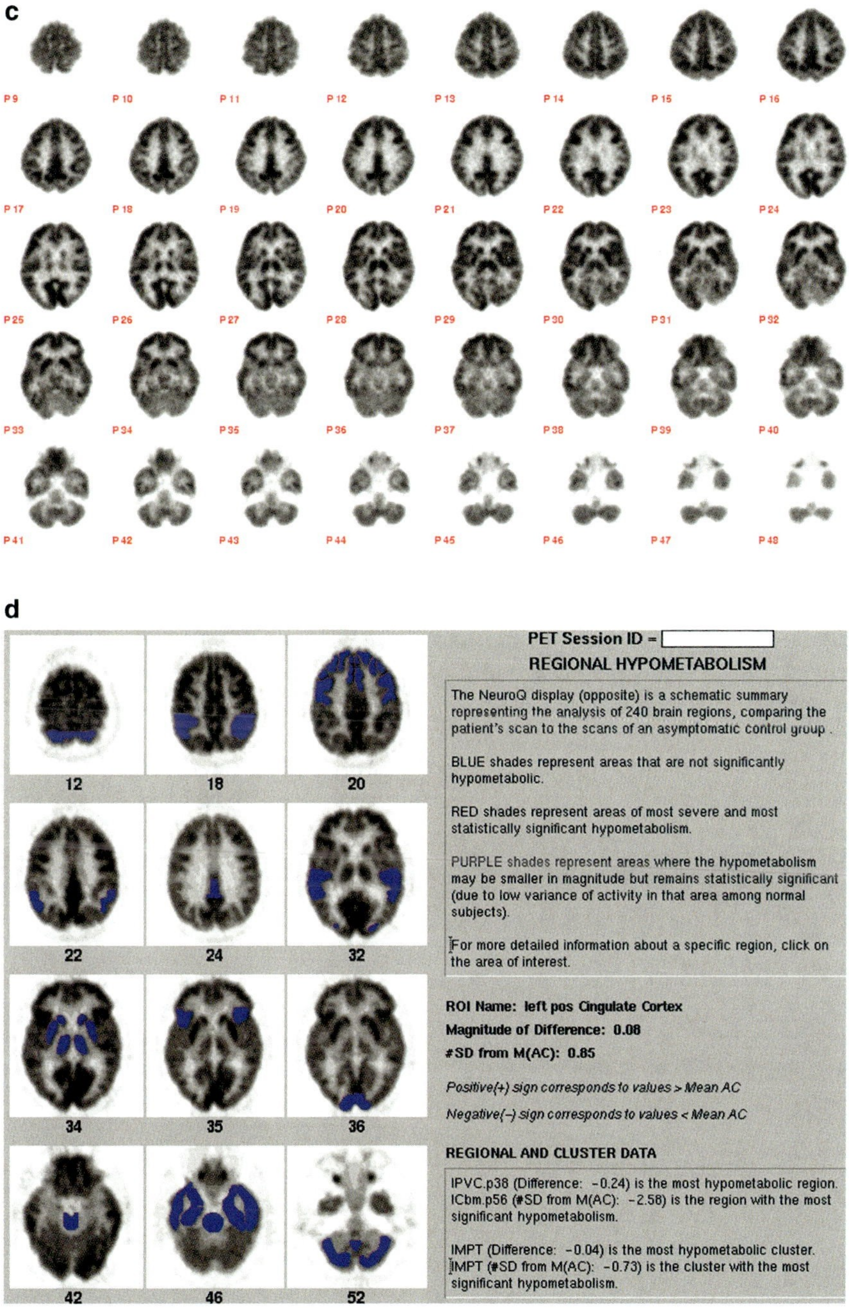

Fig. 7.4 (continued) **C.** PET scan 19 months later, with variable results on testing neuropsychological performance, along with symptoms for depression. **D.** Follow-up quantitative (NeuroQ) assessment confirming no areas of significant hypometabolism

Indication

Ms. D, a 54-year-old right-handed woman, underwent initial memory testing as a volunteer for part of a neuropsychological study. She came to the United States as a young adult after growing up in India and had been married for 30 years, with no children. In addition to English, she spoke three Indian languages. She had also obtained a law degree (19 years of education) in India. Although she never practiced law, she worked several jobs as a law clerk, stockbroker, and financial advisor, along with being a homemaker and office manager in her husband's office. Ms. D's psychiatric and medical histories were insignificant for any major illnesses or hospitalizations. She reported drinking alcohol 4–5 times per week, with no history of tobacco use or recreational drugs.

At the time of her initial examination, Ms. D expressed concern about her memory capabilities, stating that she had begun to forget things such as phone numbers, names, and titles of books and movies, which in the past had come quickly to her. In the same way, she reported that her mathematical calculations were taking longer than they had in the past. Results from a comprehensive neuropsychological examination were found to be variable. Ms. D obtained an MMSE score of 30/30 and generally performed within normal limits in areas of orientation, attention and concentration, and executive functioning. On the other hand, she demonstrated significant impairment on some measures of phonemic fluency, visuospatial functioning, and psychomotor speed. In terms of immediate and delayed recall for both visual and verbal memory, Ms. D performed consistently within age norms for 91% of the tasks, with a decreased score on only one dimension of immediate visual memory. She was diagnosed with age consistent memory impairment.

Scan 1 Interpretation

The gross structure of the brain was normal. The pattern of distribution of FDG throughout the cortex was symmetric and unremarkable, with relatively higher uptake in the posterior cingulate appropriately seen (Fig. 7.4a). The deep structures and cerebellum were also preserved. No evidence of neurodegenerative disease was seen. Quantitative (NeuroQ) assessment confirmed no areas of significant hypometabolism (Fig. 7.4b).

Follow-up Visit

Ms. D returned 19 months later for both neuropsychological and PET follow-ups. She stated that her declining memory problems were still present, although she believed that they were now comparable with her peers. In addition, she reported feeling overwhelmed with multitasking duties, and as result, had reduced her social activities. She also noted having difficulty concentrating, which had begun to affect her reading comprehension, along with symptoms of insomnia, fatigue, reduced appetite, and anhedonia. She admitted feelings of a depressed mood, likely attributed to the fact that her parents living in India had begun to suffer from poor health. These reported symptoms were apparent behaviorally, as the neurologist noted that although she did appear motivated to complete each task, she seemed "far off in thought" and directions had to be repeated. Her clinical reevaluation continued to exhibit variable results. Ms. D achieved an MMSE score of 29/30 and significantly improved on measures of psychomotor speed and visuospatial functioning on which she previously had demonstrated severe impairment. In contrast, her phonemic fluency significantly decreased, as well as her ability with confrontation naming. Memory assessments were variable.

Scan 2 Interpretation

No significant change was seen since the previous scan (Fig. 7.4c). Quantitative (NeuroQ) assessment again confirmed no areas of significant hypometabolism (Fig. 7.4d).

Teaching Point

Ms. D reported memory problems that seemed to have progressed in the 5–7 years before her most recent examination. Given her high education and estimated intelligence level, her self-reported symptoms and rote-retrieval deficits over time compared with others her age raised concern for a progressive neurodegenerative disease process. In addition, she also reported that her mother, grandfather, and sister also showed memory problems with age, revealing a possible genetic predisposition for memory decline. On the other hand, Ms. D's results from both neuropsychological evaluations over a 19-month period were variable. She obtained scores spanning the high average to impaired range on many of the subtests under each cognitive area assessed, with no clear evidence for neurodegenerative disease. In addition, confounding factors may have complicated results from her neuropsychological results. For example, Ms. D reported additional symptoms that were consistent with depression (e.g., insomnia, loss of appetite, anhedonia, anxiety),[9] which may have been heightened because of her parents' recent declining health. In her case, anxiety and depression could have contributed to memory impairment.[10] Ms. D's memory deficits, clinical symptoms, and variable neuropsychological results were almost certainly caused by factors unrelated to a progressive dementing disorder, most likely depression. This conclusion is supported by Ms. D's PET scan results over the same period, which both indicated a normal pattern of FDG uptake inconsistent with Alzheimer's or a related progressive disease process. Ms. D should seek an evaluation and subsequent treatment for anxiety/depression, and if symptoms of memory decline still persist, a clinical and metabolic follow-up could be beneficial.

Case Study 5

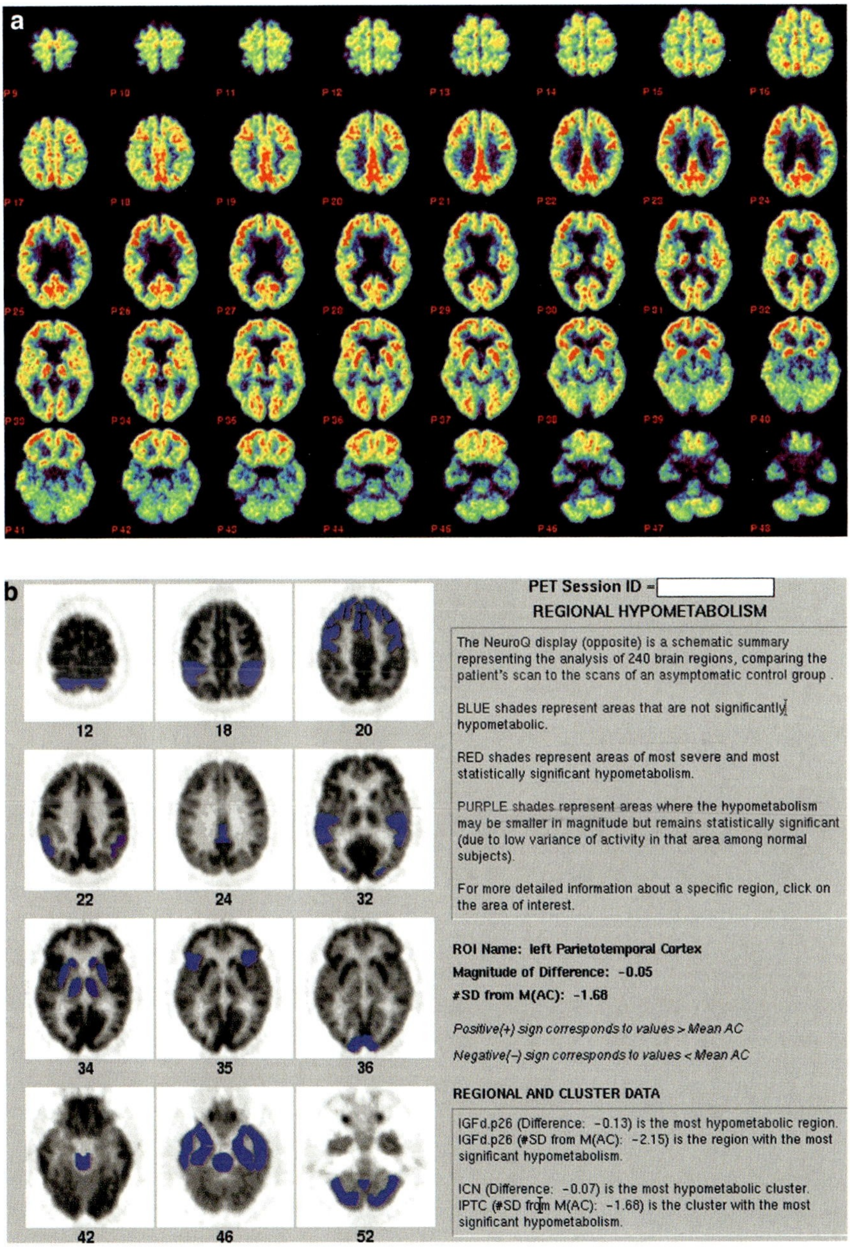

Fig. 7.5 **A.** Brain FDG PET of 76-year-old man with a diagnosis of age consistent memory impairment. **B.** Quantitative (NeuroQ) assessment showing mild hypometabolism in the parieto-temporal region.

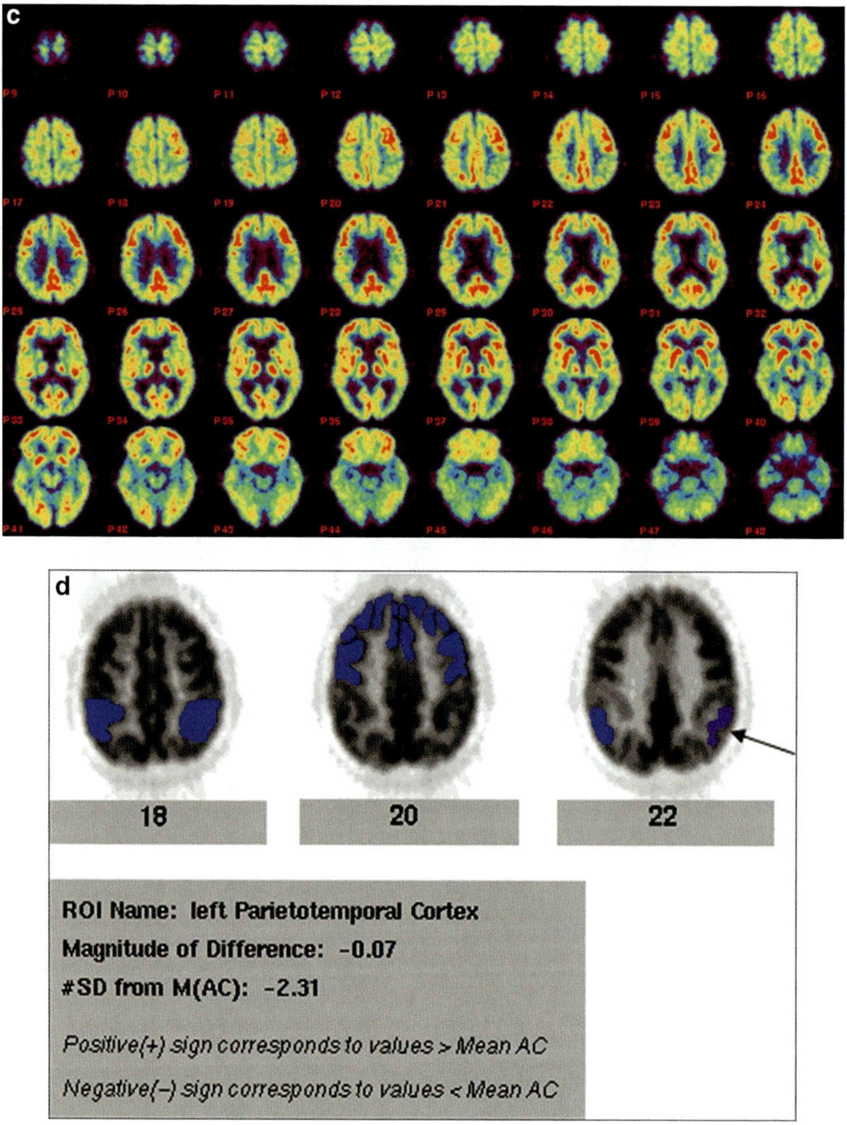

Fig. 7.5 (continued) **C.** PET scan 19 months later, with ambiguous results on testing neuropsychological performance. **D.** Quantitative (NeuroQ) assessment showing significant progression of hypometabolism in the parietotemporal region

Indication

Mr. M, a right-handed man, was 76 years old at the time of clinical evaluation. With a degree in civil engineering, he had held several high-level jobs in the private sector and public service. His family medical history was significant for cardiovascular disease, and his sister was suffering from progressive dementia. Mr. M's medical history was otherwise unremarkable, with only a lumbar laminectomy for back trouble. He reported drinking approximately five glasses of wine per week, but denied any history of tobacco or drug use. He also did not endorse any symptoms of anxiety or depression. At the time of his initial examination, Mr. M had no serious complaints of memory decline, with the exception that he had started forgetting where he placed his keys.

Comprehensive clinical and neuropsychological testing showed that he was cognitively normal for age. However, he demonstrated relative weaknesses on measures of verbal and nonverbal working memory, semantic fluency, and immediate and delayed verbal memory when his superior occupational and educational backgrounds were taken into consideration. The patient was diagnosed with age consistent memory impairment.

Scan 1 Interpretation

Initial FDG PET showed generalized atrophy with associated cortical hypometabolism (Fig. 7.5a). There was also a slight frontal-parietal gradient, at the borderline of the range of normal variation. FDG uptake in the area of the posterior cingulate cortex (the cortical region that decreases the most significantly in the earliest stages of Alzheimer's[1,11]) remained robust. Quantitative (NeuroQ) assessment (Fig. 7.5b) demonstrated left parietotemporal cortex falling approximately 5% and 1.7 standard deviations below normal mean values.

Follow-up Visit

On clinical and neuropsychological follow-up, Mr. M reported new memory problems—such as forgetting familiar movie stars and restaurant names—that had developed over the past year. He insisted that these symptoms were not "major complaints." His performance on the neuropsychological battery was generally within normal limits for age; however, these results were variable, as he had both significantly higher and significantly lower performance scores compared with those of his previous examination. For example, whereas his performances on tests of orientation, attention and concentration, and visuospatial functioning were comparable, there was marked improvement for tasks of executive functioning, and inconsistent results for tasks of immediate and delayed memory. Mr. M declined on two delayed verbal memory tasks (rote list recall, word pairs), whereas he significantly improved on tasks of delayed recall of learning paragraph stories and immediate recall of word pairs. The neurologist noted that his improvements on some tasks could result from pharmacologic intervention (i.e., donepezil)[12] or practice effects (although Mr. M could not recall when his first evaluation was and did not remember the majority of the tests). A second brain PET scan was obtained.

Scan 2 Interpretation

Follow-up FDG PET again demonstrated moderate atrophy with associated generalized cortical hypometabolism (Fig. 7.5c). In addition, there was an abnormal distribution of FDG, with mild bilateral inferior parietal and posterior cingulate cortical hypometabolism. Activity in deep cortical structures and cerebellum was preserved. Figure 7.5d shows follow-up results from quantitative (NeuroQ) analysis, demonstrating left parietotemporal hypometabolism falling approximately 7% and 2.3 standard deviations below normal mean values.

Teaching Point

The patient's clinical follow-up was ambiguous, as Mr. M showed some signs of cognitive stability, as well as of possible memory deficits. Taking into account his high premorbid abilities, family history of dementia, memory complaints, and immediate and delayed memory problems observed during his more recent evaluation, Mr. M's cognitive profile raised concern for memory decline related to the onset of the early stages of a progressive disease process such as Alzheimer's. Although his more recent clinical evaluation lacked conclusive evidence for significant cognitive changes compared with his evaluation 2 years prior, FDG PET did show progression to a representative pattern of tracer uptake most consistent with changes occurring in the early stages of Alzheimer's disease, taking advantage of the high sensitivity of PET.[1,4] In this case, FDG PET was useful in providing Mr. M the opportunity to consider possible further treatment intervention, such as supplementing his cholinesterase inhibitor regimen with memantine, as well as more accurately forecasting his future cognitive course.[13]

Case Study 6

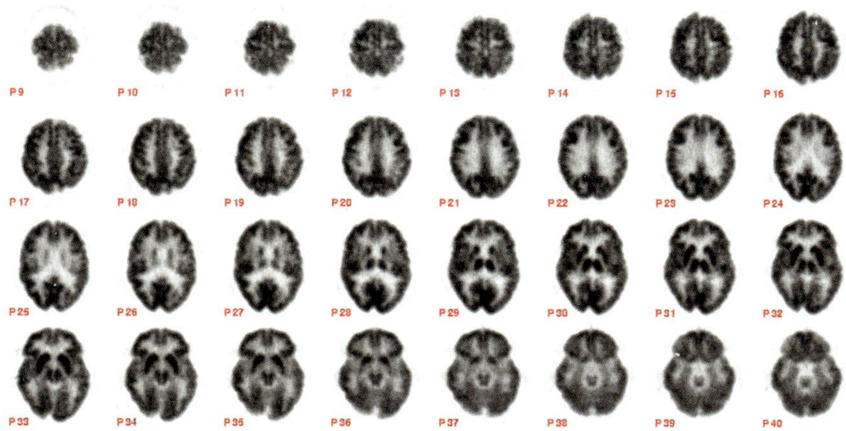

Fig. 7.6 Brain FDG PET of 71-year-old woman who denied having short-term memory difficulties

Indication

Ms. L was a retired English teacher with a Bachelor's degree in education. Ms. L believed her cognition was intact; however, her family insisted that she had difficulties with short-term memory and misplacing objects, and that her symptoms had become more noticeable over the past year. Ms. L's family and psychiatric histories were unremarkable. In a preliminary MMSE test, she scored a 22/30, including a 0/3 for short-term recall.

Scan Interpretation

Ms. L's PET scan shows normal metabolic brain activity (very mild left temporal hypometabolism, not clearly beyond the range of normal variation) (Fig. 7.6). Regions hypometabolic in patients with early Alzheimer's disease (inferior parietal cortex, parietotemporal cortex, posterior temporal cortex)[5,6] were unremarkable.

Follow-up Visit

Ms. L was treated with donepezil for her mild cognitive impairment and made frequent follow-up visits. One and a half years subsequent to her initial evaluation, Ms. L seemed active and independent in spite of her memory impairment. Her daughter reported no behavior or memory changes. Her MMSE score was 27/30.

Teaching Point

Ms. L denied having any memory problems, although her family insisted she had difficulties with short-term memory. Her MMSE score of 22/30 suggested cognitive impairment. A PET scan was thus performed to assess cognitive functioning and evaluate for the possibility of Alzheimer's disease, as autopsy series and longitudinal follow-up studies show that visual analysis of FDG PET has 90%–95% sensitivity for detecting neurodegenerative diseases causing dementia, including among patients having only mild or even questionable dementia.[5] Ms. L's PET scan revealed normal brain activity in the frontal, parietal, and temporal cortex. A follow-up clinical evaluation demonstrated a stable or reversible impairment (MMSE, 27/30), unlikely caused by Alzheimer's disease. This conclusion is consistent with her initial PET scan.

Case Study 7

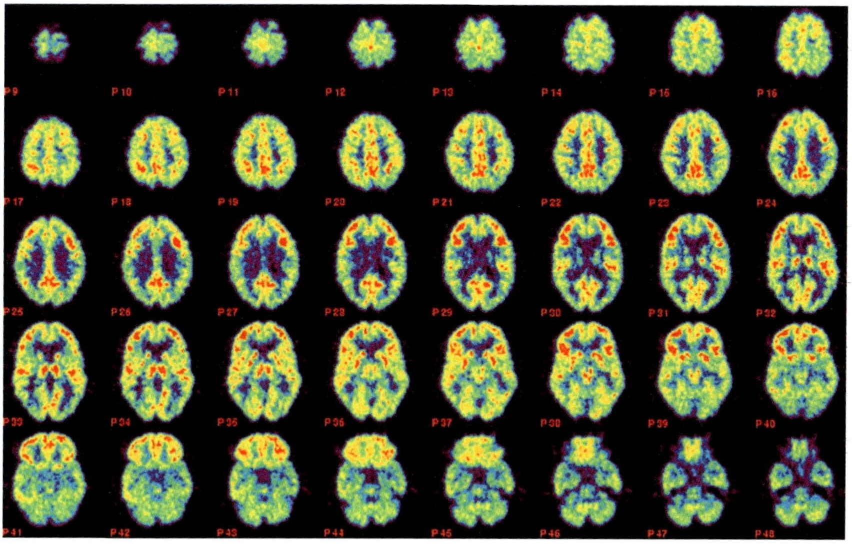

Fig. 7.7 A PET scan of 63-year-old man who had normal neuropsychological performance

Indication

Mr. K, a right-handed man, was 62 years old at the time of initial presentation. He lived alone, after being divorced with no children. He obtained a graduate degree in computer science and had worked as an aerospace engineer for 20 years before retirement. Mr. K's psychiatric and medical histories were unremarkable, with the exception of a minor surgery to remove a stone from his salivary glands and a possible concussion resulting from a fight during high school. He also reported infrequent alcohol intake and no family history of dementia.

At the time of initial clinical evaluation, Mr. K complained of minor memory difficulties, especially with auditory information, but reported that he had no difficulty remembering something if he had seen it. He claimed that these memory problems, such as forgetting where he had put his glasses and forgetting someone's name right after he had heard it, had gradually worsened over the past few years. However, on comprehensive neuropsychological testing, whereupon he obtained an MMSE score of 29/30, Mr. K was evaluated as cognitively normal, as indicated by his functioning within normal, if not superior, ranges for all areas tested: orientation, attention and concentration, psychomotor speed, visual and spatial abilities, language, executive functioning, and immediate and delayed memory.

During a clinical follow-up evaluation 14 months later, Mr. K continued to complain of memory difficulties involving language, word-finding, and remembering names. He also reported that for the past month or 2, he had been experiencing "dull headaches."

Comprehensive neuropsychological follow-up indicated that his performance on all tasks stayed relatively consistent when compared with scores acquired 14 months previously. Mr. K had an MMSE score of 30/30. He performed within normal limits in areas of concern. For example, he demonstrated intact immediate and delayed verbal memory, with relative strengths in tasks of recalling contextual information and rote word list learning.

Scan Interpretation

The patient's PET scan showed mild global hypometabolism, with superimposed inferior parietal, occipital, and posterior cingulate cortical hypometabolism (Fig. 7.7). Areas of the basal ganglia, thalamus and cerebellum auditory cortex, and brainstem were relatively preserved.

Teaching Point

Mr. K's FDG PET indicated a pattern of tracer uptake suggestive of an early neurodegenerative disease process. The pattern of posterior cingulate (the cortical region decreasing the most significantly in the earliest stages of Alzheimer's disease[1,11]) hypometabolism, along with inferior parietal hypometabolism, is most suggestive of incipient Alzheimer's disease.[5,6] In this case, whereas Mr. K's clinical and neuropsychological evaluations failed to show any signs of memory decline related to a progressive dementing disorder, FDG PET demonstrated representative patterns of a degenerative process possibly underlying his self-reported memory complaints. PET has sensitivity for detecting both early neurodegenerative disease, along with any clinical progression that would occur over the next 3 years, of approximately 95%.[1,3,4] Thus, the pattern of regional cerebral metabolism noted, and the interim development of posterior cortical hypometabolism, indicate that Mr. K deserves close follow-up to monitor for likely imminent cognitive decline, allowing early institution of an appropriate plan of management if and when such changes become more clinically evident to the patient, any close contacts, or his physician.[13,14]

Case Study 8

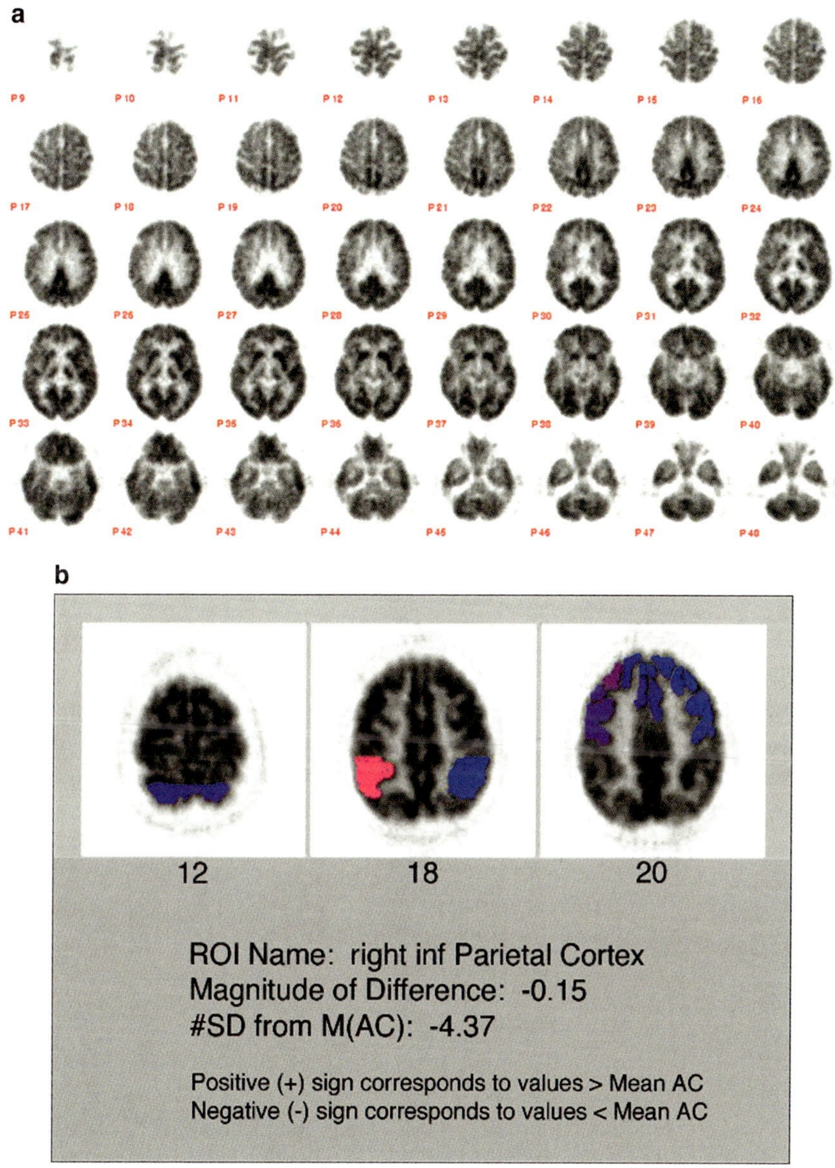

Fig. 7.8 **A.** Brain FDG PET of 74-year-old man with symptoms of memory loss, cognitive deficits, and motor deficits. **B.** Quantitative (NeuroQ) assessment showing significant hypometabolism in the right inferior parietal cortex (>4 standard deviations below normal controls)

Indication

Mr. F, a retired lawyer, was 74 years old when he first visited a neurologist for symptoms of memory loss and cognitive decline. His symptoms included "slowness and retrieval problems" associated with subcortical conditions that did not meet criteria for dementia or Lewy bodies. Mr. F demonstrated an atypical Parkinsonism, consistent with akinetic rigid form, frequent falls, and restricted eye movements. At the time of his evaluation, his medications included carbidopa-levodopa (Sinemet), pergolide, selegiline (Atapryl), vitamins B and E, and calcium supplements. The patient also had a past history of heavy alcohol use. A brain MRI obtained that same year revealed cerebral cortical atrophy, moderate cerebellar atrophy, and severe midbrain atrophy.

Scan Interpretation

FDG PET demonstrated moderate right frontal and parietal hypometabolism, not normal for age-related decline (Fig. 7.8a). Mild hypometabolism of the right thalamus and basal ganglia was also observed, as was mild left cerebellar hypometabolism secondary to cross-cerebellar diaschisis. NeuroQ analysis (Fig. 7.8b) quantified the abnormality in the right inferior parietal cortex as falling 15% and four standard deviations below normal. The posterior cingulate cortex was relatively preserved.

Follow-up Visit

Mr. F was last seen in the outpatient clinic 10 months after his initial examination, with worsening symptoms of progressive memory deficit, slowness in responsiveness, and confused speech. His motor symptoms at that time also included loss of balance not associated with vertigo, resulting in multiple falls.

Upon his death 2 months later, a brain-only autopsy was performed, which revealed "marked atrophy of the cerebral hemispheres with widening of the sulci, most prominent at the frontal and parietal lobes." In addition, the cerebellum and brainstem were also found to be mild to moderately atrophic. At autopsy, Mr. F was diagnosed with progressive supranuclear palsy.

Teaching Point

Mr. F showed symptoms of cognitive decline and motor deficits at the time of his neurologic examination that did not meet criteria for dementia or Lewy bodies. The patient's MRI was suspicious for a neurodegenerative disorder; however, a clear diagnosis was not made. FDG PET demonstrated moderate hypometabolism of the frontal and parietal lobes, and mild hypometabolism of the right thalamus, basal ganglia, and cerebellum. Such changes were consistent with the subcortical dementia type, progressive supranuclear palsy, which was confirmed at autopsy.[15] In this case, FDG PET, 12 months before Mr. F's death, accurately showed a distribution of cerebral metabolism consistent with progressive supranuclear palsy.

Case Study 9

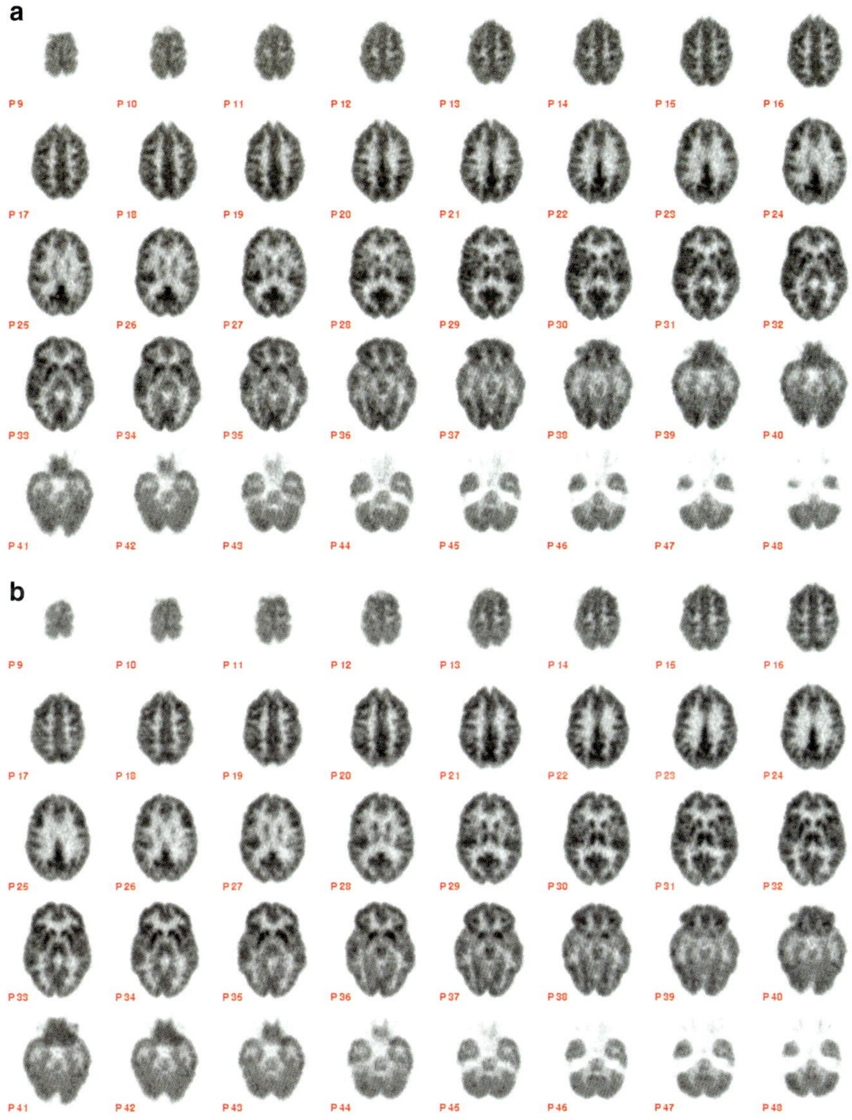

Fig. 7.9 **A.** Brain FDG PET of 54-year-old woman with impaired neuropsychological performance. **B.** PET scan 18 months later, with no change in neuropsychological performance

Indication

Ms. G was a right-handed 54-year-old woman when first evaluated. She had 13 years of education and had been working as a supervisor at a clinical appointment call center for 30 years. Her mother, who was 80 years old, had been diagnosed with both Alzheimer's and Parkinson's diseases and her father had died from Creutzfeldt-Jakob disease. Her medical history was notable for Bartholin cyst removal and back surgery. She had also recently entered menopause and had started taking fluoxetine (Prozac) to alleviate hot flashes. She reported mild alcohol consumption and no cigarette or drug use.

Ms. G noted that she had begun experiencing tension and irritability associated with her mother's care in her own home (Hamilton Anxiety Rating Scale = 10). In addition, she reported that she had begun to occasionally forget names and words that she wanted to use, although she claimed that it did not significantly affect her daily functioning. Upon neuropsychological evaluation, Ms. G was found to be functioning within normal limits in tests of orientation and psychomotor speed. MMSE score was 27/30. On the other hand, language, visuospatial functioning, executive functioning, and memory domains yielded variable results, with most of her scores falling in the mild-to-moderately impaired range. More specifically, her ability to consistently recall the same words fell within the severely impaired range (4th percentile), which raised concern for memory decline when her scores were compared with other individuals of her age group. The pattern of impaired performance on aspects of attention and concentration, phonemic fluency, visual spatial functioning, and verbal memory was thought to possibly have been reflective of hormonal imbalance. In addition, psychosocial stress because of her home situation also may have impacted her scores. Ms. G was diagnosed with age consistent memory impairment.

Scan 1 Interpretation

The gross structure of the brain was normal (Fig. 7.9a). Normal distribution of FDG was observed, and the pattern throughout the cortex was symmetric and unremarkable. Relatively higher uptake in the posterior cingulate cortex was appropriately observed, along with the typical pattern of higher uptake in the basal ganglia, thalamus, and cerebellum. There was no evidence for neurodegenerative disease.

Follow-up Visit

Ms. G returned 18 months later for a neuropsychological follow-up. At that time, she acknowledged additional symptoms of depression related to the burden of taking care of her ailing mother. She reported minimal social activity since she had begun her care-giving duties and stated that her job had started causing her considerable stress. However, she noted that her memory has remained the same since her last evaluation. Completion of the neuropsychological battery indicated that Ms. G's functioning in the domains of orientation (MMSE, 30/30), attention and concentration, psychomotor speed, language, and executive functioning had generally improved or remained consistent from her initial evaluation. On the other hand, her performance in the memory domain remained variable, with scores on immediate verbal and visual memory tasks remaining consistent, and scores on delayed memory tasks spanning the superior to severely impaired range. Ms. G was also noted to have heightened anxiety, particularly during attention and memory tasks and made comments such as, "My mind is blank," and "It's hard to concentrate."

Scan 2 Interpretation

No significant change since previous scan was observed (Fig. 7.9b).

Teaching Point

Although Ms. G reported only mild memory symptoms, her maternal family history of dementia and impaired performances on most of the subtests of the neuropsychological battery on presentation raised concern for the onset of further memory decline. However, several factors could have impacted her scores. It was unclear to what degree her heightened anxiety level, depressive symptoms from the strain of caregiving, apprehension of developing dementia herself, and altered hormonal levels because of her recent transition into menopause could be affecting her cognition. Ms. G's impairment on some tests could be attributed to her anxiety, as she appeared to become overwhelmed and complained of her mind going blank when there was too much new input. In this case, Ms. G's initial PET scan did not yield patterns reflective of a progressive neurodegenerative disease. This was reconfirmed in her follow-up PET. The use of PET aided in ruling out neurodegenerative dementia as the cause of her cognitive deficits.[6,16]

Case Study 10

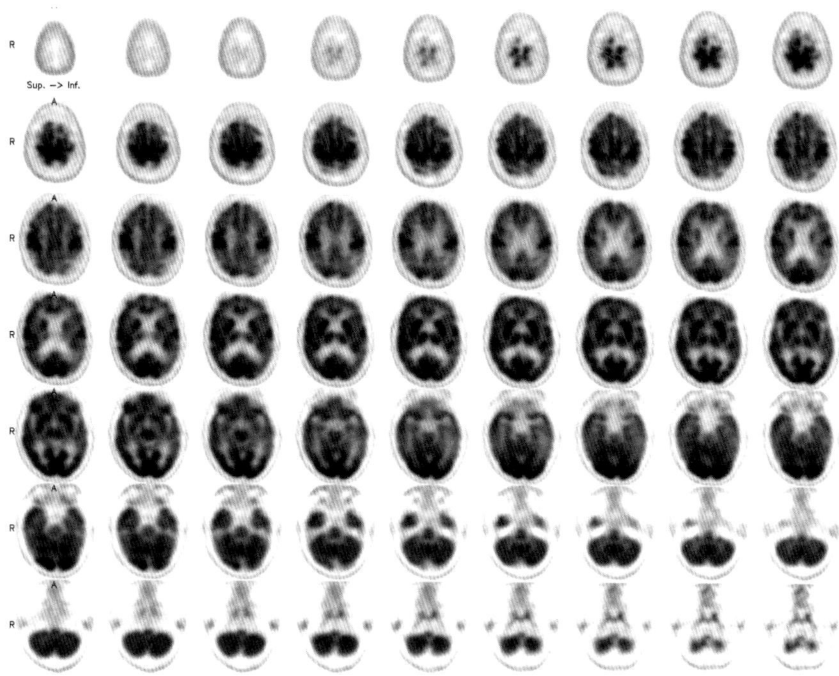

Fig. 7.10 Brain FDG PET of 55-year-old woman clinically diagnosed with frontotemporal dementia

Indication

Ms. W, a 55-year-old left-handed woman with severe progressive memory loss for more than 3 years, reported that she was sometimes depressed. She had recently given up her driver's license. The patient's working diagnosis included frontotemporal dementia. She had been treated with donepezil (Aricept) and memantine (Namenda). Her MMSE score was 3/30, and her recent MRI report showed mild generalized atrophy.

Scan Interpretation

The FDG PET scan was markedly abnormal with severe mid- and inferior parietal, posterior cingulate, and left temporal cortical hypometabolism, as well as moderately severe frontal, right temporal, and superior parietal hypometabolism (Fig. 7.10). The metabolism of the sensorimotor and occipital cortex was preserved. Basal ganglia, thalamus, and brainstem activity was unremarkable; the cerebellum showed less metabolic activity on the right, consistent with crossed-cerebellar diaschisis.

Teaching Point

Although Ms. W's working diagnosis was frontotemporal dementia, the patient was treated with donepezil and memantine, medications that have only been approved by the Food and Drug Administration for the treatment of Alzheimer's disease.[12,17,18] Although memantine is indicated for moderate-to-severe Alzheimer's disease, its value for treatment of frontotemporal dementia is unproved. Donepezil, like other cholinesterase inhibitors, has not been approved for the treatment of frontotemporal dementia and may even exacerbate the symptoms of patients with that disorder. The patient's diagnosis must be clarified so that an appropriate treatment plan may be constructed.[14] In this case, Ms. W's PET scan demonstrated posterior-predominant hypometabolism of the brain, with severe hypometabolism of the parietal, posterior cingulate, and left temporal cortex. The frontal-to-parietal gradient of diminishing activity and the degree of involvement of the posterior cingulate cortex were consistent with a diagnosis of Alzheimer's disease, making an anti-Alzheimer's pharmacologic regimen appropriate.[5,6,11] In addition, the young age of onset for this patient's presumptive Alzheimer's disease suggested that she may be suffering from one of the three familial forms known to be associated with early onset of symptoms, and her family history should be detailed.

Case Study 11

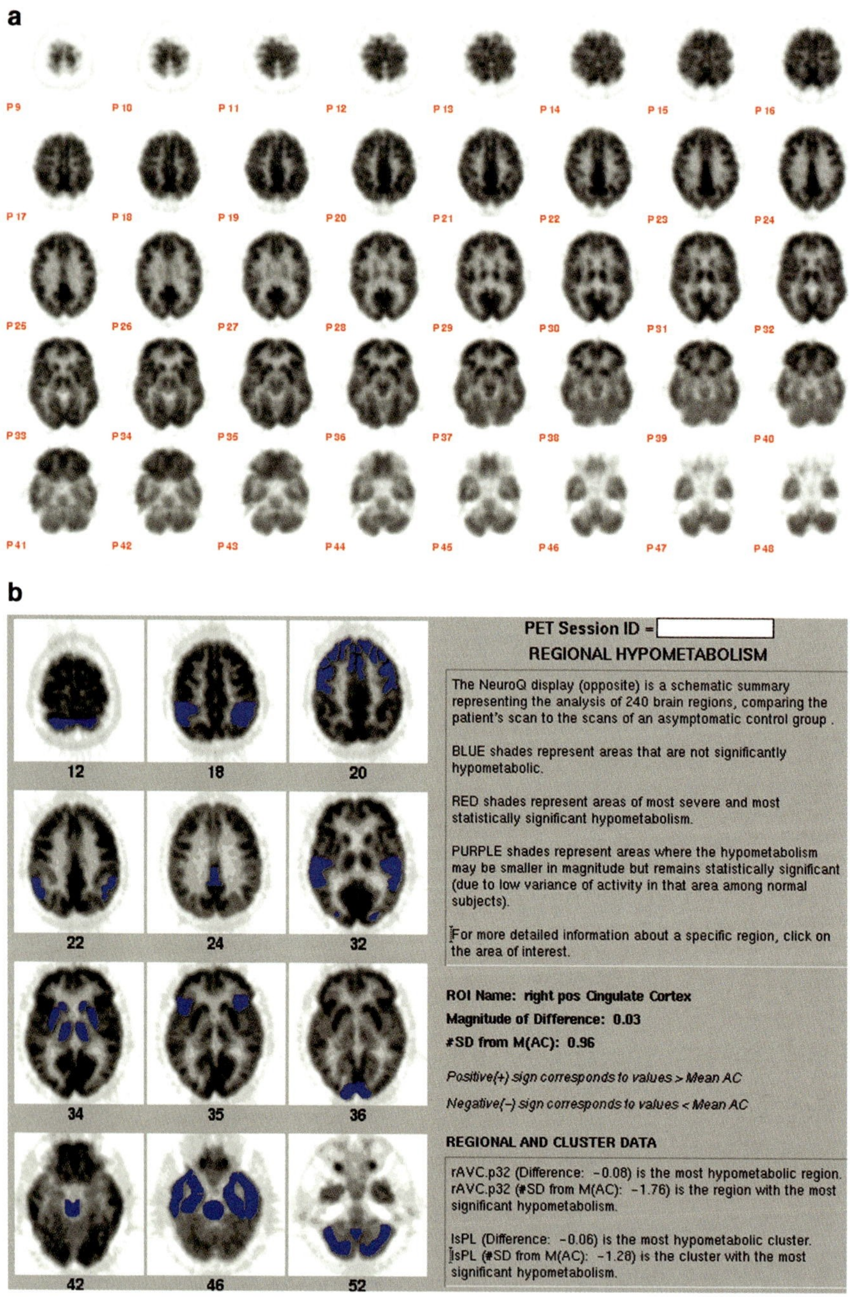

Fig. 7.11 A. Brain FDG PET of 76-year-old woman with self-reported memory complaints. **B.** Quantitative (NeuroQ) assessment showing no areas of significant hypometabolism.

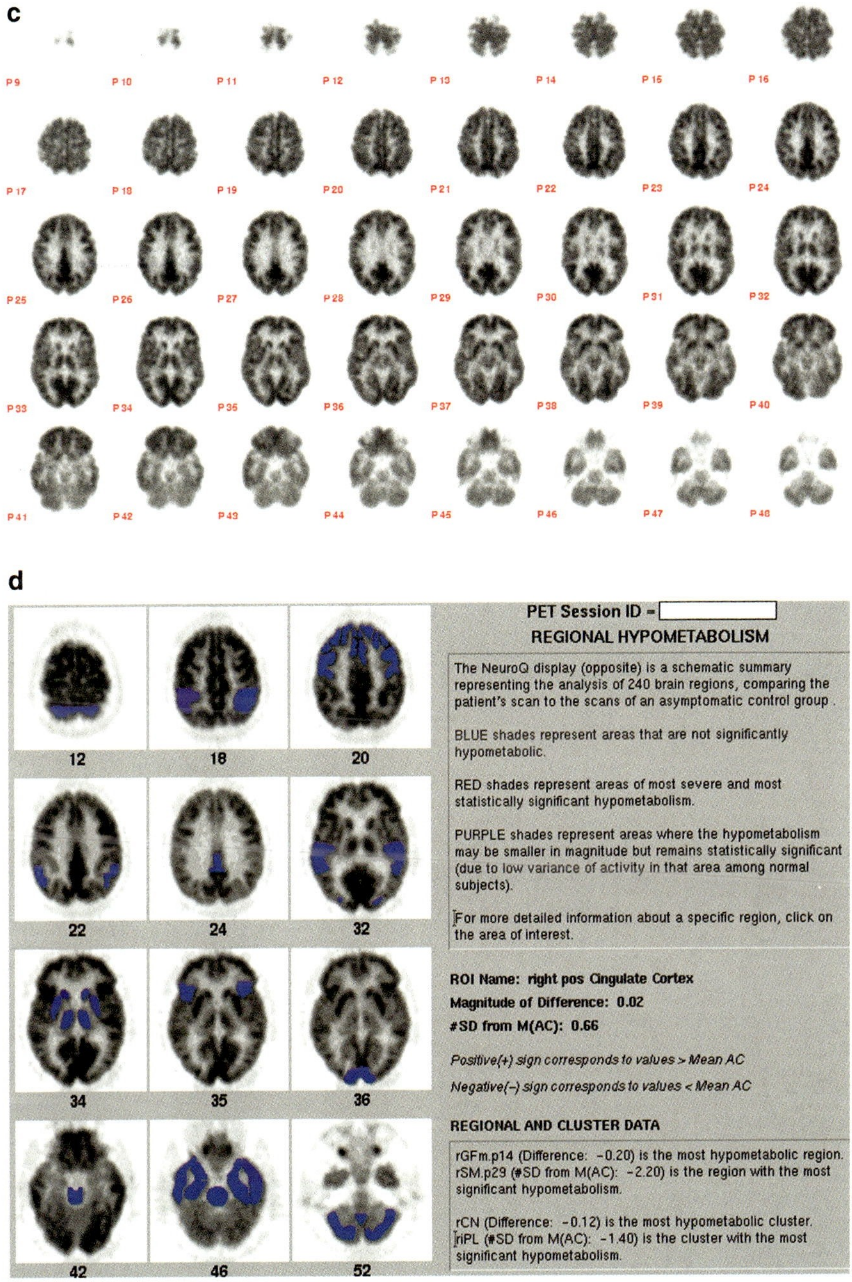

Fig. 7.11 (continued) **C.** PET scan 19 months later, with no change in cognitive functioning. **D.** Quantitative (NeuroQ) assessment showing no significant change in areas of hypometabolism

Indication

Ms. F, a right-handed woman with a high school education, was 76 years old on initial clinical evaluation. She lived with her middle-aged daughter and had been doing volunteer work for the past 7 years. She had worked in the field of electronics prior to that, but retired early in order to take care of her ailing husband, who died from complications of Parkinson's disease. Although Ms. F did not report a family history of dementia, there was a strong family history of depression, cancer, and heart disease among her siblings and parents. In terms of her personal medical history, Ms. F had a history of phlebitis, surgery for cataracts, and osteoporosis. She denied tobacco or drug use and reported having alcoholic drinks only on special occasions.

At the time of clinical evaluation, Ms. F reported some memory decline over the past several years, most notably for names, details, and some short-term loss (i.e., cannot remember what she was looking for when she gets to the next room). Comprehensive clinical and neuropsychological examination indicated overall functioning within normal limits in most cognitive domains. However, she had difficulty with visuospatial functioning in terms of organizing complex information and seemed to fail at grasping the overall gestalt of an image design she was copying. On tasks of immediate and delayed memory, her scores were variable—she seemed to have more difficulties with retrieving than encoding information—and she was diagnosed with age consistent memory impairment.

Scan 1 Interpretation

Ms. F's first FDG PET indicated normal gross structure of the brain (Fig. 7.11a). Higher FDG uptake in the posterior cingulate cortex was appropriately seen, with the pattern of uptake in basal ganglia, thalamus, and cerebellum within normal limits. No areas of hypometabolism evident for neurodegenerative disease were seen. This was confirmed by quantitative (NeuroQ analysis, Fig. 7.11b).

Follow-up Visit

During her clinical follow-up evaluation, Ms. F continued to complain of mild cognitive symptoms, reporting that she "can't remember anything." In particular, she had difficulty remembering events, things, word finding, names, and retrieving objects around the house. In addition, she seemed to have a deficit in remembering historical information, for example, providing inconsistent numbers for her daughter's age with the year that she was born. When asked about possible symptoms of depression given her significant family history, Ms. F stated, "I could be depressed, but I keep myself busy." She also had difficulty hearing and admitted that she needed to consult a doctor about it. She attained a MMSE score of 28/30, which was consistent with her previous evaluation 19 months previously. Her performance levels on tasks of psychomotor speed, attention and concentration, visuospatial functioning, and executive functioning were also not significantly changed. However, her achievement on tasks of language and memory remained variable.

Scan 2 Interpretation

Ms. F's second FDG PET indicated that a small area of the left inferior temporal cortex was slightly less metabolic than the right side, but otherwise the scan was essentially unchanged from her previous scan (Fig. 7.11c). This was again confirmed by quantitative (NeuroQ) analysis (Fig. 7.11d).

Teaching Point

Ms. F's results from her follow-up neuropsychological testing remained variable. She did not present obvious signs of a progressive neurodegenerative disorder; however, the neurologist noted that results of neuropsychological testing may have been biased because of practice effects. Furthermore, Ms. F's acknowledgment of possible depression may have complicated the finding of a clear etiologic explanation for the locus of her memory complaints, as the presence of behavioral and psychological signs, including depressive symptoms, predicts a high likelihood of cognitive decline[19] and progression to cognitive impairment as well.[20] Taking all these factors from the clinical examination into consideration, FDG PET would provide a more useful measurement of predicting whether she would likely have a clinical course marked by progressive dementia caused by factors such as Alzheimer's disease.[1,15,21] Comparing Ms. F's FDG PET scans over a 19-month period showed that there was little change in brain metabolism. In this case, her memory complaints were almost certainly related to factors unrelated to a progressive dementing disorder, most likely depression.

Case Study 12

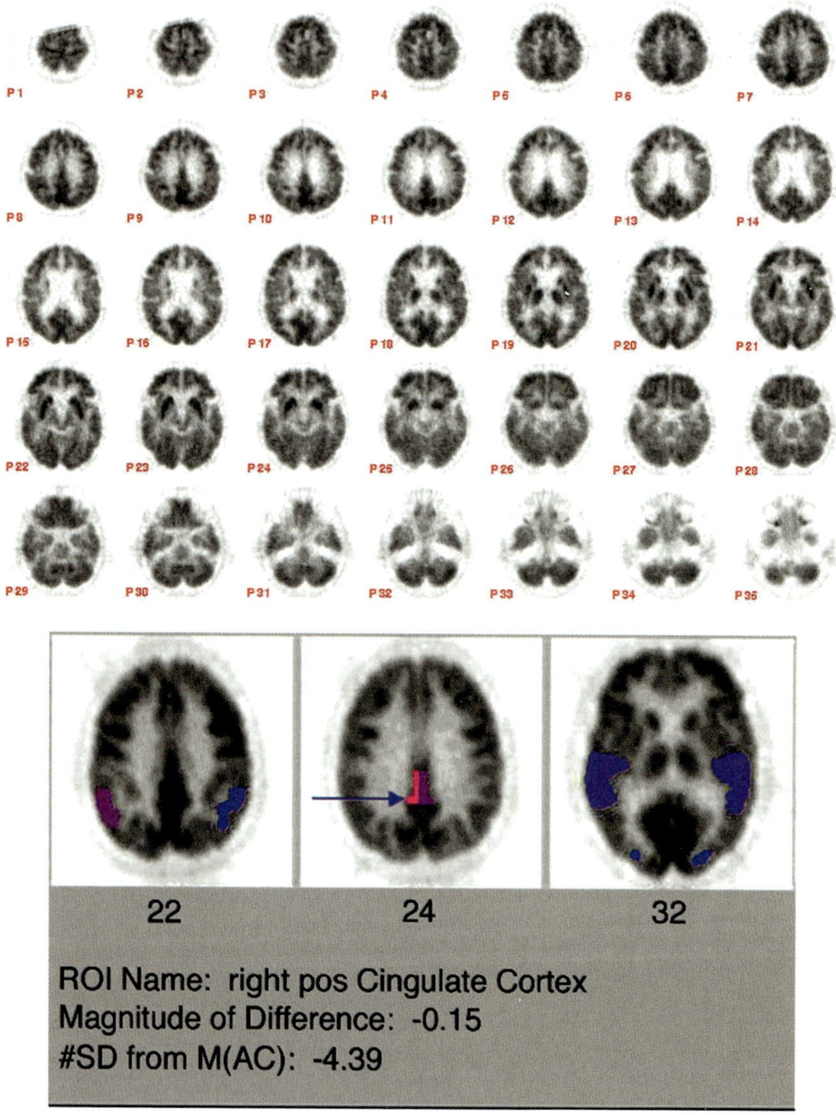

Fig. 7.12 **A.** Brain FDG PET of 79-year-old woman with questionable cognitive and neurobehavioral symptoms. **B.** Quantitative (NeuroQ) assessment identifying hypometabolism of posterior cingulate cortex (the cortical region that decreases most significantly in the earliest stages of Alzheimer's disease) to fall four standard deviations below that of normal control subjects

Indication

Ms. E was unwilling to attempt some neuropsychological tests during an initial evaluation. She performed in the below-average range for immediate and delayed recall of a rote-learned list and phonemic fluency and had a tendency to give up easily on verbal pair tasks. However, the patient performed in the above-average range in most other domains, providing a mixed picture with respect to the variety of cognitive domains tested.

Her examining neuropsychologist determined that there were no signs of dementia at the time and concluded that Ms. E had age consistent memory impairment. She recommended clinical treatment for Ms. E's memory difficulties, a prescription for Aricept, and a re-evaluation in 2 years.

Scan Indication

FDG PET demonstrated decreased tracer uptake in the inferior parietal cortex and posterior cingulate cortex, as well as preservation of the thalamus, basal ganglia, frontal cortex, visual cortex, and cerebellum (Fig. 7.12a). The pattern is most consistent with Alzheimer's disease. Quantitative (NeuroQ) assessment showed hypometabolism of posterior cingulate cortex (the cortical region that decreases the most significantly in the earliest stages of Alzheimer's disease)[11] to fall four standard deviations below normal controls (Fig. 7.12b).

Teaching Point

On initial evaluation, Ms. E demonstrated isolated areas of cognitive impairment, and results from comprehensive neuropsychological testing led to an ambiguous conclusion. In addition, anti-Alzheimer's medication was considered in the absence of a firm diagnosis of Alzheimer's disease or another dementing condition. Ms. E's PET scan demonstrated decreased activity in the inferior parietal and posterior cingulate cortex, which indicated that anticholinesterase therapy would indeed be a reasonable plan of action.[17,22–24] In this case, PET offered a more secure diagnosis of Alzheimer's disease than clinical evaluation alone, allowing for the administration of a proper therapy regimen, improvement of the patient's functional abilities, and the reduction of caregiver burdens.[12,22,24–26]

Case Study 13

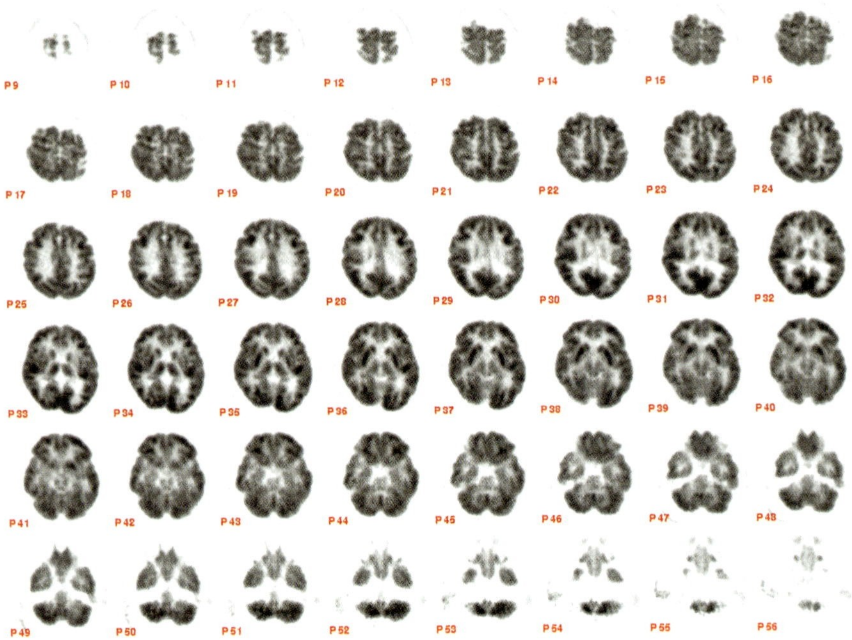

Fig. 7.13 Brain FDG PET of 71-year-old man reporting 6 months of memory loss

Indication

Mr. M was a retired musician with a high school education. His medical history was positive for cervical spondylosis, depression, and coronary artery disease. The onset of his symptoms was thought to be associated with pain killers he had taken 6 months prior for a urinary tract of prostate infection.

Since then, Mr. M was reported to be increasingly irritable, aggressive, and verbally abusive toward his family. He also reported decreased appetite and a depressed mood. The neurologist's working diagnosis at that point was early Alzheimer's versus frontotemporal dementia. Mr. M was prescribed the cholinesterase inhibitor donepezil, later switched to galantamine, and was also started on escitalopram (Lexapro) for his depression. Mr. M obtained an MMSE score of 17/30.

Scan Interpretation

FDG PET demonstrated decreased tracer uptake in only the most anterior portion of the prefrontal cortex (Fig. 7.13). The scan revealed a pattern within normal limits for the patient's age.

Follow-up Visit

Two weeks after his PET scan, Mr. M had been on Lexapro for 1 month and was reported to be in a less irritable mood. He had also regained some of his appetite. He subsequently achieved an MMSE score of 23/30 and was notably more talkative during his evaluation. Five months later, Mr. M continued to exhibit a positive mood and was continued on Lexapro. The clinician did not rule out dementia as a factor contributing to Mr. M's memory problems, but concluded that he was at least in a partial remission for major depressive disorder.

Teaching Point

Mr. M reported 6 months of memory problems, decreased appetite, and depressed mood. His family also complained of his increasing irritability and aggressive behavior. Mr. M was diagnosed with early dementia, and was started on Aricept (later switched to galantamine) and Lexapro for his depression. He subsequently improved his MMSE score from 17/30 to 23/30. Because of the coexistence of depression and dementia symptoms, the etiology of his cognitive deficit remained uncertain. However, FDG PET demonstrated that it was unlikely that Mr. M's cognitive problems were related to Alzheimer's disease (sparing of parietal, temporal, and posterior cingulate cortices) or frontotemporal dementia (sparing of frontal cortex and anterior temporal regions).[5,21] Autopsy series indicate a sensitivity for FDG PET of 90%–95% for neurodegenerative cases, even at early stages.[1,4]

Case Study 14

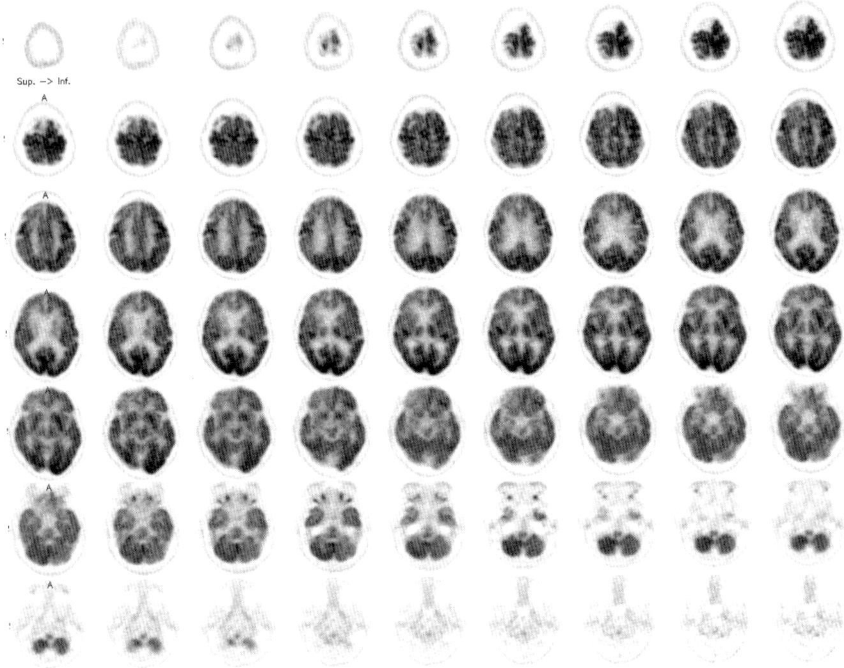

Fig. 7.14 A. Brain FDG PET of 77-year-old woman with a history of progressive cognitive decline. **B.** Quantitative assessment identifying several regions of hypometabolism, including the posterior cingulate cortex (four standard deviations below normal mean), the parietal, parietotemporal, and temporal regions (2–5 standard deviations below normal mean), right prefrontal cortical region (4–7 standard deviations below normal mean), left prefrontal cortical region (2–3 standard deviations below normal mean), and the right thalamus and right basal ganglia (2–3 standard deviations below normal mean)

Indication

Ms. C was a 77-year-old woman with a 3- to 4-year history of progressive neurocognitive slowing, as well as cerebrovascular accident. Although she had intact remote memory recall, she had increasing difficulty with short-term memory recall. For example, she was able to recall only one out of three objects after 3 min and could not recall what she had for dinner the past two nights. In addition, Ms. C often exhibited confusion, some behavioral abnormalities, sleep disorder, and difficulty with language.

Scan Interpretation

The PET scan showed moderate generalized cerebral atrophy with moderately severe right prefrontal, right temporal, and right posterior cingulate cortical

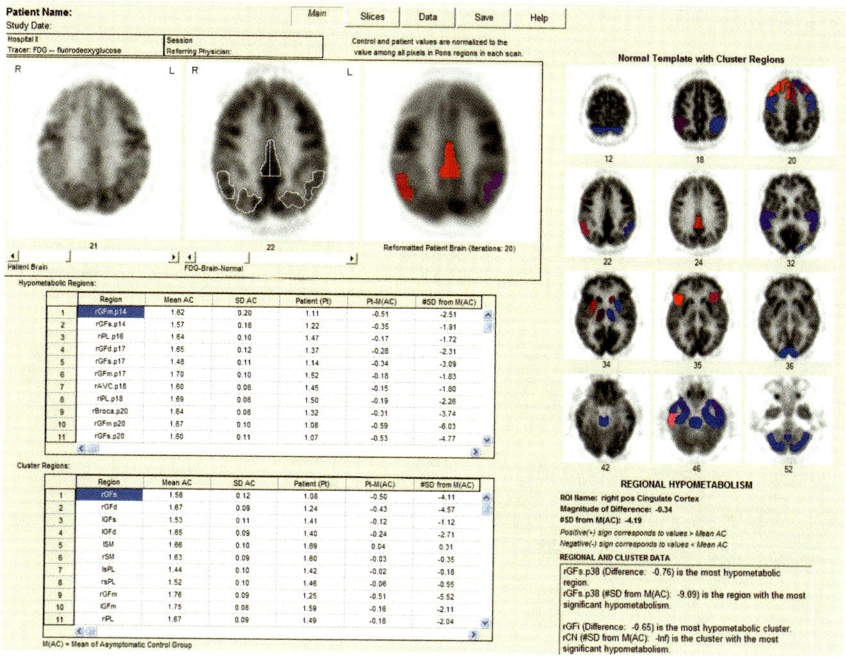

Fig. 7.14 (continued)

hypometabolism, mild hypometabolism of the right temporal and left parietal cortex, and very mild hypometabolism of the left prefrontal cortex (Fig. 7.14a). The sensorimotor and occipital cortex is preserved bilaterally. The metabolism of the right basal ganglia and right thalamus is mildly diminished and crossed-cerebellar diaschisis is seen with moderately reduced left-sided metabolism. Much of the right-sided changes are consistent with her prior cerebrovascular accident. The left-sided changes show a pattern of posterior-predominant hypometabolism and sensorimotor preservation that would be typical for Alzheimer's-type changes. Figure 7.14b depicts results from quantitative (NeuroQ) analysis.

Teaching Point

Ms. C demonstrated progressive cognitive impairment and some behavioral abnormalities. She also had a history of cerebrovascular accident. The findings of the FDG PET scan showed a pattern consistent with mixed cerebrovascular plus Alzheimer's disease. In addition, the frontal cortical involvement correlated with report of the patient's neurobehavioral abnormalities. Note that the asymmetric subcortical involvement reflected the concomitant involvement of her cerebrovascular disease.[5]

Case Study 15

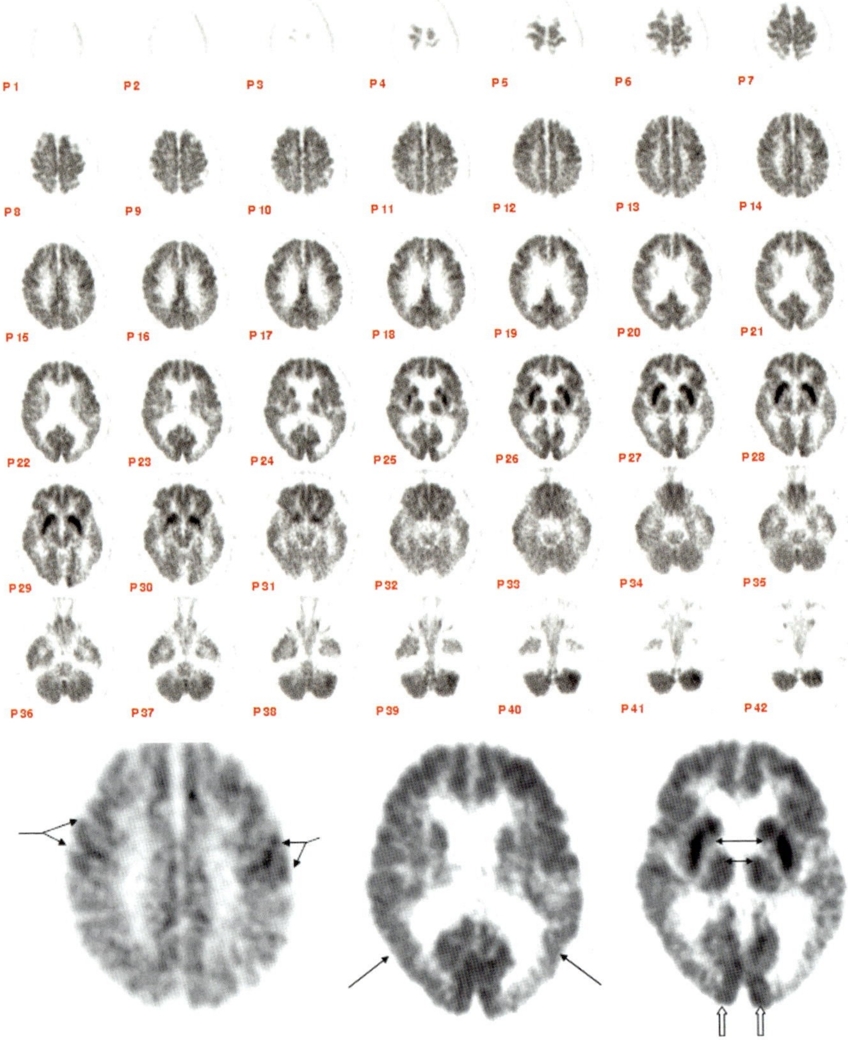

Fig. 7.15 Brain FDG PET of 88-year-old man with symptoms of cognitive decline. (see text for details of metabolic changes illustrated in individual planes.)

Indication

Mr. A was 88 years old when he first underwent FDG PET for symptoms of cognitive decline. The patient completed a high school degree and was an actor before his retirement. At the time of evaluation, he reported that his symptoms, including

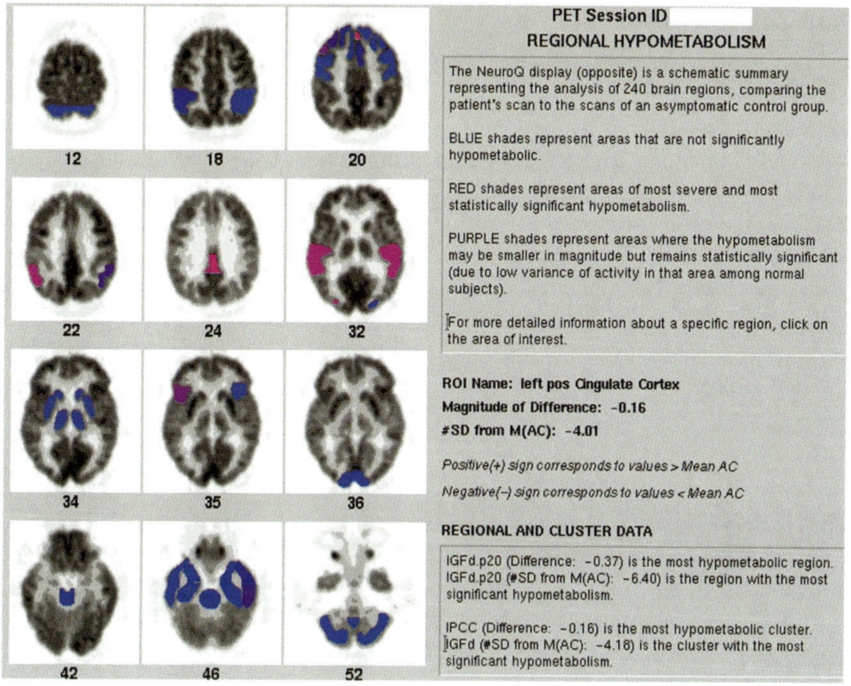

Fig. 7.15 (continued)

reduced hearing, poor memory, and difficulty with word finding, began 10 years earlier. In the 2 years leading up to the initial examination, Mr. A's memory had significantly declined. He had also been regularly seeing a psychologist for his lifelong tendency toward depression. His past medical history was positive for angioplasty and prostate carcinoma, for which he underwent prostatectomy several years prior. At the time of initial evaluation, Mr. A's laboratory results were within normal limits, with the exception of thyroid-stimulating hormone (0.2) consistent with hyperthyroidism. Mr. A reported no use of tobacco and occasional use of alcohol.

On comprehensive neuropsychological testing, the patient achieved an initial MMSE score of 23/30 and was assessed with possible dementia, characterized by reduced acquisition and recall, poor recognition, mild anomia, reduced verbal fluency, and mild visual-spatial deficits.

Brain MRI at the time of his initial evaluation also revealed "mild periventricular and periatrial white matter microvascular ischemic disease. General cerebral atrophy is present. There is no evidence of extra-axial fluid collection or cortical infarction."

Scan Interpretation

FDG PET (Fig. 7.15a) revealed bilateral parietal and temporal (see Fig. 7.15b) hypometabolism (somewhat more pronounced on the left side) consistent with Alzheimer's changes. The patient's PET scan demonstrated well-preserved basal ganglia and thalami (see double-headed arrows in Fig. 7.15c), sensorimotor (see Fig. 7.15d), and occipital cortices (see open arrows in Fig. 7.15c). Decreased activity of the right cerebellum relative to the left was also noted, a result of cross-cerebellar diaschisis. The patient's more hypometabolic left parietal and temporal regions help to explain the pattern of cerebral metabolism observed in the right cerebellum. Quantitative (NeuroQ) assessment also showed significant hypometabolism in posterior cingulate cortex (Fig. 7.15e).

Follow-up Visit

Mr. A obtained a MMSE score of 26/30 in a follow-up examination 10 months after his first evaluation and was diagnosed with mild cognitive impairment. He was placed on a regimen of vitamin E (2,000 IU/day) and Aricept (10 mg/day).

In the years following his initial examination, Mr. A's memory continued to worsen, although his performances on follow-up MMSE tests varied from visit to visit, ranging from 22/30 to 26/30. He reported continuous problems with recall and in particular, name retrieval. His companion reported a day-to-day fluctuation in his memory. Neurologic examinations revealed gait and station within normal limits. Two years after his initial scan, he was also evaluated for symptoms of chronic depression, stress, and insomnia—at which time he was prescribed sertraline (Zoloft) (50 mg/day). During his most recent neuropsychological evaluation, it was noted that the patient's speech revealed severe anomia, circumlocution, and stutter. He was finally diagnosed with early Alzheimer's disease and was continued on a regimen of vitamin E and Aricept.

Teaching Point

Mr. A reported memory decline that was unexplained by his general history, physical examination, laboratory screen, and structural neuroimaging tests. When Mr. A first underwent a comprehensive neuropsychological evaluation, he had already experienced significant cognitive decline with symptoms beginning 10 years before his initial visit and that became progressively more severe. He had an MMSE score of 23/30 and was assessed with possible dementia. PET was used to clarify the etiology of his cognitive deterioration, as there are no tests documented to be as accurate as FDG PET in the identification of progressive Alzheimer's disease.[1,5]

Although the patient's numerous earlier neuropsychological evaluations remained inconclusive for progressive neurodegeneration, and his initial MRI provided only general information regarding the patient's cerebral atrophy, FDG PET was able to detect clear patterns of cerebral metabolism consistent with Alzheimer's disease as early as the initial clinical examination.

Case Study 16

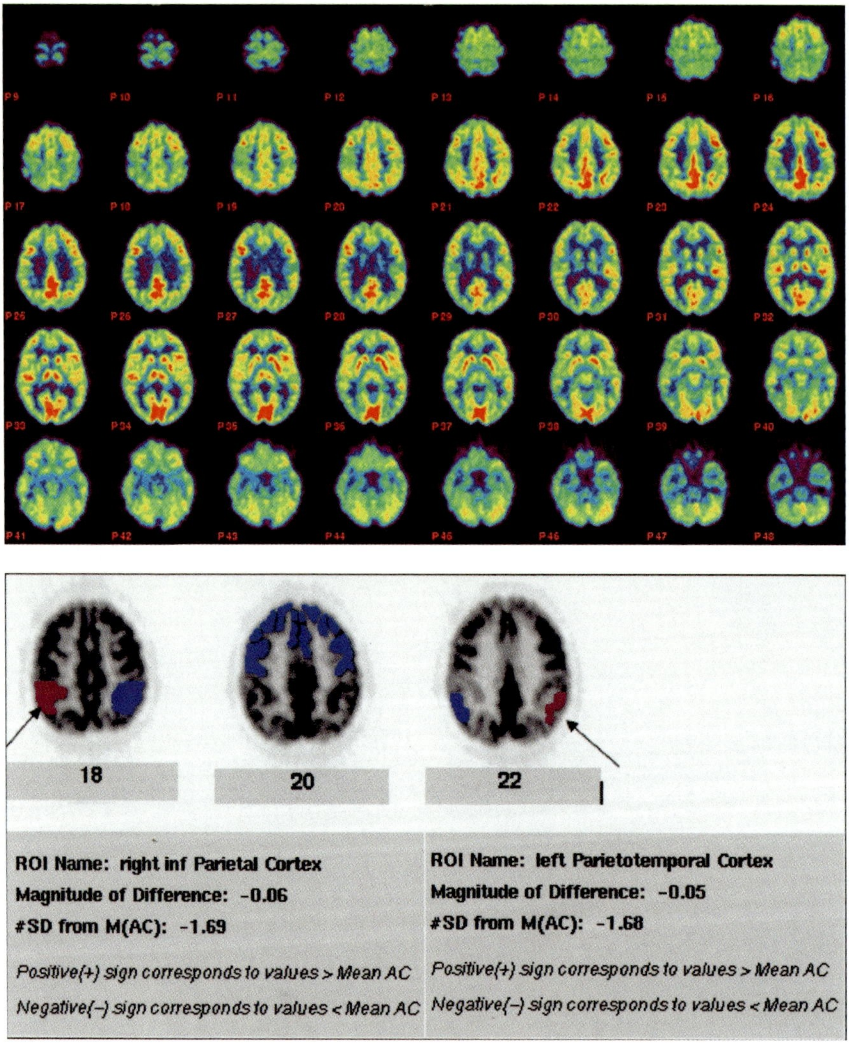

Fig. 7.16 **A.** Brain FDG PET of 56-year-old woman. **B.** Quantitative (NeuroQ) assessment quantifying mild hypometabolism in the inferior parietal and parietotemporal regions

Indication

Ms. R, a right-handed 56-year-old woman, underwent neuropsychological evaluation. She was married, with two grown children, had 17 years of education, and was employed as a travel agent. Several years previously, she had received psychiatric treatment for manifesting posttraumatic stress disorder symptoms; however, physically, she was in good health. Ms. R reported drinking only on the weekends (two glasses each night) and had used marijuana during her youth.

Ms. R underwent a complete neuropsychological evaluation, which showed that her intellectual and cognitive functioning was mainly within normal limits. She demonstrated particular strengths in general intellectual functioning, attention and concentration, language, and the immediate and delayed recall of unassociated word pairs. Her immediate and delayed recall for paragraph stories and her executive skills were also within normal limits. However, Ms. R showed moderate-to-severe impairment in her ability to copy and recall a complex figure, failing to conceptualize the gestalt of the design. In addition, Ms. R demonstrated reduced encoding and retrieval during a rote list-learning task. She was diagnosed with age consistent memory impairment.

Scan Interpretation

FDG PET showed mild biparietal and very mild bitemporal hypometabolism through extensive portions of the posterior cortex (Fig. 7.16a). Sensorimotor and primary visual cortical activity was relatively preserved. In addition, there was preservation of activity of deep structures and cerebellum. Quantitative (NeuroQ) assessment showed hypometabolism in the inferior parietal and parietotemporal regions (Fig. 7.16b).

Teaching Point

The results from Ms. R's neuropsychological evaluation showed that she had a preserved memory capacity on the majority of tasks. In addition, her family history, self-reported memory capabilities, and working clinical diagnosis raised no concern for the presence of a neurodegenerative disease process. On the other hand, an FDG PET scan administered at the time of her clinical evaluation demonstrated a pattern of brain metabolism consistent with an early Alzheimer's-type neurodegenerative process. Previous literature has indicated that regional cerebral hypometabolism detected by PET,[5,6] such as the mild biparietal and bitemporal hypometabolism observed in the case of Ms. R, is 95%,[1,4] sensitive to changes associated with neurodegenerative disease, including changes occurring years before the emergence of overt symptoms.[1,2] In addition, it is likely that Ms. R would manifest deterioration of mental status in the 2- to 3-year period following the abnormal PET scan,[3] as evidence has suggested that among patients with nonprogressive working diagnoses, the decline in patients' performance scores (i.e., MMSE) was significantly greater for those with progressive PET patterns than for those with nonprogressive PET patterns[5] and 18 times more likely to be detected in the former group. Taking into consideration her abnormal pattern of brain metabolism observed with PET alone, Ms. R may take advantage of an earlier clinical diagnosis of Alzheimer's disease, to receive appropriate treatment (e.g., anticholinesterase inhibitors [17,22,23]) and delay cognitive decline by 9–12 months on average relative to untreated patients[18,24,27] and institutionalization by 18 months on average.[14]

Case Study 17

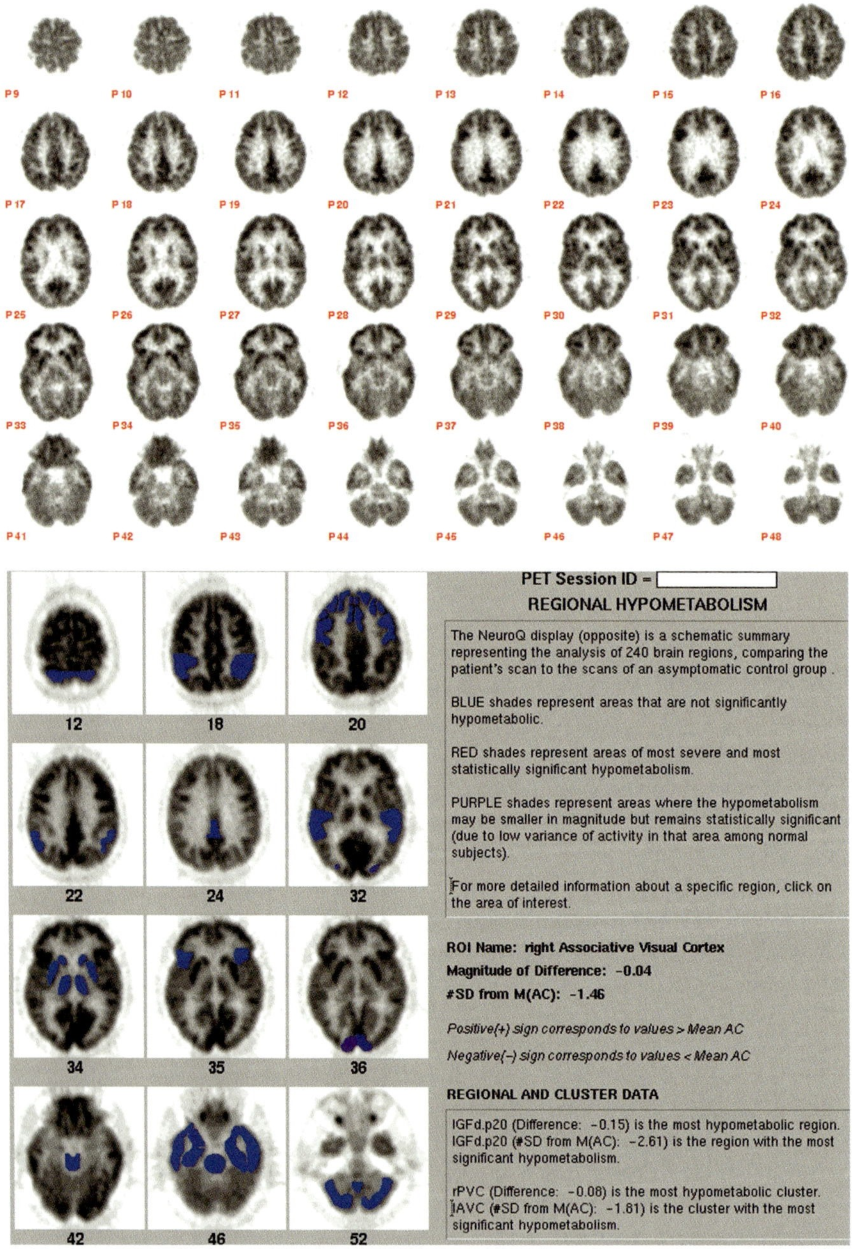

Fig. 7.17 A. Brain FDG of 52-year-old man with age consistent memory impairment. **B.** Quantitative (NeuroQ) assessment showing slight hypometabolism in the associative visual cortex

Indication

Mr. H, a right-handed man, was 52 years old when first evaluated. He had obtained his bachelor's degree (16 years of education) and had been working in real estate for approximately 25 years. He had recently begun thyroid and testosterone replacement therapy, but his medical history was insignificant for any major illnesses or head trauma. Mr. H reported a past history of marijuana and cocaine use in his early thirties. He denied tobacco use and reported consuming approximately five glasses of wine per month.

Mr. H endorsed no symptoms of depression, with the exception of mild work-related fatigue. In addition, he reported difficulty concentrating, with mild symptoms of anxiety because of work-related stress. Results from comprehensive clinical and neuropsychological evaluation demonstrated that Mr. H presented no signs of dementia, and he performed within normal limits on all measures of orientation (MMSE, 30/30), attention and concentration, language, visuospatial functioning, executive functioning, and immediate and delayed verbal and visual memory. These findings were supported with results from FDG PET, which showed no patterns of abnormal brain metabolism, with the exception of slight age-appropriate atrophy (Fig. 7.17a). Quantitative analysis using NeuroQ confirmed a largely unremarkable pattern of cortical metabolism (Fig. 7.17b).

Follow-up Visit

Mr. H returned 13 months later, whereupon he presented with new concerns of mild consistent forgetfulness. He reported that he had begun to have trouble remembering the plots of movies and details about the context of recent events (e.g., weather and date). He noted that these complaints had become gradually worse in the past year, although he stated that he had no difficulty remembering important information about the distant past or significant details of major events. Re-administration of the neuropsychological battery showed that Mr. H had few significant deviations from his previous performances in the areas of orientation (MMSE, 30/30), attention and concentration, psychomotor speed, language, and visuospatial abilities. In terms of executive functioning, he demonstrated relative stability across testing sessions, with the exception of showing significant decline on a task of blocking out interference and inhibiting automatic responses, upon which he fell in the severely impaired range. Mr. H's scores on tasks of immediate verbal memory showed that he declined slightly in performance across testing sessions on some tasks (rote-list learning; word retrieval), although remaining stable (long-term storage on rote memorization task; paragraph stories) or even improving on others (word pairs). In terms of delayed verbal memory, Mr. H demonstrated no change from his previous performance. Furthermore, Mr. H's scores showed relative improvement on all tasks of delayed visual memory.

Teaching Point

Mr. H's clinical follow-up evaluation garnered no suspicion for dementia. His functioning remained within normal limits, with few significant deviations from his previous examination, which was unremarkable for any clinical or metabolic abnormality. Moreover, his performance on the majority of immediate and delayed memory assessments remained consistent, with a trend for improvement, as well as superior scores even on the more difficult tasks (e.g., delayed rote recall). These findings were consistent with the PET scan obtained at the time of his initial evaluation.

Case Study 18

Indication

Mr. P, a 60-year-old man with 14 years of education, worked with investment properties. On clinical evaluation, he complained of persistent memory impairment and had MMSE scores of 23/30 and 26/30. His family history was positive for Alzheimer's disease and revealed that he carried a single allele of each ApoE3 and ApoE4. Mr. P's primary care physician's working diagnosis was early dementia, suggestive of Alzheimer's disease.

Scan 1 Interpretation

FDG PET administered at the time of presentation indicated moderate hypometabolism in the right parietal and temporal cortices, along with mild hypometabolism in the posterior cingulate cortex (Fig. 7.18a).

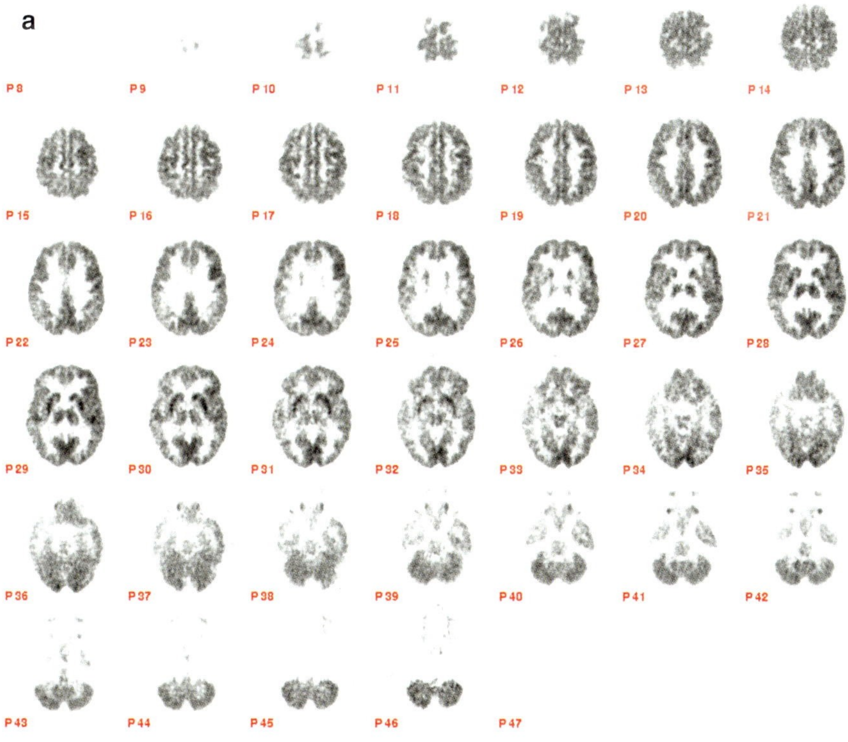

Fig. 7.18 A. Brain FDG PET of 60-year-old man reporting 2 years of impaired memory.

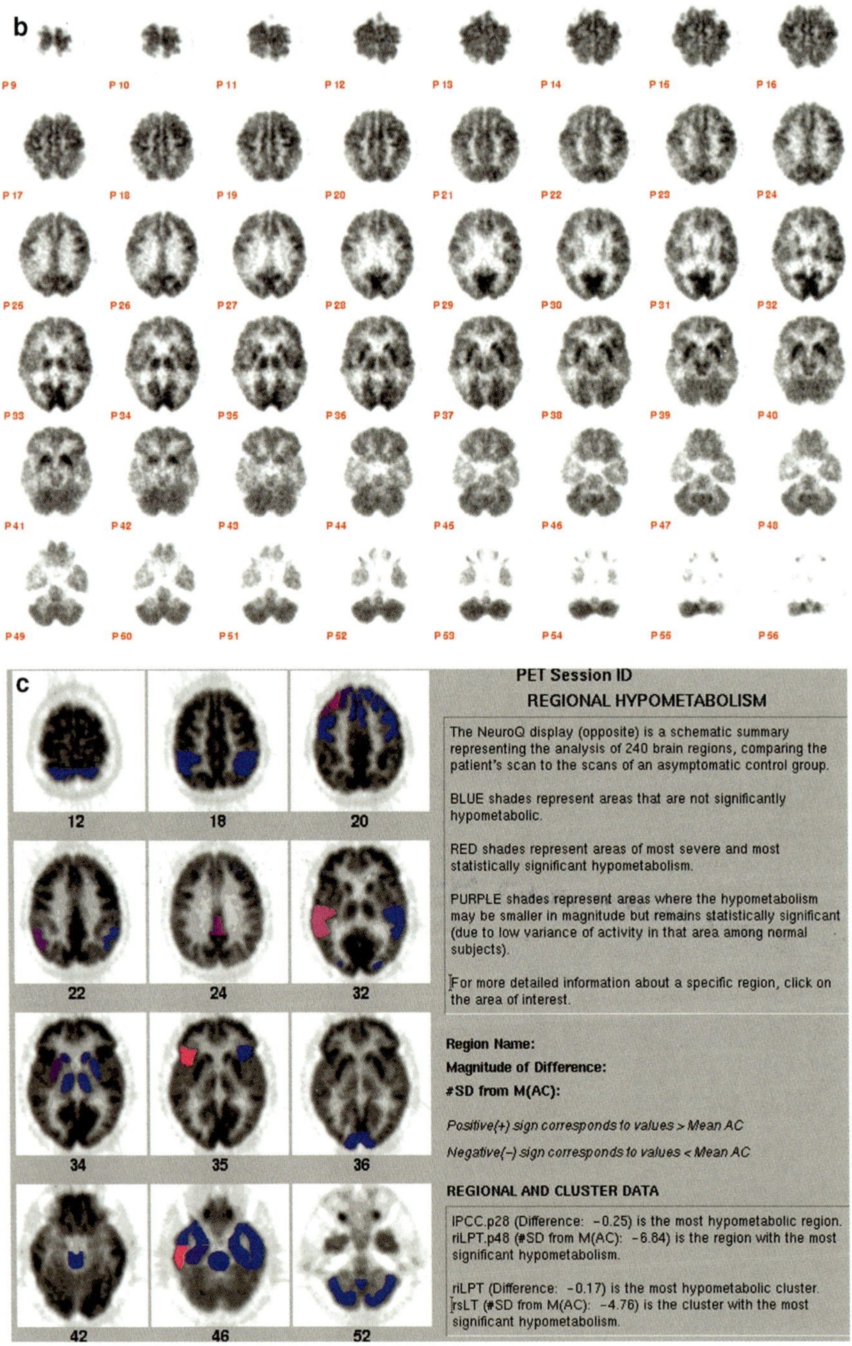

Fig. 7.18 (continued) **B.** PET scan 2 years later, with no change in neuropsychological performance. **C.** Quantitative (NeuroQ) assessment showing hypometabolism in the right lateral temporal areas (four standard deviations below normal mean), the right parietotemporal regions (three standard deviations below normal mean), and the posterior cingulate cortex (2.5–3.5 standard deviations below normal mean)

Scan 2 Interpretation

FDG PET administered 2 years after his first scan indicated bilateral hypometabolism in the parietal and temporal regions (more pronounced on right side), and revealed hypometabolism in the posterior cingulate cortex (Fig. 7.18b). The basal ganglia appeared relatively preserved, as expected in Alzheimer's disease. NeuroQ assessment was used to quantify hypometabolism (Fig. 7.18c).

Follow-up Visit

Two years later, Mr. P was found to have progressive difficulty with memory. He demonstrated an overall decline across all cognitive domains and seemed disoriented and confused on neuropsychological testing.

Teaching Point

Mr. P reported memory difficulties on initial clinical evaluation, during which he received MMSE scores of 23/30 and 26/30. Subsequently, an FDG PET scan was performed to evaluate the possibility of Alzheimer's disease, which had been clinically suspected. Whereas a preliminary MRI revealed only "normal age-appropriate brain," a concurrent PET scan identified multiple abnormalities reflective of early neurodegenerative disease. Mr. P's follow-up PET scan, again demonstrated bilateral parietal and temporal hypometabolism, along with hypometabolism in the posterior cingulate cortex, clearly consistent with a diagnosis of Alzheimer's disease.[5,6,11]

Case Study 19

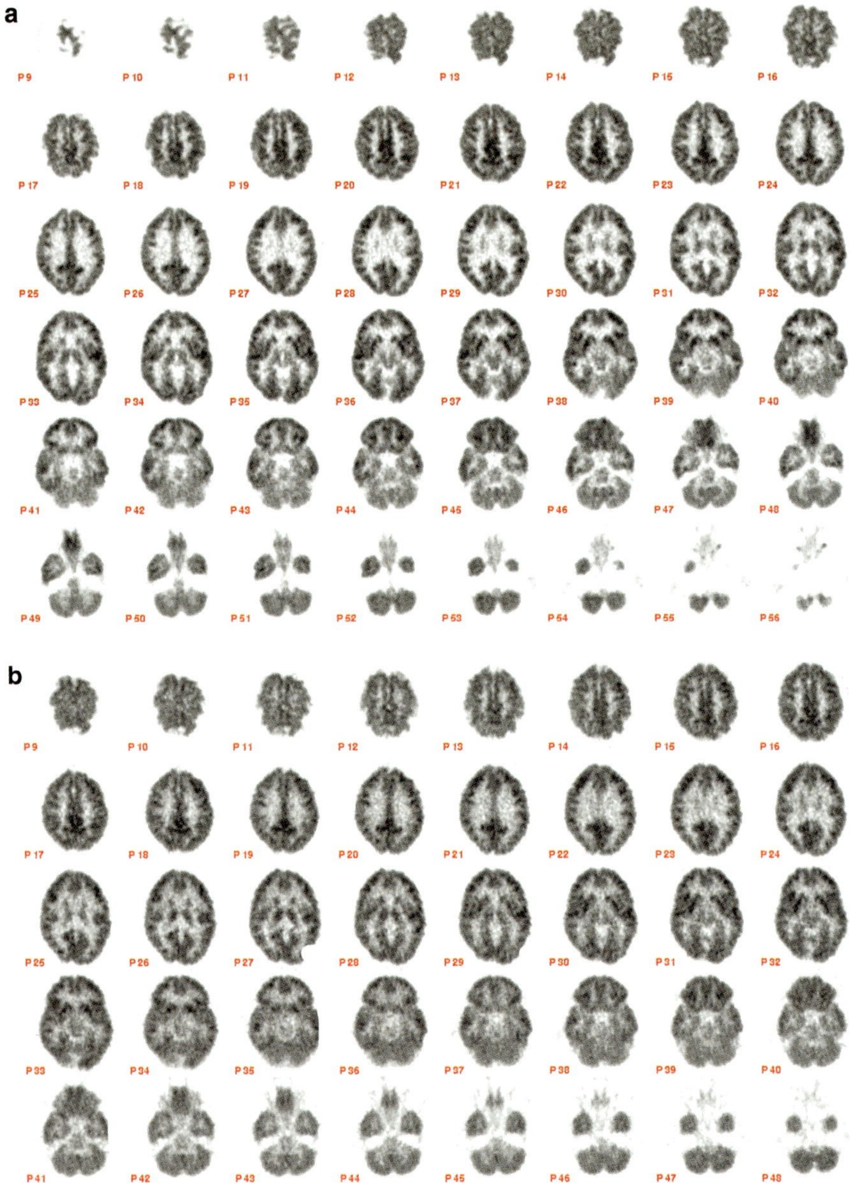

Fig. 7.19 **A.** Brain FDG of 56-year-old man with age consistent memory impairment. **B.** PET scan 2 years later, with a re-diagnosis of age associated memory impairment

Indication

Mr. S, a right-handed man with 15 years of education, was 56 years old when clinically evaluated. He was married, with three adolescent children, and had worked as a financial planner for 13 years. Mr. S's medical and psychiatric histories were insignificant, with the exception of high cholesterol and two hip replacement surgeries. He reported mild alcohol intake, but no history of substance abuse or cigarette use.

At the time of his evaluation, Mr. S reported difficulty recalling names. He also found it difficult to concentrate when doing more than one thing at once. The results of Mr. S's neuropsychological performance indicated that he was normal in areas of attention and concentration, language, and visuospatial functioning. Whereas his phonemic fluency, abstract reasoning, and set shifting were also all within normal limits, he had variable scores pertaining to executive functioning and demonstrated impairment on tasks of semantic fluency and psychomotor speed. Mr. S generally scored within average ranges on most measures of immediate and delayed memory; however, he scored within the mild-moderately impaired ranges on tests of immediate rote-list learning and delayed visual memory. His scores placed him within the criteria for age consistent memory impairment.

Scan 1 Interpretation

FDG PET administered at the time of initial presentation indicated mild generalized cortical atrophy (Fig. 7.19a). The pattern of FDG throughout the cortex was symmetric and unremarkable, with the relatively higher uptake in the posterior cingulate cortex, as expected. In addition, the pattern of FDG uptake in the basal ganglia, thalamus, and cerebellum was within normal limits. No evidence of neurodegenerative disease was seen. This was a normal scan.

Follow-up Visit

Mr. S returned approximately 2 years later for a clinical reevaluation. At that time, he reported no change in memory since his initial evaluation. However, he stated that he was experiencing a considerable amount of stress, anxiety, and depression because of his recent divorce from his wife after 15 years of marriage. After comprehensive clinical and neuropsychological reevaluation, Mr. S was found to have performed within normal limits on all tasks. All of his scores actually improved significantly since his initial evaluation, even raising scores that were previously in the impaired ranges, placing him one standard deviation above the mean for his age group on 82% of all memory tasks. In this regard, Mr. S's diagnosis was revised from age consistent memory impairment to age associated memory impairment.

Scan 2 Interpretation

No significant change was seen since the previous scan (Fig. 7.19b).

Teaching Point

Mr. S's working diagnosis indicated no clear signs of dementia. However, his self-reported memory and concentration difficulties, along with the variable results obtained from the initial neuropsychological evaluation, could not have confidently ruled out the possibility of a dementia process as an underlying factor. The patient's clinical follow-up 2 years later showed relative improvement on all tasks, including all memory tasks. This finding was consistent with Mr. S's brain scans over a 2-year period, both of which suggested that there was no indication of neurodegenerative disease. In this case, whereas his initial clinical examination remained ambiguous for performance deficits attributed to a disease process, both PET scans were consistent in ruling out Alzheimer's disease/neurodegenerative disease as the underlying mechanism for his self-perceived memory complaints, owing to FDG PET's 95% sensitivity in detecting the early stages of neurodegenerative disease and predicting clinical progression occurring over the subsequent 2- to 3-year period.[1,3,4]

Case Study 20

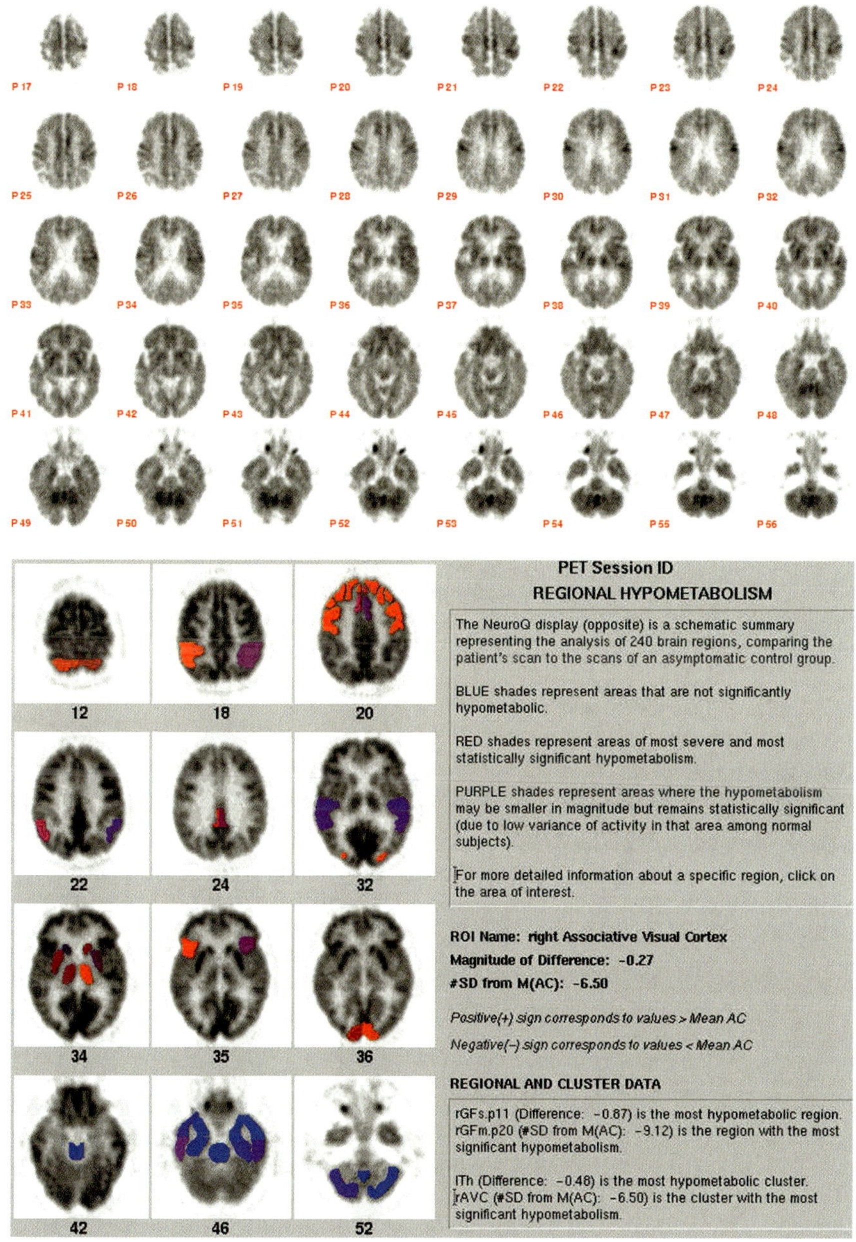

Fig. 7.20 **A.** Brain FDG PET of 59-year-old woman reporting 4 years of cognitive impairment and motor deficits. **B.** Quantitative (NeuroQ) assessment identifying hypometabolism involving the visual cortex (six standard deviations below normal mean) and the anterior basal ganglia

Indication

Ms. P was first seen for the onset of a chorea athetosis-like disorder. Huntington's disease had been ruled out by DNA analysis. Four years later, her symptoms included intermittent fevers associated with cognitive impairment. An MRI obtained 18 months prior to PET was negative. Ms. P was placed on amantadine therapy and had shown considerable improvement, but was discontinued because of concern about its side effects. Because cognitive decline and motor deficits were noted on neurologic examination, FDG PET was implemented to evaluate for possible abnormal patterns of cerebral metabolism in the face of normal structural neuroimaging results.

Scan Interpretation

FDG PET demonstrated atrophy-associated global hypometabolism as well as more severe focal hypometabolism in subcortical structures (Fig. 7.20a). The scan also showed generalized atrophy of the frontal and parietal cortices, but prominently preserved metabolism of the primary sensorimotor cortex, suggesting a neurodegenerative dementing disorder. Quantitative (NeuroQ) assessment showed hypometabolism involving the visual cortex (six standard deviations below normal mean) and the basal ganglia (Fig. 7.20b).

Follow-up Visit

In the 4 years before her death, Ms. P experienced stiffness of gait, dystonia, choreoathetoid movements, and progressive mental degeneration. At autopsy, Ms. P was diagnosed with Hallervorden-Spatz syndrome, with iron deposition found in her brain.

Teaching Point

Ms. P demonstrated cognitive and motor deficits after the onset of a chorea athetosis–like disorder. Her PET scan demonstrated hypometabolism of the basal ganglia and visual cortex (along with frontal, parietal, and temporal cortices). On autopsy, the patient was diagnosed with Hallervorden-Spatz syndrome, with iron deposition found in her brain.[28,29] The hypometabolism of the basal ganglia revealed by PET was most likely attributed to the iron accumulation in the area of the globus pallidus and substantia nigra identified at autopsy.

References

1. Silverman DHS, Small GW, Chang CY, et al. Positron emission tomography in evaluation of dementia. JAMA 2001;286:2120–2127.
2. Herholz K, Nordberg A, Salmon E, et al. Impairment of neocortical metabolism predicts progression in AD. Dement Geriatr Cogn Disord 1999;10:494–504.
3. Silverman DHS, Truong CT, Kim SK, et al. Prognostic value of regional cerebral metabolism in patients undergoing dementia evaluation: comparison to a quantifying parameter of subsequent cognitive performance and to prognostic assessment without PET. Molec Genet Metab 2003;80:350–355.
4. Hoffman JM, Welsh-Bohmer KA, Hanson M, et al. FDG PET imaging in patients with pathologically verified dementia. J Nucl Med 2000;41:1920–1928.
5. Silverman DHS. Brain ^{18}F-FDG PET in the diagnosis of neurodegenerative dementias: comparison with perfusion SPECT and with clinical evaluations lacking nuclear imaging. J Nucl Med 2004;45:594–606.
6. Hoffman JM, Hanson MW, Welsh KA, et al. Interpretation variability of 18 FDG positron emission tomography studies in dementia. Invest Radiol 1996;31:316–322.
7. Diehl-Schmid J, Grimmer T, Drzezga A, et al. Decline of cerebral glucose metabolism in frontotemporal dementia: a longitudinal 18F-FDG-PET-study. Neurobiol Aging 2007;28:42–50.
8. Ishii K, Sakmoto S, Sasaki M, et al. Cerebral glucose metabolism in patients with frontotemporal dementia. J Nucl Med 1998;39:1875–1878.
9. Frank L, Matza LS, Hanlon J, et al. The patient experience of depression and remission: focus group results. J Nerv Ment Dis 2007;195:647–654.
10. Copeland MP, Daly E, Hines V, et al. Psychiatric symptomatology and prodromal Alzheimer's disease. Alz Dis Assoc Disord 2003;17:1–8.
11. Minoshima S, Giordani B, Berent S, et al. Metabolic reduction in the posterior cingulate cortex in very early AD. Ann Neurol 2004;42:85–94.
12. Weiner MF, Martin-Cook K, Foster BM, et al. Effects of donepezil on emotional/behavioral symptoms in Alzheimer's disease patients. J Clin Psychiatry 2000;61:487–492.
13. Silverman DHS, Cumming JL, Small GW, et al. assessment of the added clinical benefit of incorporating FDG-PET into the clinical evaluation of patients with cognitive impairment. Mol Imaging Biol 2002;4:283–293.
14. Fago JP. Dementia: causes, evaluation, and management. Hosp Pract (Minneap) 2001;36: 59–66, 69.
15. Whitehouse PJ, Friedland RP, Strauss ME. Neuropsychiatric aspects of degenerative dementias associated with motor dysfunction. The American Psychiatric Press Textbook of Neuropsychiatry, 2nd ed. Washington, DC: American Psychiatric Press, 1992, pp 585–604.
16. Silverman DHS, Gambhir SS, Huang HC, et al. Evaluating early dementia with and without assessment of regional cerebral metabolism by PET: a comparison of predicted costs and benefits. J Nucl Med 2002;43:253–266.
17. Doody RS, Geldmacher DS, Gordon B, et al. Open-label, multicenter, phase 3 extension study of the safety and efficacy of donepezil in patients with Alzheimer disease. Arch Neurol 2001;58:427–433.
18. Rogers SL, Friedhoff LT. Long-term efficacy and safety of donepezil in the treatment of Alzheimer's disease: an interim analysis of the results of a US multicentre open label extension study. Eur Neuropsychopharmacol 1998;8:67–75.
19. Butters MA, Whyte EM, Nebes RD, et al. The nature and determinants of neuropsychological functioning in late-life depression. Arch Gen Psychiatry 2004;61:587–595.
20. Chodosh J, Kado DM, Seeman TE, et al. Depressive symptoms as a predictor of cognitive decline: MacArthur studies of successful aging. Am J Geriatr Psychiatry 2007;15:406–415.
21. Foster NL, Heidebrink JL, Clark CM, et al. FDG-PET improves accuracy in distinguishing frontotemporal dementia and Alzheimer's disease. Brain 2007;130:2616–2635.

22. Raskind MA, Peskind ER, Wessel T, et al. Galantamine in AD: A 6-month randomized, placebo-controlled trial with a 6-month extension. The Galantamine USA-1 Study Group. Neurology 2000;54:2261–2268.
23. Corey-Bloom J, Anand R, Veach J. A randomized trial evaluating the efficacy and safety of ENA 713 rivastigmine tartrate, a new acetylcholinesterase inhibitor, in patients with mild to moderately severe Alzheimer's disease: the ENA 713 B352 Study Group. Int J Geriatr Psychopharmacol 1998;1:55–65.
24. Coyle J, Kershaw P. Galantamine, a cholinesterase inhibitor that allosterically modulates nicotinic receptors: effects on the course of Alzheimer's disease. Biol Psychiatry 2001;49:289–299.
25. Morris JC, Cyrus PA, Orazem J, et al. Metrifonate benefits cognitive, behavioral, and global function in patients with Alzheimer's disease. Neurology 1998;50:1222–1230.
26. Tariot PN, Solomon PR, Morris JC, et al. A 5-month, randomized, placebo-controlled trial of galantamine in AD. The Galantamine USA-10 Study Group. Neurology 2000;54:2269–2276.
27. Imbimbo BP, Verdelli G, Martelli P, et al. Two-year treatment of Alzheimer's disease with eptastigmine. The Eptastigmine Study Group. Dement Geriatr Cogn Disord 1999;10:139–147.
28. Gregory A, Hayflick SJ. Neurodegeneration with brain iron accumulation. Folia Neuropathol 2005;43:286–296.
29. Clement F, Devos D, Moreau C. Neurodegeneration with brain iron accumulation: clinical, radiographic and genetic heterogeneity and corresponding therapeutic options. Acta Neurol Belg 2007;107:26–31.**Fig. 7.13** Brain FDG PET of 71-year-old man reporting 6 months of memory loss

Index